Diagnosis, Pathology and Management of Bovine Infectious Diseases

Diagnosis, Pathology and Management of Bovine Infectious Diseases

Editor: George Allen

Callisto Reference
www.callistoreference.com

Callisto Reference,
118-35 Queens Blvd., Suite 400,
Forest Hills, NY 11375, USA

Visit us on the World Wide Web at:
www.callistoreference.com

ISBN: 978-1-64116-770-3 (Hardback)

Cataloging-in-Publication Data

Diagnosis, pathology and management of bovine infectious diseases / edited by George Allen.
p. cm.
Includes bibliographical references and index.
ISBN 978-1-64116-770-3
1. Cattle--Infections. 2. Cattle--Diseases. 3. Cattle--Infections--Diagnosis. 4. Cattle--Diseases--Treatment.
5. Communicable diseases in animals. I. Allen, George.
SF961 .D53 2023
636.208 96--dc23

Table of Contents

Preface

The world is advancing at a fast pace like never before. Therefore, the need is to keep up with the latest developments. This book was an idea that came to fruition when the specialists in the area realized the need to coordinate together and document essential themes in the subject. That's when I was requested to be the editor. Editing this book has been an honour as it brings together diverse authors researching on different streams of the field. The book collates essential materials contributed by veterans in the area which can be utilized by students and researchers alike.

Bovine infections refer to the group of infectious diseases affecting the cattle which are caused by pathogens. The most common symptoms of acute infection are the loss of appetite, fever, lethargy, ocular discharge, nasal discharge, oral lesions, diarrhea, and a decreased level of milk production. Some of the common types of bovine infections include bovine viral diarrhea (BVD), anaplasmosis, anthrax, black quarter, bovine anemia, coccidiosis, and enterotoxemia. Bovine viral diarrhea (BVD) is a viral disease of cattle caused by the bovine viral diarrhea virus (BVDV). Management of bovine infectious diseases depends on the specific type of disease affecting the cattle. There are two categories of vaccines available for the prevention of these diseases, namely, modified live virus (MLV) vaccines and killed virus (KV) vaccines. This book includes some of the vital pieces of works being conducted across the world, on the diagnosis, pathology and management of bovine infectious diseases. Researchers and students actively engaged in the field of veterinary science will be greatly assisted by it.

Each chapter is a sole-standing publication that reflects each author´s interpretation. Thus, the book displays a multi-facetted picture of our current understanding of application, resources and aspects of the field. I would like to thank the contributors of this book and my family for their endless support.

Editor

1

Current Developments in the Epidemiology and Control of Enzootic Bovine Leukosis as Caused by Bovine Leukemia Virus

Paul C. Bartlett [1,*], Vickie J. Ruggiero [1], Holden C. Hutchinson [2], Casey J. Droscha [3], Bo Norby [1], Kelly R. B. Sporer [3] and Tasia M. Taxis [4]

1 College of Veterinary Medicine, Michigan State University, East Lansing, MI 48824, USA; woodsvi1@msu.edu (V.J.R.); norby@msu.edu (B.N.)
2 USDA, Fort Collins, CO 80526, USA; holdenhutchinson@gmail.com
3 CentralStar Cooperative, East Lansing, MI 48910, USA; Casey.Droscha@mycentralstar.com (C.J.D.); Kelly.Sporer@mycentralstar.com (K.R.B.S.)
4 Department of Animal Science, Michigan State University, East Lansing, MI 48824, USA; taxistas@msu.edu
* Correspondence: bartle16@msu.edu

Abstract: Enzootic Bovine Leukosis (EBL) caused by the bovine leukemia virus (BLV) has been eradicated in over 20 countries. In contrast, the U.S. and many other nations are experiencing increasing prevalence in the absence of efforts to control transmission. Recent studies have shown that BLV infection in dairy cattle has a greater impact beyond the long-recognized lymphoma development that occurs in <5% of infected cattle. Like other retroviruses, BLV appears to cause multiple immune system disruptions, affecting both cellular and humoral immunity, which are likely responsible for increasingly documented associations with decreased dairy production and decreased productive lifespan. Realization of these economic losses has increased interest in controlling BLV using technology that was unavailable decades ago, when many nations eradicated BLV via traditional antibody testing and slaughter methods. This traditional control is not economically feasible for many nations where the average herd antibody prevalence is rapidly approaching 50%. The ELISA screening of cattle with follow-up testing via qPCR for proviral load helps prioritize the most infectious cattle for segregation or culling. The efficacy of this approach has been demonstrated in at least four herds. Breeding cattle for resistance to BLV disease progression also appears to hold promise, and several laboratories are working on BLV vaccines. There are many research priorities for a wide variety of disciplines, especially including the need to investigate the reports linking BLV and human breast cancer.

Keywords: epidemiology; dairy; beef; retrovirus

1. Introduction

Enzootic Bovine Leukosis caused by the bovine leukemia virus (BLV) has been eradicated in over 20 countries, while many other nations are experiencing increased prevalence. Recent recognition of BLV's economic impact has led to increased interest in controlling BLV in our cattle populations. In the last several years, major advancements have improved our understanding of BLV epidemiology, diagnosis and disease control methods, and this review will summarize those advancements and suggest areas for further research.

2. Increasing Prevalence

Recent surveys in most nations outside of Europe have reported continuous increases in BLV prevalence in both beef and dairy cattle. Prevalence is generally higher in dairy cattle, with the U.S. Japan, Canada, Brazil, China and Argentina reporting that most herds are infected and are approaching a situation where almost half of their dairy cattle are showing serologic evidence of infection. The following countries and regions around the world are reporting moderate increases in BLV: China [1], Columbia [2,3], Costa Rica [4], Iran [5,6], Japan [7], Mongolia [8], Philippines [9], South Africa [10], Turkey [11] and West Africa [12]. Other nations report higher increases: Argentina [13], Canada [14] and the USA [15,16]. As a result of this increasing prevalence, many areas have implemented BLV-control programs, which include tightened trade restrictions to protect their herds [17].

3. Transmission

Most transmission of BLV is through the provirus-infected lymphocyte. Many modes of BLV transmission are possible, but the most important means of transmission likely varies greatly by geography and agricultural system. For example, transmission via fly bites is thought to be important in some parts of the world but not in other parts. Bloodborne transmission is the most recognized route of transmission, but direct contact may be very important in most all management systems. The importance of milk-borne spread is still unknown, as is the potential role of the free RNA-virus. It is unknown if early exposure as a calf or even in utero may lead to a latent infection which later becomes activated, perhaps at times of stress such as pregnancy, first calving and lactation.

4. Economic Impact in Dairy Cattle

The economic loss from BLV-induced lymphoma was previously the only known impact of BLV in cattle. Reportedly occurring in <5% of BLV-infected cattle, lymphomatous tumors remain the top cause of condemnation for U.S. dairy cattle carcasses [18]. Like its retrovirus cousin HIV of humans, BLV appears to show most of its impact by facilitating a wide variety of opportunistic pathogens and causes of suboptimal performance. For example, BLV has been associated with infectious diseases such as mastitis, hoof problems and mucosal diseases [19], as well as failure to clear ringworm infection [20,21]. This indirect influence through facilitating other disease conditions probably delayed the cattle industry's recognition of BLV's full impact.

BLV-infected dairy cattle may reduce milk production and shorten cow lifespan [18,22]. The impact of BLV infection on milk production has been difficult to measure, since cows which drop in production are usually quickly removed from the herd. Oftentimes, cows that are still present, but designated to be culled, are often excluded from herd production calculations. Some have reported that infected cattle make more milk than BLV-negative cattle [23], or about the same [20,24,25]. However, most researchers have found BLV infection to be associated with lower milk production [1,16,19,26–29]. In addition, for every 10% increase in BLV prevalence, a loss of 115 kg in rolling herd average was observed [29]. Three large studies (Figure 1) showed a dose-response between rolling herd average milk production and herd BLV prevalence.

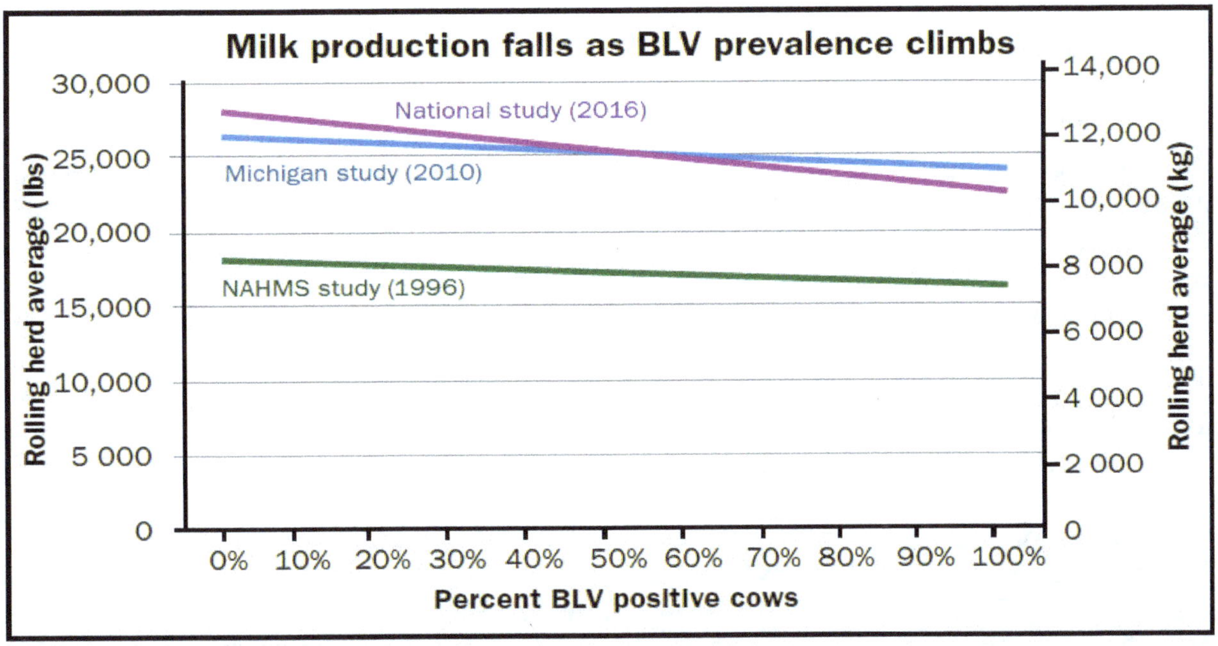

Figure 1. Milk production rolling herd average vs the prevalence of bovine leukemia virus (BLV) ELISA-antibodies from three US studies: LaDronka [16], Erskine [29] and USDA [15].

One study [29] showing substantial decreased production among older cows showed no decreased production when ELISA-positive animals were compared to their ELISA-negative peers. An analysis of genetic potentials by Wu et al. [30] found that, regardless of blood lymphocyte count, seropositive cattle had a higher genetic potential for milk production than did seronegative herd mates.

BLV-infected cattle were reported to have a shorter lifespan in the herd when compared to their ELISA-negative herd mates [19,23,31,32]. In one analysis, BLV-infected dairy cattle were 23% more likely to be culled than their negative herd mates [31]. A dose-response was seen in cattle with higher ELISA optical density values experienced greater culling. The reasons for the increased culling of BLV-infected cattle are difficult to study because culling decisions are affected by so many issues (such as production, age, disease, market and stocking rates) that are simultaneously and subjectively assessed by the herd managers.

5. Altered Immunity

BLV-associated disease and production inefficiencies are thought to be due to a disrupted immune system. A 2015 review by Frie and Coussens [33] outlines several of the altered immune responses reported in BLV-infected cattle. Many of these immune disruptions have clear negative implications for individual and herd health due to infectious disease, especially BLV-associated decreases in systemic immunity (IgG2, IgM), altered activation of immune cells, disrupted T:B cell ratios [21,34–36] and diminished response to vaccination [34,37] as indicative of diminished response to naturally presented antigens. BLV infection has also been associated with decreased neutrophil and monocyte function, such as reduced phagocytosis and inhibited apoptosis [38]. Della Libera et al. [39] reported that milk leukocytes (neutrophils and B-lymphocytes) are similarly affected, raising concerns about mammary gland immunity.

The effects of BLV infection on mucosal immunity are not well-characterized despite the importance of mucosal immunity in preventing many cattle diseases. BLV provirus has been detected in a variety of mucosal secretions, including milk, saliva, nasal secretions [40], vaginal secretions and feces [1,41], which raises concerns both for transmission risk and immune function. In a recent report on a small group of cows, average total IgA concentrations were unchanged in serum but were 34% and 24% lower in milk and saliva samples, respectively, in ELISA-positive cows, although neither result reached statistical significance [41]. In contrast, average total IgM concentrations did not differ in milk or saliva but were decreased in serum, as has been observed in other studies [42].

6. Proviral Load (PVL)

Multiple copies of the BLV provirus can integrate into the host cell genome at multiple sites [43]. Quantitative PCR (qPCR) tests have recently been developed to determine the PVL which is the number of copies of provirus detected per one of several denominators, such as the microgram of extracted genomic DNA [44]. The PVL measures the actual concentration of provirus in the blood sample rather than the BLV-induced antibodies, which are measured by serological tests such as ELISA [45,46]. Viral load or PVL are used in retroviral diagnosis and management as a measure of infectivity, as they reflect the number of infectious particles per unit of blood. For example, viral load is commonly used for monitoring the risk of transmission for humans infected with the related retrovirus human T-cell lymphotrophic virus 1 (HTLV-1) [47,48]. It is, therefore, consistent that BLV PVL is now being used as a measure of BLV infectivity [49,50].

The correlation between ELISA antibodies and PVL is generally weak, but there is a strong correlation ($r = 0.855$) between BLV PVL and blood lymphocyte counts [51]. Previous studies have demonstrated that cattle with high lymphocyte counts are more efficient at transmitting BLV [52,53]. Molloy et al. [54] ran experiments in which they reduced the incidence of new BLV infections by selectively culling cows based on viral antigen expression, which they associated with PVL. More recently, Gutiérrez et al. [55] reported increased periparturient transmission of BLV in cows with high PVL, and other investigators have demonstrated that cows with low PVL present a low transmission risk of BLV transmission to their susceptible herd-mates [56,57].

Recently, Hutchinson modeled lymphocyte counts and proviral load over 6-month intervals and measured a small average increase over time [58]. However, this increase was surprisingly small in most cows, and supports the idea that perhaps annual testing is sufficient to identify the most infectious cattle for removal.

7. BLV in Beef Cattle

Compared with dairy cattle, much less is known about the epidemiology of BLV in beef cattle. A US Midwest survey completed by Benitez et al. in 2019 showed that 78% of 28 cow-calf herds had at least one ELISA-positive animal, with 36% ELISA-positive cattle among the 3175 tested [59]. A 24-month survival analysis in these herds found that ELISA-positive cattle faced a borderline significant ($P = 0.06$) 18% greater hazard of being culled compared to their ELISA-negative herdmates. In contrast, cattle with a higher proviral load had an 84% greater hazard of leaving the herd as compared with ELISA-negative cattle ($P = 0.01$).

Among breeding beef bulls in the Midwest US, 49% of 39 farms had at least one ELISA-positive bull, and 45% of the 121 bulls tested were ELISA-positive in a recent study [60]. Proviral DNA was identified in the smegma of 7.4% (4/54) of bulls tested in this study, raising the possibility of BLV transmission during natural breeding.

8. Controlling BLV

Early control efforts were based on culling cattle with high blood lymphocyte counts [61]. More recently, targeted culling to control BLV has been based on an BLV antibody response. However, eradicating BLV by culling antibody-positive cattle is usually economically impossible for farms with high prevalence rates. Management interventions such as single-use hypodermic needles and examination gloves have not always been effective in reducing transmission [62]. Alternative control approaches are being sought such as vaccination and host genetic selection. Recent development of qPCR tests to measure BLV proviral load are showing efficacy in identifying the most infectious cattle so they can be removed via segregating or culling. Researchers were able to demonstrate in three small herds that selectively segregating or culling of cows with high PVL and high blood lymphocyte counts led to a dramatic decrease in BLV incidence and prevalence within a few years (Figure 2) [63]. Output from the testing laboratory (Central Star Cooperative, E. Lansing, MI, USA) now shows how much each cow contributes to the herd's total PVL. For example, the manager of one particular farm can see that the 28 cows with the highest PVL accounted for 43% of the herd's total PVL. This output is proving useful to producers in identifying the most infectious cows to prioritize for removal in order to reduce the incidence of new infections.

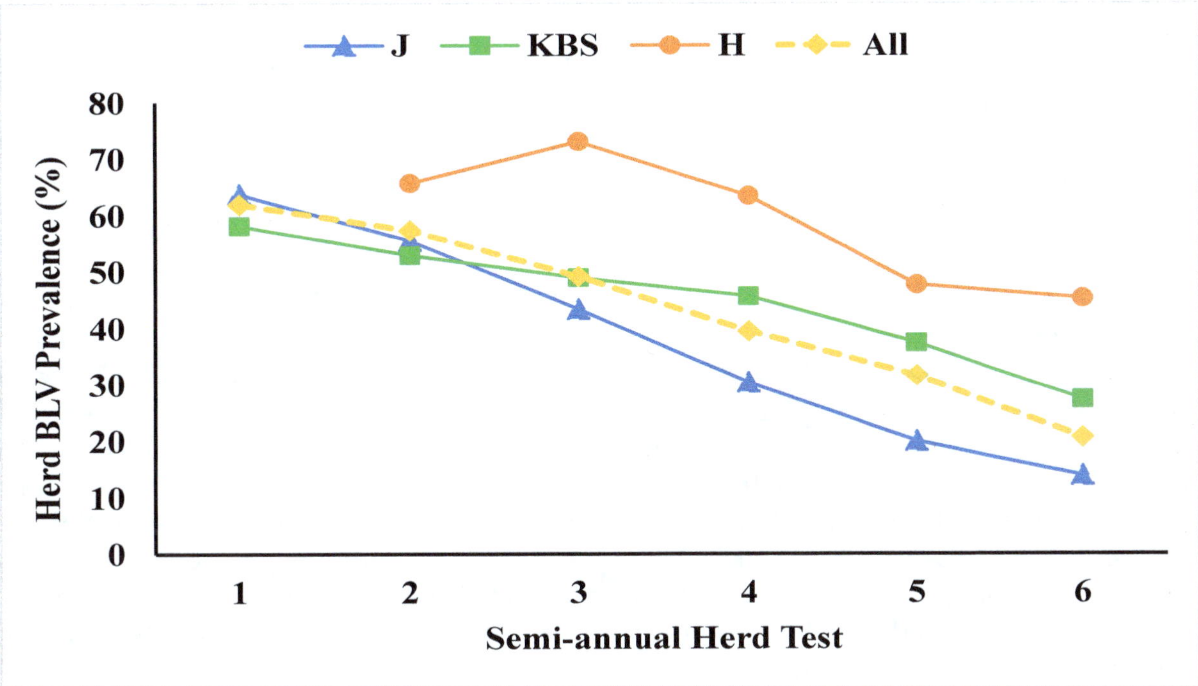

Figure 2. Decrease in herd BLV prevalence among three herds, culling or segregating those cows with the highest lymphocyte counts and/or BLV proviral loads, from Ruggiero [63].

One 3000-cow herd in the Midwest U.S. has had great success in screening cows with the ELISA test and measuring PVL on ELISA-positive cows. Cows with the highest PVL were then segregated and prioritized for culling. As of 27 October 2020, only 10 cows with a PVL > 0 remained in a separate pen awaiting culling. Because BLV in the heifers had been controlled via ELISA testing, this large herd is on the verge of eradicating BLV [64].

9. Host Genetics

Genetic diversity within a population is directly linked to that population's ability to respond to specific pathogens, reflecting the high degree of heterogeneity within genes involved in the innate and adaptive immune system. The major histocompatibility complex (MHC) is a cluster of genes that are responsible for self and non-self-antigen recognition for proper immune function in mammals. While the general structure of the MHC is conserved amongst species, specific exons encoding MHC molecules are highly polymorphic to provide a diversity of adaptive immune responses to emerging pathogens within a population. The Bovine leukocyte antigen (BoLA) in cattle is orthologous to the human MHC or Human Leukocyte Antigen (HLA) complex. Within this cluster of evolutionarily conserved genes, the BoLA Class IIa subregion houses the DR and DQ genes, which have undergone extensive genetic characterization within the context of BLV susceptibility and disease progression [65–68].

Specifically, DRB3 and DQA1 sequence-based typing (SBT) is becoming a requisite component of BLV cohort studies in order to better understand the propensity of individual disease trajectory. The DRB3 gene has 130 identified alleles to date [69] and is the only functional locus within the DR gene; thus, it is the strongest expressed gene within this cluster. In contrast, there are numerous functional DQ genes, including five DQA genes, DQA1 being the most polymorphic with 31 different identified alleles. The second exon of the II BoLA-DRB3 and DQA1 alleles encodes the extracellular portion of the molecule and is polymorphic in nature, which provides antigen-presenting cells with variability in the immune response to particular pathogens for individuals.

Pedigree analysis first demonstrated that bovine lymphosarcoma and persistent lymphocytosis track with family lineages, providing the first evidence for genetic influence on susceptibility to BLV [70]. Originally, serologically defined BoLA Class I alleles were found to be associated with BLV-resistance phenotype [71]; however, MHC class II alleles were later identified as playing a stronger role in BLV outcome in cattle [72]. More recently, SBT of BoLA alleles has found specific BoLA Class II DRB3 and DQA1 alleles to be associated with resistance or susceptibility to the development of BLV-associated disease. Over the last 30 years, a substantial amount of evidence has demonstrated that BoLA class II allele associates with BLV PVL. Although numerous alleles have been classified as leading to a resistant or susceptible BLV phenotype, DRB3*0902 has been most notably associated with the resistant phenotype [65,66,68,72–74]. More recently, polymorphism within the DRB3 gene has been identified as having a stronger association with the BLV phenotype than the DQA1 gene [75].

Initial approaches to BoLA typing involved restriction enzyme digestion and analysis of resulting fragments to identify alleles (RFLP). BoLA-allele identification is now accomplished via different sequencing approaches such as PCR followed by Sanger sequencing. Presently, research groups are utilizing multiplex barcoded primers in order to systematically tag hundreds of animals prior to next generation sequencing and bioinformatic analysis, enabling a wider scope of animals. This approach will enable studies to analyze a much larger number of animals to determine how various BoLA-DRB3 alleles associate with disease state. Due to the high degree of heterogeneity of this genetic locus, SNP-based genotyping is unable to resolve the identity via hybridization probes. This genetic analysis would allow bull studs to determine the BoLA status of their young sires and potentially market BLV-resistance as an economically important trait. Use of this approach as an in-herd selection tool may not be as useful, as cattle do not persist within modern commercial dairy herds long enough to recover an economic benefit. Current studies are under way to determine if colostrum from BoLA-DRB3*0902 dams provide additional protection to their young over non-BoLA-DRB3*0902 dams, which may be a useful management strategy for producers. Though selection for this important gene may not resolve the high rate of BLV prevalence in North America, it may be a useful tool for understanding virus-host interaction and BLV's impact on profitability.

10. The BLV Viral Genome

BLV is a retrovirus closely related to HTLV-1, whereby definition, it encodes a reverse-transcribed DNA copy of its RNA genome into the host cell that it invades. Once integrated, the proviral genome is propagated via mitosis. Expression of BLV proviral genes occurs through endogenous transcription and translation mechanisms. The BLV genome consists of a common 5′–gag–pro–pol–env–3′ gene cassette encoding the viral capsid, protease and envelope proteins required for viral repackaging. Additionally, the BLV viral genome encodes its own reverse transcriptase (pol) required for creating the DNA version of the virus for integration accomplished via the virally encoded integrase also located within the pol gene. Accessory genes, including the U3 region within the 3′ untranslated region (UTR) and U5 within the 5′ UTR, enhance viral gene transcription via transcription factor binding sites. Two protein coding genes, Tax and Rex, are considered CIS-transcriptional activators that bind to the 3′ LTR and are commonly implicated in viral oncogenesis [76,77]. Unlike other retroviruses, BLV also encodes 10 microRNAs and other long non-coding RNAs, in which their expression levels are now being shown to associate with BLV pathogenesis [78,79]. Though the genomic architecture is not unique to other retroviruses, such as HTLV-1 and HIV, many knowledge gaps still remain as to how genetic variation within accessory genes may confer differences in transmissibility, virulence and pathogenicity.

11. Human Health

The zoonotic potential of BLV has long been debated, but the understanding of retrovirus biology developed for the AIDS/HIV epidemic has led to more recent findings for the BLV retrovirus [80]. Approximately 70% of humans have been reported to have anti-BLV antibodies [81,82], and 25% have detectable BLV provirus in their blood [82,83]. These studies are in contrast to those conducted in the 1970s, which failed to detect BLV antibodies in people with high cattle exposure, such as farmers, veterinarians, meat inspectors and creamery workers [84].

Evidence for human infection has not been reported from any investigator. Whole genome sequencing of 51 breast cancer tumors showed no evidence of BLV DNA [85]. A query of the Cancer Genome atlas failed to identify BLV proviral DNA among 750 breast carcinomas [86] or BLV transcripts among 810 breast cancer samples [87]. However, case-control studies have reported finding BLV DNA in cancerous breast tissue at higher rates than in benign, non-cancerous tissue [88–90]. The relationship between BLV and breast cancer was reported to have an attributable risk of between 37–52% [88,91].

Potential routes of transmission between cattle and people are numerous, including direct contact with infected animals and the consumption of unpasteurized or undercooked dairy and beef products, which have been shown to contain the BLV provirus [92]. The detection of the DNA provirus is more suggestive of an actual infection than are anti-BLV antibodies, which may only indicate exposure and not necessarily infection. Clearly, more work is needed to determine all possible human health effects of BLV exposure. It is worth noting that northern European countries that eradicated BLV many years ago are currently experiencing somewhat higher rates of mammary cancer than in the U.S. A more careful ecological study should be conducted once the European women born post-eradication reach adulthood.

12. Vaccines

Vaccination of cattle for BLV is still being investigated. Unlike some other retroviruses, such as HIV, BLV has a relatively stable genome, and thus, an efficacious vaccine may be possible. However, many previous attempts at developing a vaccine for BLV have been unsuccessful [93]. Several research groups are currently working on BLV vaccines. One group has developed an attenuated vaccine by targeted mutations and deletions and is seeking regulatory approval for use [93].

Genetically modified vaccine candidates must contend with additional regulatory requirements. Hopefully any developed vaccine will enable vaccinates to be distinguished from cattle with natural infection, and thus, enhance rather than deter any ongoing BLV control efforts.

13. Issues for Future Inquiry

1. What causes a minority of cattle to develop extremely high proviral load and to what extent is this determined by their genetics or the time at which they become infected (in utero or very early in life via colostrum)?
2. How important are host genetics, whereby certain alleles predispose an animal to a high or low proviral load, antibody titer and/or severity of pathology?
3. Why do first lactation animals seemingly avoid the milk production loss and increased risk of culling that are associated with older ELISA-positive cows?
4. The severe inbreeding of Holstein dairy cattle is such that the effective population size is <50 animals, and they would be considered critically endangered if they were a wild animal species [94]. This raises the question of how long a provirus-infected lymphocyte could survive and propagate upon being introduced into an almost genetically identical cow compared to a genetically distinct cow.
5. Attribution studies are needed to determine the percentage of new BLV infections that come from direct contact, biting fly transmission, shared hypodermic needles, etc.
6. The role of free BLV RNA in disease transmission should be definitively established.

7. Controlled studies are required to measure the extent to which BLV infection contributes to the causation of the major dairy diseases such as mastitis, lameness, infertility, etc.
8. Longitudinal studies should determine how commonly animals are infected with BLV as calves, but the virus becomes sequestered until the stress of birth and lactation. Genetic methods should be developed to determine if newly recognized infections in cows are usually caused by the same strain found in their dams over two years ago, or the same strains found in their contemporaries.
9. The role of BLV in the induction and pathogenesis of human breast cancer and other human diseases should be definitively established.
10. What role does microRNA play in the pathogenesis of BLV, and can it be used for diagnosis or prognosis?
11. A safe and efficacious BLV vaccine should be developed that allows differentiation between vaccinates and natural infection.
12. The likely return on investment for BLV control and eradication should be determined for test and removal using ELISA and by using ELISA screening with proviral load follow-up testing.

14. BLV and the Future of Animal Agriculture

BLV control measures must be targeted to the needs of the future, rather than the needs of the present. A recent Rethinkx analysis of animal agriculture predicts a rapid contraction in the dairy and beef industries as alternative methods of producing protein are developed, e.g., fermentation of specific proteins and tissue culture [95]. They predict that demand for cow products will have fallen by 70% by 2030. If the Rethinkx predictions are even close to accurate, then efforts to control BLV would be occurring in a market of rapidly declining numbers of herds and cows. The future cattle industry would need to survive competition with the molecular-food industry, which presumably avoids animal welfare concerns, excessive water and land use, serious environmental contamination with manure or generation of excessive greenhouse gases. Supposedly antibiotic residues can be prevented in the food product and in any waste material. Contamination with our common foodborne pathogens such as *E. coli, Campylobacter* and *Salmonella* will become an issue unique to animal agriculture, as it will be much easier to produce a pathogen-free food product coming out of a controlled fermentation or tissue culture process than it will be to produce such a product from a pathogen-abundant farm environment. As the public's immune systems become increasingly naïve to our common foodborne pathogens, progressively lower pathogen doses will be capable of causing clinical disease.

To compete with these new food products, the surviving animal industry will need to have adequately solved the previously mentioned issues. Future consumers may not want animal products from herds infected with BLV, which may become recognized as a possible public health hazard and also a cause of animal suffering. If the predicted contraction of herd and cow numbers becomes a reality, many producers will likely forgo controlling BLV if they do not expect their herd to survive for many more years. However, herd managers wanting to reduce the size of their herd may take this as an opportunity for selectively culling BLV-infected cows in the belief that BLV-free herds will be more profitable and appealing to consumers. However, in these uncertain times for the animal industries, many producers may not want to invest funds to eradicate BLV. Some may even decide to wait in the hope that a vaccine is developed that will serve as a useful tool for BLV eradication.

15. Conclusions

Heightened BLV research activity has been driven by BLV's increasing prevalence in many nations and recent recognition of its impact on milk production, cow lifespan and possible public health implications. The means by which BLV disrupts the cow's immune system are being described in greater detail than was possible before. It must be determined how newly available BLV diagnostic tools can best be used to control this infection. Many important research questions must be addressed regarding BLV epidemiology, immunology and control. It is likely that the future of the animal industries will see a continued effort to control BLV.

References

1. Yang, Y.; Fan, W.; Mao, Y.; Yang, Z.; Lu, G.; Zhang, R.; Zhang, H.; Szeto, C.; Wang, C. Bovine leukemia virus infection in cattle of China: Association with reduced milk production and increased somatic cell score. *J. Dairy Sci.* **2016**, *99*, 3688–3697. [CrossRef] [PubMed]
2. Benavides, B.B.; Quevedo, D.A.C.; de La Cruz, M.F.S. Epidemiological study of bovine leukemia virus in dairy cows in six herds in the municipality of Pasto, Nariño. *Rev. Lasallista Investig.* **2013**, *10*, 18–23.
3. Úsuga-Monroy, C.; Echeverri, J.; López-Herrera, H. Molecular diagnosis of bovine Leukemia Virus in a population of Holstein cows, Colombia. *Arch. Zootec.* **2015**, *64*, 383–388. [CrossRef]
4. Jimenez, C.; Bonilla, J.A.; Dolz, G.; Rodriguez, L.R.; Herrero, L.; Bolaños, E.; Cortéz, M.R.; Moreno, E. Bovine Leukaemia-virus Infection in Costa Rica. *J. Veter. Med. Ser. B* **1995**, *42*, 385–390. [CrossRef] [PubMed]
5. Mousavi, S.; Haghparast, A.; Mohammadi, G.; Tabatabaeizadeh, S.-E. Prevalence of bovine leukemia virus (BLV) infection in the northeast of Iran. *Veter. Res. Forum Int. Q. J.* **2014**, *5*, 135–139.
6. Nekoei, S.; Hafshejani, T.T.; Doosti, A.; Khamesipour, F. Molecular detection of bovine leukemia virus in peripheral blood of Iranian cattle, camel and sheep. *Pol. J. Veter. Sci.* **2015**, *18*, 703–707. [CrossRef]
7. Murakami, K.; Kobayashi, S.; Konishi, M.; Kameyama, K.-I.; Tsutsui, T. Nationwide Survey of Bovine Leukemia Virus Infection among Dairy and Beef Breeding Cattle in Japan from 2009–2011. *J. Veter. Med. Sci.* **2013**, *75*, 1123–1126. [CrossRef]
8. Ochirkhuu, N.; Konnai, S.; Odbileg, R.; Nishimori, A.; Okagawa, T.; Murata, S.; Ohashi, K. Detection of bovine leukemia virus and identification of its genotype in Mongolian cattle. *Arch. Virol.* **2015**, *161*, 985–991. [CrossRef]
9. Polat, M.; Ohno, A.; Takeshima, S.-N.; Kim, J.; Kikuya, M.; Matsumoto, Y.; Mingala, C.N.; Onuma, M.; Aida, Y. Detection and molecular characterization of bovine leukemia virus in Philippine cattle. *Arch. Virol.* **2014**, *160*, 285–296. [CrossRef]
10. Ndou, R.V.; Sejesho, F.; Dzoma, B.M.; Motsei, L.; Nyirenda, M.; Bakunzi, F.R. A Serosurvey of the Prevalence of Enzootic Bovine Leukosis in the Mafikeng Area of the North West Province of South Africa. *J. Hum. Ecol.* **2011**, *36*, 53–55. [CrossRef]
11. Şevik, M.; Avcı, O.; Ince, Ö.B. An 8-year longitudinal sero-epidemiological study of bovine leukaemia virus (BLV) infection in dairy cattle in Turkey and analysis of risk factors associated with BLV seropositivity. *Trop. Anim. Health Prod.* **2015**, *47*, 715–720. [CrossRef] [PubMed]
12. Walrand, F.; Fumoux, F.; Roelants, G.; Parodi, A.-L.; Levy, D. Incidence of bovine leukemia virus-specific antibodies in west african cattle. *Int. J. Cancer* **1986**, *37*, 619–621. [CrossRef]
13. Monti, G.; Schrijver, R.; Beier, D. Genetic diversity and spread of Bovine leukaemia virus isolates in Argentine dairy cattle. *Arch. Virol.* **2004**, *150*, 443–458. [CrossRef] [PubMed]
14. Nekouei, O.; VanLeeuwen, J.; Sanchez, J.; Kelton, D.; Tiwari, A.; Keefe, G. Herd-level risk factors for infection with bovine leukemia virus in Canadian dairy herds. *Prev. Veter. Med.* **2015**, *119*, 105–113. [CrossRef] [PubMed]
15. USDA Bovine Leukosis Virus (BLV) on U.S. Dairy Operations 2007. Available online: https://web.archive.org/web/20190205034903/https://www.aphis.usda.gov/animal_health/nahms/dairy/downloads/dairy07/Dairy07_is_BLV.pdf (accessed on 4 February 2019).
16. LaDronka, R.M.; Ainsworth, S.; Wilkins, M.J.; Norby, B.; Byrem, T.M.; Bartlett, P.C. Prevalence of Bovine Leukemia Virus Antibodies in US Dairy Cattle. *Veter. Med. Int.* **2018**, *2018*, 1–8. [CrossRef] [PubMed]
17. The European Commission. Commission Implementing Decision 2016/168. *Off. J. Eur. Union* **2016**, *32*, 153–157.
18. White, T.L.; Moore, D.A. Reasons for whole carcass condemnations of cattle in the United States and implications for producer education and veterinary intervention. *J. Am. Veter. Med. Assoc.* **2009**, *235*, 937–941. [CrossRef]
19. Emanuelson, U.; Scherling, K.; Pettersson, H. Relationships between herd bovine leukemia virus infection status and reproduction, disease incidence, and productivity in Swedish dairy herds. *Prev. Veter. Med.* **1992**, *12*, 121–131. [CrossRef]
20. Brenner, J.; Van-Haam, M.; Savir, D.; Trainin, Z. The implication of BLV infection in the productivity, reproductive capacity and survival rate of a dairy cow. *Veter. Immunol. Immunopathol.* **1989**, *22*, 299–305. [CrossRef]

21. Trainin, Z.; Brenner, J.; Meirom, R.; Ungar-Waron, H. Detrimental effect of bovine leukemia virus (BLV) on the immunological state of cattle. *Veter. Immunol. Immunopathol.* **1996**, *54*, 293–302. [CrossRef]
22. Haredasht, S.A.; Vidal, G.; Edmondson, A.; Moore, D.; Silva-Del-Río, N.; Martínez-López, B. Characterization of the Temporal Trends in the Rate of Cattle Carcass Condemnations in the US and Dynamic Modeling of the Condemnation Reasons in California With a Seasonal Component. *Front. Veter. Sci.* **2018**, *5*. [CrossRef]
23. Pollari, F.L.; Wangsuphachart, V.L.; Digiacomo, R.F.; Evermann, J.F. Effects of bovine leukemia virus infection on production and reproduction in dairy cattle. *Can. J. Veter. Res.* **1992**, *56*, 289–295.
24. Huber, N.L.; Digiacomo, R.F.; Evermann, J.F.; Studer, E. Bovine leukemia virus infection in a large Holstein herd: Prospective comparison of production and reproductive performance in antibody-negative and antibody-positive cows. *Am. J. Veter. Res.* **1981**, *42*, 1477–1481.
25. Sorge, U.S.; Lissemore, K.; Cantin, R.; Kelton, D.F. Short communication: Milk ELISA status for bovine leukosis virus infection is not associated with milk production in dairy cows. *J. Dairy Sci.* **2011**, *94*, 5062–5064. [CrossRef]
26. Nekouei, O.; VanLeeuwen, J.; Stryhn, H.; Kelton, D.; Keefe, G. Lifetime effects of infection with bovine leukemia virus on longevity and milk production of dairy cows. *Prev. Veter. Med.* **2016**, *133*, 1–9. [CrossRef]
27. Norby, B.; Bartlett, P.C.; Byrem, T.M.; Erskine, R.J. Effect of infection with bovine leukemia virus on milk production in Michigan dairy cows. *J. Dairy Sci.* **2016**, *99*, 2043–2052. [CrossRef]
28. Ott, S.L.; Johnson, R.; Wells, S.J. Association between bovine-leukosis virus seroprevalence and herd-level productivity on US dairy farms. *Prev. Veter. Med.* **2003**, *61*, 249–262. [CrossRef]
29. Erskine, R.J.; Bartlett, P.C.; Byrem, T.M.; Render, C.L.; Febvay, C.; Houseman, J.T. Association between bovine leukemia virus, production, and population age in Michigan dairy herds. *J. Dairy Sci.* **2012**, *95*, 727–734. [CrossRef]
30. Wu, D.; Murakami, K.; Morooka, A.; Jin, H.; Inoshima, Y.; Sentsui, H. In vivo transcription of bovine leukemia virus and bovine immunodeficiency-like virus. *Virus Res.* **2003**, *97*, 81–87. [CrossRef]
31. Bartlett, P.C.; Norby, B.; Byrem, T.M.; Parmelee, A.; Ledergerber, J.T.; Erskine, R.J. Bovine leukemia virus and cow longevity in Michigan dairy herds. *J. Dairy Sci.* **2013**, *96*, 1591–1597. [CrossRef]
32. Rhodes, J.K.; Pelzer, K.D.; Johnson, Y.J. Economic implications of bovine leukemia virus infection in mid-Atlantic dairy herds. *J. Am. Veter. Med. Assoc.* **2003**, *223*, 346–352. [CrossRef] [PubMed]
33. Frie, M.C.; Coussens, P.M. Bovine leukemia virus: A major silent threat to proper immune responses in cattle. *Veter. Immunol. Immunopathol.* **2015**, *163*, 103–114. [CrossRef] [PubMed]
34. Erskine, R.J.; Bartlett, P.C.; Sabo, K.M.; Sordillo, L.M. Bovine Leukemia Virus Infection in Dairy Cattle: Effect on Serological Response to Immunization against J5Escherichia coliBacterin. *Veter. Med. Int.* **2011**, *2011*, 1–5. [CrossRef] [PubMed]
35. Frie, M.C.; Sporer, K.R.; Wallace, J.C.; Maes, R.K.; Sordillo, L.M.; Bartlett, P.C.; Coussens, P.M. Reduced humoral immunity and atypical cell-mediated immunity in response to vaccination in cows naturally infected with bovine leukemia virus. *Veter. Immunol. Immunopathol.* **2016**, *182*, 125–135. [CrossRef]
36. Frie, M.C.; Sporer, K.R.B.; Benitez, O.J.; Wallace, J.C.; Droscha, C.J.; Bartlett, P.C.; Coussens, P.M. Dairy Cows Naturally Infected with Bovine Leukemia Virus Exhibit Abnormal B- and T-Cell Phenotypes after Primary and Secondary Exposures to Keyhole Limpet Hemocyanin. *Front. Veter. Sci.* **2017**, *4*, 112. [CrossRef]
37. Puentes, R.; De Brun, L.; Algorta, A.; Da Silva, V.; Mansilla, F.; Sacco, G.; Llambí, S.; Capozzo, A.V. Evaluation of serological response to foot-and-mouth disease vaccination in BLV infected cows. *BMC Veter. Res.* **2016**, *12*, 1–7. [CrossRef]
38. Blagitz, M.G.; Souza, F.N.; Batista, C.F.; Azevedo, L.F.F.; Sanchez, E.M.R.; Diniz, S.A.; Silva, M.X.; Haddad, J.P.; Della Libera, A.M.M.P. Immunological implications of bovine leukemia virus infection. *Res. Veter. Sci.* **2017**, *114*, 109–116. [CrossRef]
39. Della Libera, A.M.M.P.; Souza, F.N.; Batista, C.F.; Santos, B.P.; De Azevedo, L.F.F.; Ramos-Sanchez, E.M.; Diniz, S.A.; Silva, M.X.; Haddad, J.P.; Blagitz, M.G. Effects of bovine leukemia virus infection on milk neutrophil function and the milk lymphocyte profile. *Veter. Res.* **2015**, *46*, 2. [CrossRef]
40. Yuan, Y.; Kitamura-Muramatsu, Y.; Saito, S.; Ishizaki, H.; Nakano, M.; Haga, S.; Matoba, K.; Ohno, A.; Murakami, H.; Takeshima, S.-N.; et al. Detection of the BLV provirus from nasal secretion and saliva samples using BLV-CoCoMo-qPCR-2: Comparison with blood samples from the same cattle. *Virus Res.* **2015**, *210*, 248–254. [CrossRef]

41. Ruggiero, V.J. Field Studies on the Control of Bovine Leukemia Virus in Dairy Cows. Ph.D. Thesis, Michigan State University, East Lansing, MI, USA, 2019.
42. Ruggiero, V.J.; Dziuba, M.; Bartlett, P.C.; Coussens, P.M. Untitled BLV-Immunoglobulin Paper. Unpublished manuscript in preparation, 2020.
43. Onuma, M.; Sagata, N.; Okada, K.; Ogawa, Y.; Ikawa, Y.; Oshima, K. Integration of Bovine Leukemia Virus DNA in the Genomes of Bovine Lymphosarcoma Cells. *Microbiol. Immunol.* **1982**, *26*, 813–820. [CrossRef]
44. Juliarena, M.A.; Gutierrez, S.E.; Ceriani, C. Determination of proviral load in bovine leukemia virus–infected cattle with and without lymphocytosis. *Am. J. Veter. Res.* **2007**, *68*, 1220–1225. [CrossRef]
45. Fechner, H.; Kurg, A.; Geue, L.; Blankenstein, P.; Mewes, G.; Ebner, D.; Beier, D. Evaluation of Polymerase Chain Reaction (PCR) Application in Diagnosis of Bovine Leukaemia Virus (BLV) Infection in Naturally Infected Cattle. *J. Veter. Med. Ser. B* **1996**, *43*, 621–630. [CrossRef]
46. Klintevall, K.; Ballagi-Pordány, A.; Näslund, K.; Belák, S. Bovine leukaemia virus: Rapid detection of proviral DNA by nested PCR in blood and organs of experimentally infected calves. *Veter. Microbiol.* **1994**, *42*, 191–204. [CrossRef]
47. Kaplan, J.E.; Khabbaz, R.F.; Murphy, E.L.; Hermansen, S.; Roberts, C.; Lal, R.; Heneine, W.; Wright, D.; Matijas, L.; Thomson, R.; et al. Male-to-Female Transmission of Human T-Cell Lymphotropic Virus Types I and II: Association with Viral Load. *J. Acquir. Immune Defic. Syndr. Hum. Retrovirol.* **1996**, *12*, 193–201. [CrossRef]
48. Percher, F.; Jeannin, P.; Martin-Latil, S.; Gessain, A.; Afonso, P.V.; Vidy, A.; Ceccaldi, P.-E. Mother-to-Child Transmission of HTLV-1 Epidemiological Aspects, Mechanisms and Determinants of Mother-to-Child Transmission. *Viruses* **2016**, *8*, 40. [CrossRef]
49. Gutiérrez, G.; Álvarez, I.; Politzki, R.; Lomónaco, M.; Santos, M.J.D.; Rondelli, F.; Fondevila, N.; Trono, K. Natural progression of Bovine Leukemia Virus infection in Argentinean dairy cattle. *Veter. Microbiol.* **2011**, *151*, 255–263. [CrossRef]
50. Rodríguez, S.M.; Florins, A.; Gillet, N.; De Brogniez, A.; Sánchez-Alcaraz, M.T.; Boxus, M.; Boulanger, F.; Gutiérrez, G.; Trono, K.; Alvarez, I.; et al. Preventive and Therapeutic Strategies for Bovine Leukemia Virus: Lessons for HTLV. *Viruses* **2011**, *3*, 1210–1248. [CrossRef]
51. Ohno, A.; Takeshima, S.-N.; Matsumoto, Y.; Aida, Y. Risk factors associated with increased bovine leukemia virus proviral load in infected cattle in Japan from 2012 to 2014. *Virus Res.* **2015**, *210*, 283–290. [CrossRef]
52. Buxton, B.A.; Schultz, R.D. Factors affecting the infectivity of lymphocytes from cattle with bovine leukosis virus. *Can. J. Comp. Med. Rev. Can. Med. Comp.* **1984**, *48*, 365–369.
53. Mammerickx, M.; Portetelle, D.; De Clercq, K.K.; Burny, A. Experimental transmission of enzootic bovine leukosis to cattle, sheep and goats: Infectious doses of blood and incubation period of the disease. *Leuk. Res.* **1987**, *11*, 353–358. [CrossRef]
54. Molloy, J.B.; Dimmock, C.K.; Eaves, F.W.; Bruyeres, A.G.; Cowley, J.A.; Ward, W.H. Control of bovine leukaemia virus transmission by selective culling of infected cattle on the basis of viral antigen expression in lymphocyte cultures. *Veter. Microbiol.* **1994**, *39*, 323–333. [CrossRef]
55. Gutiérrez, G.; Alvarez, I.; Merlini, R.; Rondelli, F.; Trono, K. Dynamics of perinatal bovine leukemia virus infection. *BMC Veter. Res.* **2014**, *10*, 82. [CrossRef]
56. Juliarena, M.A.; Barrios, C.N.; Ceriani, M.C.; Esteban, E.N. Hot topic: Bovine leukemia virus (BLV)-infected cows with low proviral load are not a source of infection for BLV-free cattle. *J. Dairy Sci.* **2016**, *99*, 4586–4589. [CrossRef]
57. Mekata, H.; Sekiguchi, S.; Konnai, S.; Kirino, Y.; Horii, Y.; Norimine, J. Horizontal transmission and phylogenetic analysis of bovine leukemia virus in two districts of Miyazaki, Japan. *J. Veter. Med. Sci.* **2015**, *77*, 1115–1120. [CrossRef]
58. Hutchinson, H.C. Transmission and Progression of Bovine Leukemia Virus. Ph.D. Thesis, Michigan State University, East Lansing, MI, USA, 2020.
59. Benitez, O.J.; Norby, B.; Bartlett, P.C.; Maeroff, J.E.; Grooms, D.L. Impact of bovine leukemia virus infection on beef cow longevity. *Prev. Veter. Med.* **2020**, *181*, 105055. [CrossRef]
60. Benitez, O.J.; Roberts, J.N.; Norby, B.; Bartlett, P.C.; Takeshima, S.-N.; Watanuki, S.; Aida, Y.; Grooms, D.L. Breeding bulls as a potential source of bovine leukemia virus transmission in beef herds. *J. Am. Veter. Med. Assoc.* **2019**, *254*, 1335–1340. [CrossRef]

61. Bendixen, H.J. Preventive measures in cattle leukemia: Leukosis enzootica bovis*. *Ann. N. Y. Acad. Sci.* **2006**, *108*, 1241–1267. [CrossRef]
62. Ruggiero, V.J.; Bartlett, P.C. Single-use hypodermic needles and obstetric sleeves failed to reduce bovine leukemia virus transmission in three dairy herds. *Bov. Pract.* **2019**, *53*, 128–133. [CrossRef]
63. Ruggiero, V.; Norby, B.; Benitez, O.; Hutchinson, H.; Sporer, K.; Droscha, C.; Swenson, C.; Bartlett, P. Controlling bovine leukemia virus in dairy herds by identifying and removing cows with the highest proviral load and lymphocyte counts. *J. Dairy Sci.* **2019**, *102*, 9165–9175. [CrossRef]
64. Taxis, T.M.; Sporer, K.R.B.; Droscha, C.J.; Niles, D.; DeJong, T.; Swenson, C.L.; Bartlett, P.C. Reducing bovine leukemia virus prevalence on a large midwestern dairy farm by using lymphocyte counts, ELISA antibody testing, and proviral load. *Bov. Pract.* **2020**. under review.
65. Hayashi, T.; Mekata, H.; Sekiguchi, S.; Kirino, Y.; Mitoma, S.; Honkawa, K.; Horii, Y.; Norimine, J. Cattle with the BoLA class II DRB3*0902 allele have significantly lower bovine leukemia proviral loads. *J. Veter. Med. Sci.* **2017**, *79*, 1552–1555. [CrossRef]
66. Miyasaka, T.; Takeshima, S.-N.; Jimba, M.; Matsumoto, Y.; Kobayashi, N.; Matsuhashi, T.; Sentsui, H.; Aida, Y. Identification of bovine leukocyte antigen class II haplotypes associated with variations in bovine leukemia virus proviral load in Japanese Black cattle. *Tissue Antigens* **2013**, *81*, 72–82. [CrossRef]
67. Lo, C.-W.; Borjigin, L.; Saito, S.; Fukunaga, K.; Saitou, E.; Okazaki, K.; Mizutani, T.; Wada, S.; Takeshima, S.-N.; Aida, Y. BoLA-DRB3 Polymorphism is Associated with Differential Susceptibility to Bovine Leukemia Virus-Induced Lymphoma and Proviral Load. *Viruses* **2020**, *12*, 352. [CrossRef]
68. Carignano, H.; Beribe, M.J.; Caffaro, M.E.; Amadio, A.; Nani, J.P.; Gutierrez, G.; Alvarez, I.; Trono, K.; Miretti, M.M.; Poli, M. BOLA-DRB3gene polymorphisms influence bovine leukaemia virus infection levels in Holstein and Holstein × Jersey crossbreed dairy cattle. *Anim. Genet.* **2017**, *48*, 420–430. [CrossRef]
69. Maccari, G.; Robinson, J.; Ballingall, K.; Guethlein, L.A.; Grimholt, U.; Kaufman, J.; Ho, C.-S.; De Groot, N.G.; Flicek, P.; Bontrop, R.E.; et al. IPD-MHC 2.0: An improved inter-species database for the study of the major histocompatibility complex. *Nucleic Acids Res.* **2017**, *45*, D860–D864. [CrossRef]
70. Abt, D.A.; Marshak, R.R.; Kulp, H.W.; Pollock, R.J. Studies on the Relationship Between Lymphocytosis and Bovine Leukosis. In Proceedings of the Comparative Leukemia Research 1969, 4th Inernational Symposium, Cherry Hill, NJ, USA, September 1969; Dutcher, R., Ed.; Karger Publishers: New York, NY, USA, 1970; pp. 527–536.
71. Lewin, H.A.; Bernoco, D. Evidence for BoLA-linked resistance and susceptibility to subclinical progression of bovine leukaemia virus infection. *Anim. Genet.* **1986**, *17*, 197–207. [CrossRef]
72. Xu, A.; van Eijk, M.J.; Park, C.; Lewin, H.A. Polymorphism in BoLA-DRB3 exon 2 correlates with resistance to persistent lymphocytosis caused by bovine leukemia virus. *J. Immunol.* **1993**, *151*, 6977–6985.
73. Udina, I.G.; Karamysheva, E.E.; Turkova, S.O.; Orlova, A.R.; Sulimova, G.E. Genetic mechanisms of resistance and susceptibility to leukemia in Ayrshire and black pied cattle breeds determined by allelic distribution of gene Bola-DRB3. *Генетика* **2003**, *39*, 306–317. [CrossRef]
74. Juliarena, M.A.; Poli, M.; Sala, L.; Ceriani, C.; Gutierrez, S.; Dolcini, G.L.; Rodrguez, E.M.; Mario, B.; Rodrguez-Dubra, C.; Esteban, E.; et al. Association of BLV infection profiles with alleles of theBoLA-DRB3.2gene. *Anim. Genet.* **2008**, *39*, 432–438. [CrossRef]
75. Takeshima, S.-N.; Ohno, A.; Aida, Y. Bovine leukemia virus proviral load is more strongly associated with bovine major histocompatibility complex class II DRB3 polymorphism than with DQA1 polymorphism in Holstein cow in Japan. *Retrovirology* **2019**, *16*, 1–6. [CrossRef]
76. Pluta, A.; Willems, L.; Douville, R.N.; Kuźmak, J. Effects of Naturally Occurring Mutations in Bovine Leukemia Virus 5′-LTR and Tax Gene on Viral Transcriptional Activity. *Pathogens* **2020**, *9*, 836. [CrossRef] [PubMed]
77. Zyrianova, I.M.; Kovalchuk, S. Bovine leukemia virus tax gene/Tax protein polymorphism and its relation to Enzootic Bovine Leukosis. *Virulence* **2020**, *11*, 80–87. [CrossRef] [PubMed]
78. Frie, M.C.; Droscha, C.J.; Greenlick, A.E.; Coussens, P.M. MicroRNAs Encoded by Bovine Leukemia Virus (BLV) Are Associated with Reduced Expression of B Cell Transcriptional Regulators in Dairy Cattle Naturally Infected with BLV. *Front. Veter. Sci.* **2018**, *4*, 245. [CrossRef] [PubMed]
79. Safari, R.; Jacques, J.-R.; Brostaux, Y.; Willems, L. Ablation of non-coding RNAs affects bovine leukemia virus B lymphocyte proliferation and abrogates oncogenesis. *PLOS Pathog.* **2020**, *16*, e1008502. [CrossRef]

80. Cuesta, L.M.; Lendez, P.A.; Farias, M.V.N.; Dolcini, G.L.; Ceriani, M.C. Can Bovine Leukemia Virus Be Related to Human Breast Cancer? A Review of the Evidence. *J. Mammary Gland. Biol. Neoplasia* **2018**, *23*, 101–107. [CrossRef]
81. Buehring, G.C.; Philpott, S.M.; Choi, K.Y. Humans Have Antibodies Reactive with Bovine Leukemia Virus. *AIDS Res. Hum. Retrovir.* **2003**, *19*, 1105–1113. [CrossRef]
82. Buehring, G.C.; Delaney, A.; Shen, H.; Chu, D.L.; Razavian, N.; Schwartz, D.A.; Demkovich, Z.R.; Bates, M.N. Bovine leukemia virus discovered in human blood. *BMC Infect. Dis.* **2019**, *19*, 1–10. [CrossRef]
83. Khalilian, M.; Hosseini, S.M.; Madadgar, O. Bovine leukemia virus detected in the breast tissue and blood of Iranian women. *Microb. Pathog.* **2019**, *135*, 103566. [CrossRef]
84. Burridge, M.J. The zoonotic potential of bovine leukemia virus. *Veter. Res. Commun.* **1981**, *5*, 117–126. [CrossRef]
85. Gillet, N.A.; Willems, L. Whole genome sequencing of 51 breast cancers reveals that tumors are devoid of bovine leukemia virus DNA. *Retrovirology* **2016**, *13*, 1–7. [CrossRef]
86. Khoury, J.D.; Tannir, N.M.; Williams, M.D.; Chen, Y.; Yao, H.; Zhang, J.; Thompson, E.J.; Meric-Bernstam, F.; Medeiros, L.J.; Weinstein, J.N.; et al. Landscape of DNA Virus Associations across Human Malignant Cancers: Analysis of 3775 Cases Using RNA-Seq. *J. Virol.* **2013**, *87*, 8916–8926. [CrossRef] [PubMed]
87. Tang, K.-W.; Alaei-Mahabadi, B.; Samuelsson, T.; Lindh, M.; Larsson, E. The landscape of viral expression and host gene fusion and adaptation in human cancer. *Nat. Commun.* **2013**, *4*, 2513. [CrossRef] [PubMed]
88. Baltzell, K.; Shen, H.M.; Krishnamurthy, S.; Sison, J.D.; Nuovo, G.J.; Buehring, G.C. Bovine leukemia virus linked to breast cancer but not coinfection with human papillomavirus: Case-control study of women in Texas. *Cancer* **2017**, *124*, 1342–1349. [CrossRef] [PubMed]
89. Buehring, G.C.; Shen, H.; Schwartz, D.A.; Lawson, J.S. Bovine leukemia virus linked to breast cancer in Australian women and identified before breast cancer development. *PLoS ONE* **2017**, *12*, e0179367. [CrossRef]
90. Schwingel, D.; Andreolla, A.P.; Erpen, L.M.S.; Frandoloso, R.; Kreutz, L.C. Bovine leukemia virus DNA associated with breast cancer in women from South Brazil. *Sci. Rep.* **2019**, *9*, 1–7. [CrossRef]
91. Buehring, G.C.; Shen, H.M.; Jensen, H.M.; Jin, D.L.; Hudes, M.; Block, G. Exposure to Bovine Leukemia Virus Is Associated with Breast Cancer: A Case-Control Study. *PLoS ONE* **2015**, *10*, e0134304. [CrossRef]
92. Olaya-Galán, N.N.; Corredor-Figueroa, A.P.; Guzmán-Garzón, T.C.; Ríos-Hernandez, K.S.; Salas-Cárdenas, S.P.; Patarroyo, M.A.; Gutierrez, M.F. Bovine leukaemia virus DNA in fresh milk and raw beef for human consumption. *Epidemiol. Infect.* **2017**, *145*, 3125–3130. [CrossRef]
93. Abdala, A.; Alvarez, I.; Brossel, H.; Calvinho, L.; Carignano, H.; Franco, L.; Gazon, H.; Gillissen, C.; Hamaidia, M.; Hoyos, C.; et al. BLV: Lessons on vaccine development. *Retrovirology* **2019**, *16*, 1–6. [CrossRef]
94. O'Hagan, M.; Undark. From Two Bulls, Nine Million Dairy Cows. *Sci. Am.* **2019**. Available online: https://www.scientificamerican.com/article/from-two-bulls-nine-million-dairy-cows/ (accessed on 17 December 2020).
95. RethinkX Food and Agriculture Report—RethinkX. Available online: https://www.rethinkx.com/food-and-agriculture (accessed on 29 July 2020).

2

Veterinarians' Knowledge, Attitudes and Practices Associated with Bovine Viral Diarrhoea Virus Control and Prevention in South-East Australia

Claire McMorrow [1,2], Allan J. Gunn [1,2], Shahid Khalfan [1], Marta Hernandez-Jover [1,2] and Victoria J. Brookes [1,2,*]

1 School of Animal and Veterinary Sciences, Charles Sturt University, Wagga Wagga, NSW 2650, Australia; cv.mcmorrow@gmail.com (C.M.); algunn@csu.edu.au (A.J.G.); shahid.khalfan@gmail.com (S.K.); mhernandez-jover@csu.edu.au (M.H.-J.)

2 Graham Centre for Agricultural Innovation (NSW Department of Primary Industries and Charles Sturt University), Wagga Wagga, NSW 2650, Australia

* Correspondence: vbrookes@csu.edu.au

Abstract: In Australia, the responsibility and associated costs for the control and prevention of Bovine Viral Diarrhoea Virus (BVDV) rest solely with producers. Veterinarians provide producers with farm-specific options for BVDV management and support BVDV control and elimination in their region. We surveyed veterinarians to determine their knowledge, attitudes and practices (KAP) associated with BVDV control in south-east Australia. We found that veterinarians' recommendations do not always align with producers' control measures. Veterinarians were uncertain about BVDV prevalence and the proportion of producers using BVDV control measures in their regions. Veterinarians generally promoted biosecurity and vaccination, and were concerned about the welfare and additional disease risks associated with persistently infected (PI) cattle. Veterinarians highlighted concerns about disease risks associated with a previously undocumented practice in which producers collect blood from PI cattle to administer to BVDV naïve cattle; termed "vampire vaccination" in this study. A greater understanding of the burden, impact and economics of BVDV is needed to align veterinarians' and producers' KAP to improve BVDV management on farms, and more appreciation of veterinarians' and producers' values is needed before BVDV control could be implemented at a regional or country level.

Keywords: bovine viral diarrhoea virus; Australia; control; persistently infected; welfare

---

1. Introduction

Bovine Viral Diarrhoea Virus (BVDV/Pestivirus) is a globally endemic, infectious disease of cattle that causes immunosuppression and substantial production losses, including reproductive losses, such as reduced conception rates, embryonic death, congenital deformities, abortions and stillbirths [1,2]. When infected with the non-cytopathic strain, the disease is often mild and subclinical.

During transient viraemia (4–7 days), infected animals might suffer diarrhoea, pyrexia, nasal discharge and immunosuppression [3,4]. However, infection of dams with the non-cytopathic strain in early to mid-gestation, can result in the production of a persistently infected (PI) calf [5]. These calves are often chronically ill-thrifty, with reduced growth and survival rates due to prolonged immunosuppression and other infection-associated effects [1]. Infection of a PI with the cytopathic strain of BVDV can lead to mucosal disease with animals presenting with anorexia, diarrhoea, nasal discharge and ulcerative lesions [3].

The Australian cattle industry has been estimated to incur financial losses of AUD 114 million annually due to the impacts of BVDV infection [6]. Despite the substantial financial consequences of BVDV, there are no formally structured and freely accessible BVDV control programs coordinated by producer groups, or state and federal governments in Australia. This is most likely because BVDV losses are indirect, making them difficult to observe at an individual farm level. There is also limited information about regional BVDV prevalence in Australia because the available literature is limited and is often not herd-type specific or climate specific [7–10]. Additionally, many producers are unaware of the BVDV status of cattle on their property [11]. Diagnosis of BVDV infection is necessary to establish and then implement control practices, and it is especially important to detect PI cattle [12]. Such cattle are the primary source of BVDV transmission, due to life-long, abundant viral shedding [2,13,14]. The virus persists in the calf's tissues following birth, and naïve cattle directly exposed to its bodily secretions can become infected. Some producers introduce PI cattle to their herd to maintain herd-immunity to BVDV [2,13]. Such cattle might carry and transmit other pathogens, which can lead to further disease in an immunologically naïve herd; therefore, losses might exceed those expected solely from BVDV [15]. These additional losses are also increased by the immunosuppressive nature of transient BVDV infection [16].

The implementation of control and management practices at farm level is not common in Australia [11], even though producers have indicated a willingness to implement management practices, particularly if they are economically beneficial [17]. Such practices can include herd surveillance (for example, to eliminate PI calves), increasing herd immunity, and improved biosecurity. Biosecurity is defined as actions that are implemented to prevent pathogens from entering a herd and minimise the spread of pathogens within a herd [18–20]. Increased herd immunity can be achieved by vaccination or exposure of naïve cattle to PI cattle (often termed "deliberate exposure" when used as a control method) [21–23]. Pestigard®, an inactivated vaccine, is the only commercially available vaccine within Australia [24]. It is effective against strains of subgenotypes BVDV-1a and BVDV-1c [22]; however, in Australia, BVDV-2is believed to be absent, with 97% of isolates within Australia confirmed as BVDV-1c [16,25].

Climatic differences, as well as herd size, also influence herd management practices which can influence BVDV risk; therefore, these must also be accounted for when implementing BVDV control [7,26]. Although the responsibility for control rests solely with producers, veterinarians are important in their capacity as advisers and clinicians on livestock properties and could provide farm-specific information to producers to reduce BVDV associated losses, as well as support regional or country-wide control programs.

The success of control and elimination of BVDV in other countries (for example, Ireland, France, Norway and Scotland) has highlighted different approaches to country-wide elimination. Differing perceptions of the importance of the impacts of BVDV mean that policies and attitudes relating to BVDV elimination vary between countries [9,10,27–29]. Countries in which BVDV has been eliminated introduced compulsory control programs based on the identification and subsequent removal of PI animals (the 'test and eliminate' method), leading to a reduction in both PI prevalence and herd-level incidence [23,30]. This was successful in Switzerland, in which steps initially aimed to improve the education of the industry and producers, followed by antigen testing of the entire cattle population and subsequent elimination of PIs [29,31].

Sweden and Norway implemented movement restrictions on BVDV antibody positive animals, while countries such as the United Kingdom and Ireland (countries in which BVDV control programs have yet to lead to elimination) use vaccination as well as the test and eliminate method [30].

Challenges exist in relation to control and elimination programs; for example, who should pay, and whether they should be voluntary or compulsory [27]. These challenges highlight a need for country or region-specific assessment of current knowledge, attitudes and practices of industry stakeholders, as well as bio-economic assessments to evaluate the benefits of eradication [9]. Such assessments in Sweden and Norway suggest the benefits of BVDV include elimination, improved animal welfare and production, enhanced industry reputation, and advantages in overseas markets [10,30,32]. However, there are substantial differences in the structure of cattle industries, including herd management and government regulations, as well as differing climates between Australia and the European countries that have successfully implemented BVDV control.

To assess the feasibility of improving the control of BVDV in Australia, we need to understand the current levels of knowledge, as well as attitudes and practices associated with BVDV management [33]. Veterinarians play a key role in disease control. However, to provide adequate advice to producers on BVDV management, veterinarians require knowledge of the prevalence, disease risks, efficacy of control measures and the associated costs and benefits. Veterinarians' values also need to align with those of producers. Therefore, the objective of this study was to describe veterinarians' knowledge, attitudes and practices (KAP) associated with BVDV control, relative to the practices and perceived attitudes of producers in their regions in south-east Australia. We aimed to demonstrate the range of KAPs of veterinarians (rather than determine majority opinions)—with a particular focus on the use of PI calves and deliberate exposure—to assess alignment of veterinarians' and producers' KAPs regarding BVDV control.

2. Materials and Methods

A survey of cattle veterinarians currently practising in south-east Australia was conducted. The study region was defined as the temperate climate zone in south-east Australia according to the Köppen climate classification of Australia [34]. The study was approved by the Charles Sturt University Human Research Ethics Committee (H19149).

2.1. Questionnaire Design and Implementation

The questionnaire design was informed by individual discussions with six industry and veterinary experts, including cattle veterinarians and past and current beef and dairy producers. Researchers used a semi-structured interview approach for these discussions, to gain background information to guide the questionnaire design. Topics included in these discussions were recommendations for BVDV control and practices, including those associated with PI calves such as deliberate exposure, and whether producers tested for BVDV and other diseases.

The questionnaire included 35 questions about veterinarians' knowledge, attitudes and recommended practices and their perceptions of producers' attitudes and practices associated with BVDV control. Initially, demographic information was collected, followed by the type of properties visited (beef, dairy farms or both), and the frequency of visits. Questions then differentiated BVDV management on beef and dairy properties, and on BVDV infected and uninfected properties.

Positive herds were those with a known presence of recently BVDV seropositive cattle (due to natural exposure) or presence of PI cattle, and negative herds had a perceived negative status. Finally, questions focused on deliberate exposure using PI calves, the biosecurity risks that this might pose, and the health and welfare of PI calves. The questionnaire was piloted on the previously mentioned group of experts to improve clarity and refine questions.

2.2. Distribution

The questionnaire was distributed in electronic form via an online provider (Survey Monkey®, Australia, https://www.surveymonkey.com, accessed 9 September 2020). Cattle veterinarians were invited to participate by email if they were currently registered with the Australian Veterinary Association (Australian Cattle Veterinarians Special Interest Group) or the Australian and New Zealand College of Veterinary Scientists (Cattle Chapter) organisations. The questionnaire was available to these groups from 24 July 2019 to 28 August 2019. Although each distributor invited participation once, members of both organisations may have received two invitations.

2.3. Data Analysis

Data from the questionnaire was downloaded into Excel (Microsoft Corporation, version 16.16.13 (190811)) and analysed in the statistical platform, R [35]. All responses from practitioners in local government areas (LGAs) that extended over the temperate climate zone were included in analysis. Quantitative data were summarised using descriptive statistics and plots of distributions. Statistical calculations were completed with different denominators because the number of responses for each question varied; responses were not compulsory, and some questions were specific to participants' type of work. Data from quantitative responses which included minimum, maximum and most likely estimates were combined as PERT distributions. Statistical significance between distributions was tested using Kruskal-Wallis tests. Qualitative responses were reviewed and discussed by all authors to summarise participants' opinions.

3. Results

3.1. Demographics

The questionnaire was completed by 48 veterinarians, of whom eight were excluded because they were not currently practising cattle veterinarians ($n = 3$), or were either not within the climate zone for this study or did not state their workplace postcode ($n = 5$). Of the remaining veterinarians ($n = 40$) who described their type of practice ($n = 35$), 48% worked with beef producers ($n = 19$), 15% worked with dairy producers ($n = 6$), and 25% worked with both beef and dairy producers ($n = 10$). Veterinarians most commonly visited one to five cattle producers each week (43%, $n = 17$; Supplementary Materials Figure S1). Most of the veterinarians were male (70%, $n = 28$), but in the youngest age group (<30 years old) there were more females than males (71% female, $n = 5$; data are presented in Supplementary Materials Figure S2). Most veterinarians were from New South Wales (56%, $n = 24$) and Victoria (28%, $n = 12$; Figure 1). The response rate for the questionnaire was not available because we did not have access to the databases of the distributing organisations.

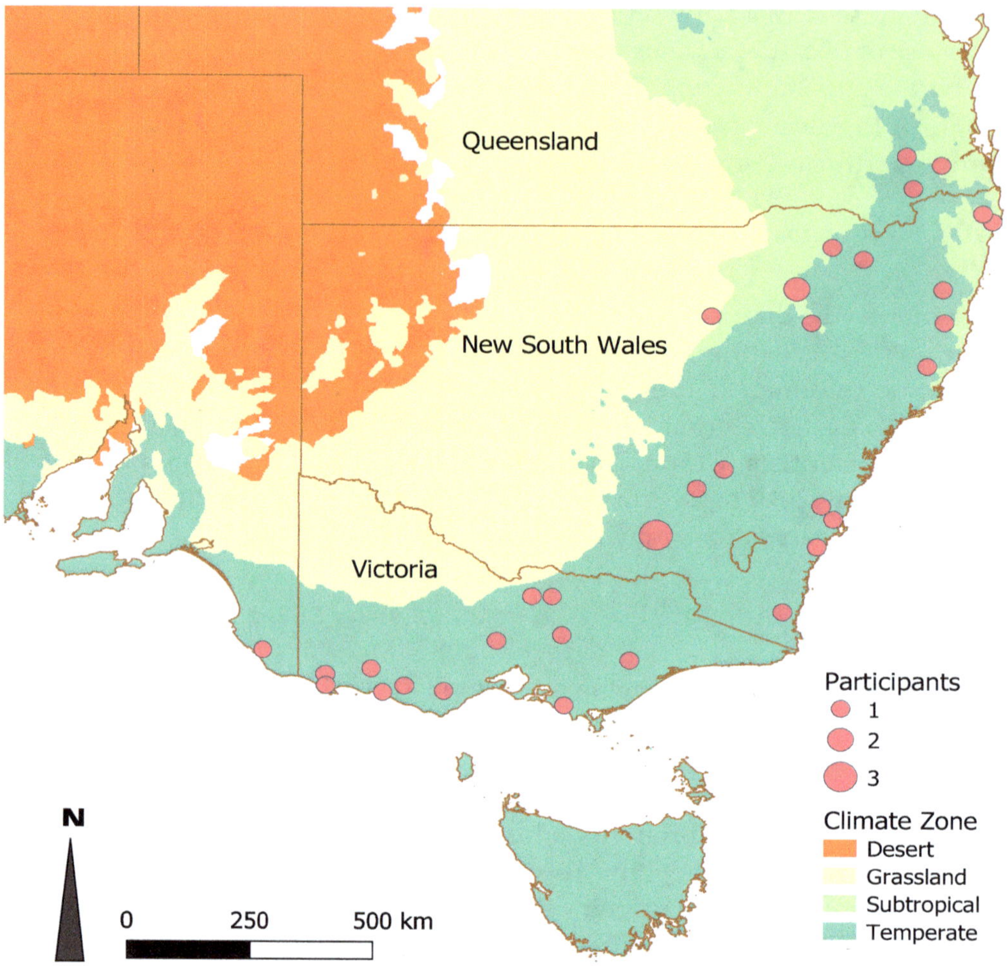

Figure 1. Location of participating veterinarians in a survey of veterinarians' knowledge, attitudes and practices associated with bovine viral diarrhoea virus management on farms in the temperate zone of south-east Australia in 2019. Each dot is located on the centroid of the participant's local government area (LGA); all LGSs extended into the temperate climate zone.

3.2. Estimates of Herd-Level Prevalence of BVDV

There was no significant difference in the veterinarians' estimated herd-level prevalence of BVDV on beef breeder (median 57%, 95% range 4–91%) and beef rearer (median 64%, 95% range 2–94%) properties throughout the veterinarians' areas ($p = 0.50$) (Figure 2). For all property types, veterinarians' estimates of herd-level prevalence in their areas appeared to follow a bimodal distribution of either low (approximately 5–10%), or, more commonly, high (approximately 80–90%) prevalence. The combined breeder and rearer beef properties' median estimated herd-level prevalence was 61% (95% range 3–93%). Veterinarians estimated a median herd-level prevalence of 53% (95% range 2–95%) on dairy properties. Although the median estimated herd-level prevalence of BVDV was greater for beef properties than dairy properties, this was not a statistically significant difference ($p = 0.50$).

Most vets were moderately uncertain about the herd-level prevalence in their area of work (median 39%; 95% range 5–74%; Figure 3). The main tests reported to be used by veterinarians were Agarose Gel Immunodiffusion (AGID; $n = 15$), PCR ($n = 17$) and ELISA ($n = 27$) (Supplementary Materials Figure S3).

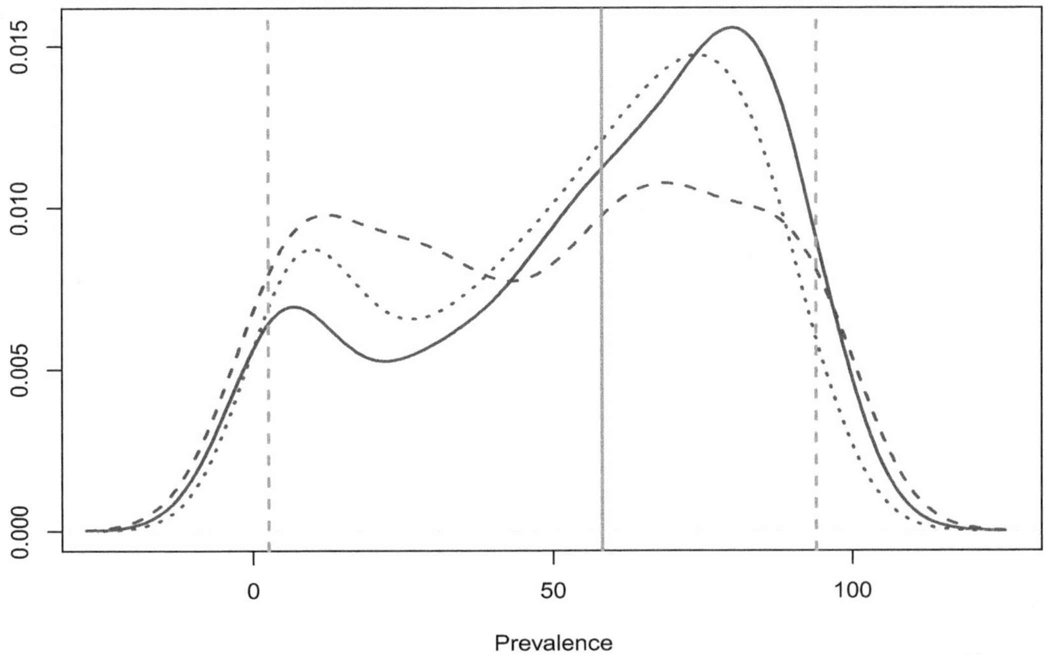

Figure 2. Density plot of the distribution of the estimated herd-level prevalence of bovine viral diarrhoea virus (BVDV) in beef breeder (black dotted line), beef rearer (black solid line) and dairy properties (dashed line) in a survey of veterinarians' knowledge, attitudes and practices associated with BVDV management on properties in the temperate zone of south-east Australia in 2019. Vertical lines: grey solid = median combined between-property prevalence; grey dashed = 95% range of between-property prevalence. The extents of the plot <0 and >100 should not be interpreted; line extension is due to the smoothing process in constructing density plots.

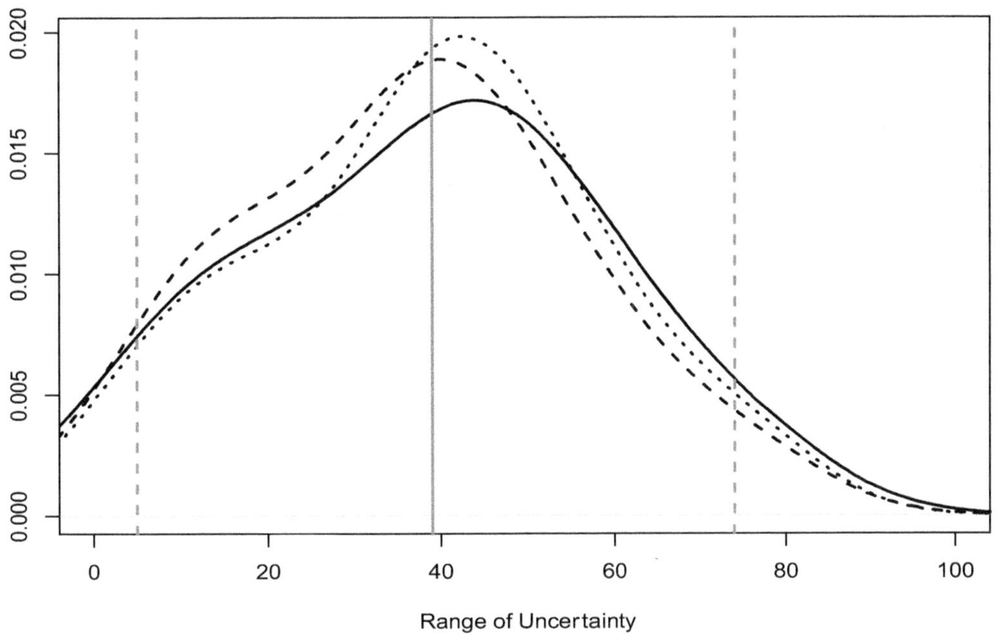

Figure 3. Density plot of the range of uncertainty about between-farm prevalence of bovine viral diarrhoea virus (BVDV) in beef breeder (dotted line), beef rearer (solid line) and dairy properties (dashed line) in a survey of veterinarians' knowledge, attitudes and practices associated with BVDV management on properties in the temperate zone of south-east Australia in 2019. Vertical lines: grey solid = median combined between-property prevalence; grey dashed = 95% range of between-property prevalence. The extents of the plot <0 and >100 should not be interpreted; line extension is due to the smoothing process in constructing density plots.

3.3. Control and Prevention Practices

Veterinarians estimated that the proportion of BVDV positive properties on which control measures were implemented was 32%, although this varied widely (95% range 1–92%). Veterinarians similarly estimated that the proportion of BVDV negative properties on which preventive measures were implemented was 26% (95% range 2–87%).

Vaccination was reported as more commonly used on BVDV positive properties than BVDV negative properties, and "no prevention" was relatively commonly reported on BVDV negative properties (Figure 4). Biosecurity on BVDV positive properties was estimated as "rarely" used on dairy properties and "often" used on beef properties (Figure 4), and "sometimes" used on BVDV negative properties (beef and dairy; Figure 5).

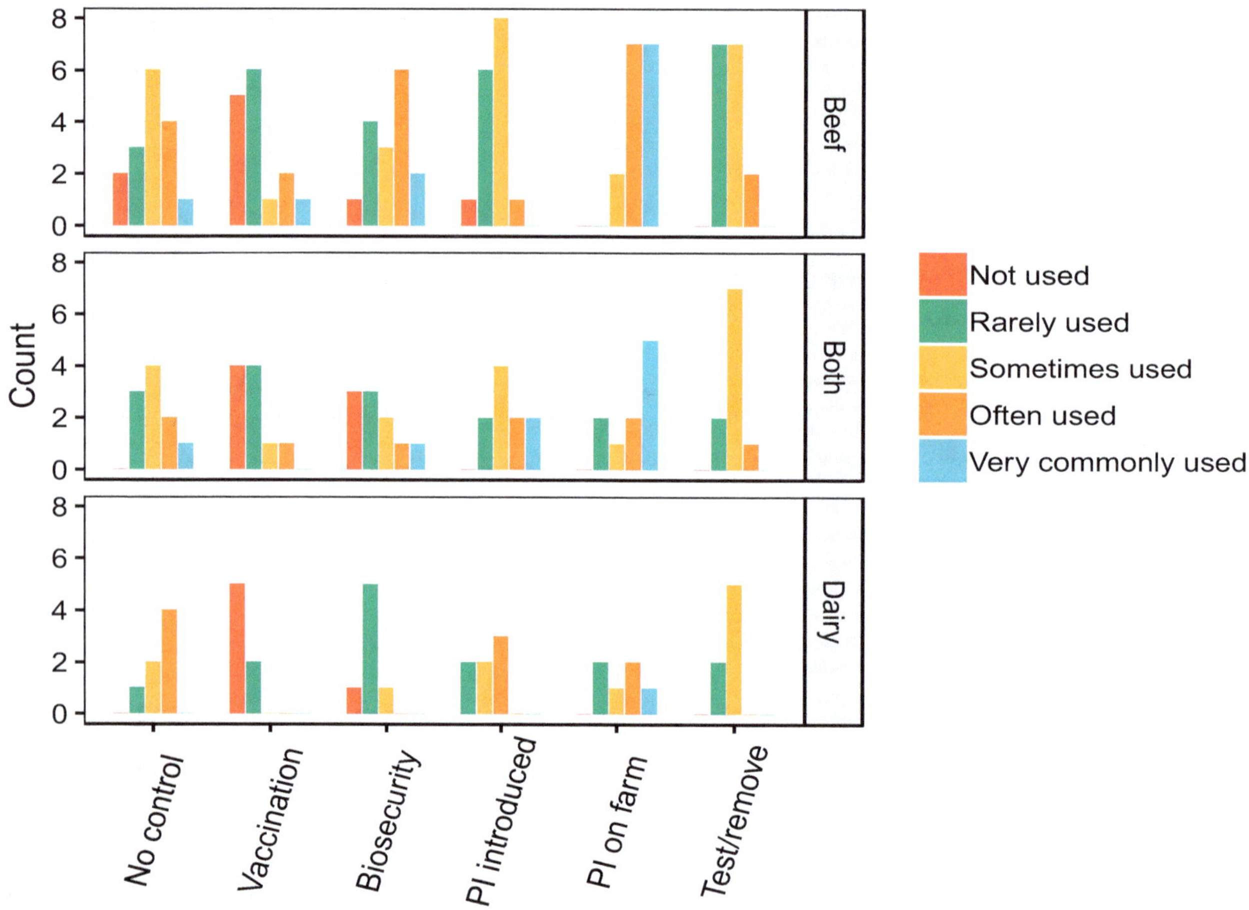

Figure 4. Barplots of the frequency of management practices used on bovine viral diarrhoea virus (BVDV) positive properties reported by veterinarians, in a survey of veterinarians' knowledge, attitudes and practices associated with BVDV management on properties in the temperate climate zone of south-east Australia in 2019. PI = persistently infected cattle. Both = veterinarians working with both beef and dairy properties.

When asked how biosecurity was achieved on BVDV positive properties (an open question), veterinarians reported that producers used a range of measures. These included testing and quarantine of introduced stock, avoiding introducing pregnant stock, segregation of introduced and pregnant stock and improved perimeter fence control. While quarantine of acute infections was suggested to occur, there was little suggested in regard to determining PI status.

In response to an open question describing how producers employ preventive biosecurity practices (on perceived negative properties), veterinarians stated that it was achieved through bioexclusion, which included maintaining closed herds, testing of any introduced stock, and fencing.

Veterinarians reported that maintaining a closed herd was more frequently associated with BVDV negative than BVDV positive properties. However, selective purchasing was sometimes practised and included only purchasing tested cattle (e.g., bulls) and obtaining a vaccination history before purchase. While determining the efficacy of prevention strategies was not an objective of this study, some veterinarians suggested that producers who had an awareness of the disease consequences tended to employ adequate biosecurity measures.

Veterinarians also reported that the use of PIs that were sourced on farm were "often" and "very commonly" used on BVDV positive properties, especially beef properties (Figure 4). In contrast, the introduction of PIs was reported less frequently overall on all positive property types. As expected, the use of PI cattle, vaccination and "test and remove" strategies were generally rarely used on BVDV negative properties (Figure 5).

When asked what measures veterinarians would recommend for BVDV control, veterinarians recommended vaccination ($n = 20$), and combined biosecurity and vaccination ($n = 9$). For prevention of BVDV, veterinarians most commonly recommended vaccination ($n = 16$) and biosecurity ($n = 7$). Deliberate exposure ($n = 2$), and the opposite strategy, the identification and removal of PIs ($n = 7$), were less often recommended overall.

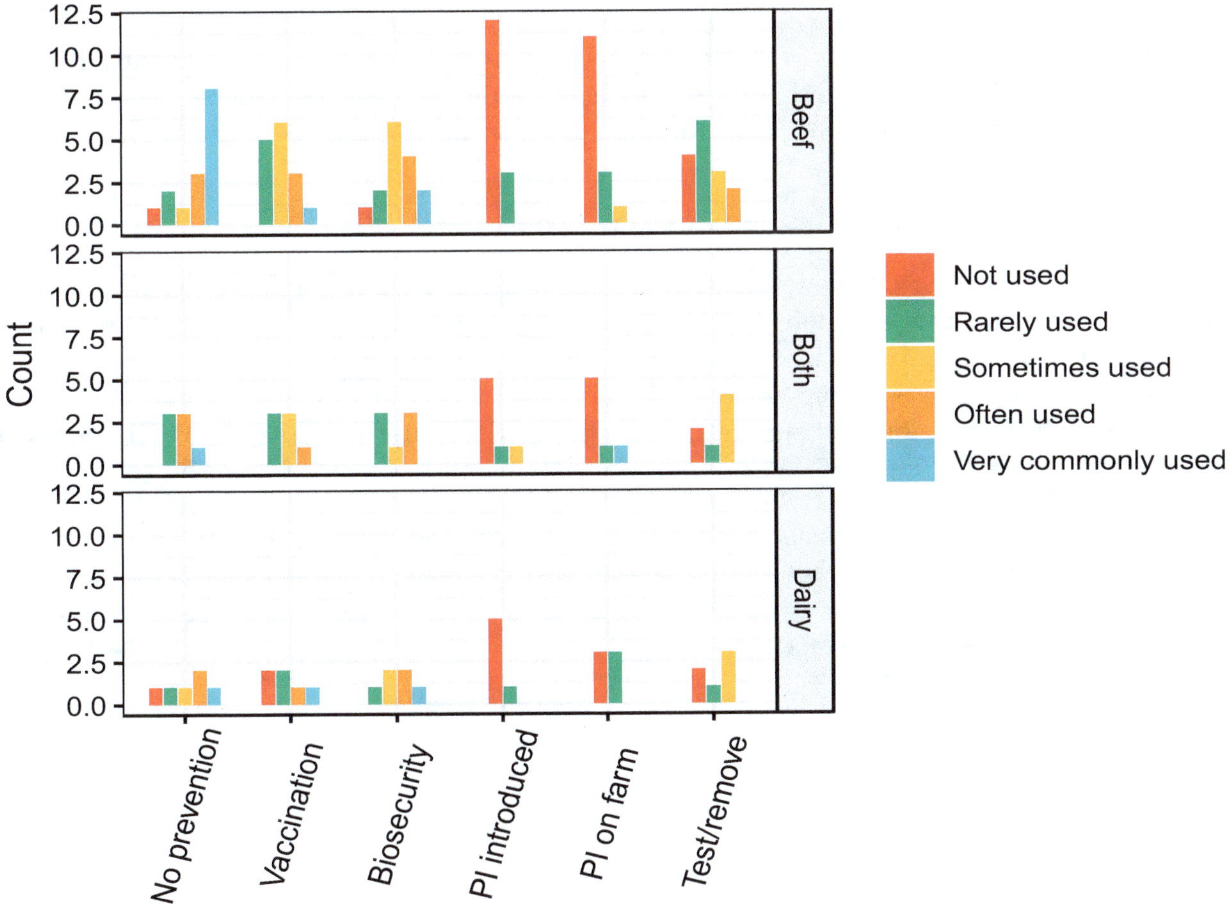

Figure 5. Barplots of the frequency of management practices used on bovine viral diarrhoea virus (BVDV) negative properties reported by veterinarians, in a survey of veterinarians' knowledge, attitudes and practices associated with BVDV management on farms in the temperate zone of south-east Australia in 2019. PI = persistently infected cattle.

3.4. *Deliberate Exposure*

Overall, veterinarians did not support the use of deliberate exposure to control BVDV (supporters = 2; non-supporters = 11), but some veterinarians said support of deliberate exposure was dependent on the producer's circumstances ($n = 16$). Most veterinarians ($n = 21$) were willing to work with producers who used deliberate exposure, regardless of their own personal support for the practice, although two were not willing to do so because of welfare concerns.

There were mixed responses to open questions about the use of deliberate exposure that gave more insights about veterinarians' attitudes and practices relating to deliberate exposure. Although most veterinarians recommended biosecurity and vaccination, some veterinarians suggested the use of deliberate exposure instead of vaccination. Others said that vaccination was an alternative when deliberate exposure was not feasible ($n = 2$) and deliberate exposure was termed "auto vaccination" by some veterinarians ($n = 3$). Some veterinarians also suggested that advice from veterinarians about BVDV control was influenced by producers' willingness to control the disease. For example, by working with producers using deliberate exposure, veterinarians can "educate and harness their [producers'] enthusiasm into the right direction". Two veterinarians specifically recommended education to improve producers' understanding of BVDV to achieve effective control on BVDV positive properties.

When asked about PI acquisition, veterinarians reported a range of methods. Some producers actively sought PIs from within their own or other properties. Some inadvertently introduced PIs from newly acquired pregnant stock. Veterinarians also reported that young stock were more likely to be deliberately exposed to PI cattle than older stock (Supplementary Materials Figure S4). Veterinarians perceived that a driver for using PI cattle by producers was economic pressure ($n = 12$) and thought that producers perceived deliberate exposure as a cost-effective control method ($n = 11$) compared to vaccination. Some veterinarians ($n = 3$) also suggested that the longer lasting immunity generated from natural infection was a reason that producers used deliberate exposure. Some veterinarians also stated that producers used deliberate exposure due to "ignorance of the costs of disease" and "poor veterinary advice".

3.5. Infectious Pathogen Risks Associated with PI Cattle

Most veterinarians ($n = 26$) believed that the introduction of PI cattle posed disease risks other than BVDV to a herd. Pathogens mentioned by veterinarians were grouped by researchers according to body system affected during clinical disease (Table 1). The combined (beef and dairy) median prevalence of enteric diseases within herds and the prevalence in PI cattle was estimated as 30% and 40%, respectively (distributions not significantly different; Kruskal-Wallis $X^2 = 11.65$, df = 9, $p = 0.23$; Supplementary Materials Figure S5).

Table 1. Cattle pathogens suggested as having an increased prevalence in herds in which a PI is introduced, grouped by affected body system, reported by veterinarians in a survey of veterinarians' knowledge, attitudes and practices associated with bovine viral diarrhoea virus management on farms in the temperate zone of south-east Australia in 2019.

Body System	Pathogen or Disease
Enteric	Coccidiosis
	Colibacillosis
	Cryptosporidiosis
	Neonatal Diarrhoea
	Salmonellosis Rotavirus
Respiratory	Bovine Respiratory Disease
	Mycoplasmosis Pneumonia
Systemic	BVDV
	Leptospirosis Septicaemia
	Theileriosis
Other	Lice
	Pinkeye (infectious bovine keratoconjunctivitis)

The prevalence of respiratory diseases was estimated with combined medians of 27.5% within herds and 50% in PIs (distributions not significantly different; Kruskal-Wallis $X^2 = 12.11$, df = 9,

$p = 0.21$). Systemic diseases were reported as a potential risk by 18 veterinarians. Combined estimated prevalence both within herds and in PIs was low (median 17.5% and 3.5%, respectively, distributions not significantly different; Kruskal-Wallis $X^2 = 3$, df = 3, $p = 0.39$). While only reported by three veterinarians, "other" diseases (infectious kerato-conjunctivitis [pinkeye] and lice) on beef properties were estimated to have a high within herd and PI prevalence (median 80% and 70%, respectively).

Veterinarians reported that producers generally did not test for the presence of diseases other than BVDV in PIs (combined median proportion of producers who test for diseases other than BVDV = 10%, 95% range 5–85%).

3.6. Welfare and PI Cattle

Most veterinarians ($n = 19$) thought that PI cattle had compromised welfare, but only a small number ($n = 3$) believed that producers were concerned about PI welfare. Veterinarians considered the cost of disease and production losses caused by active BVDV infections were producers' main concerns. When asked to describe their concerns about PI cattle, veterinarians ($n = 13$) stated that PI cattle were clinically unhealthy and likely to have early and painful deaths. Due to increased susceptibility to pathogens, they are subject to other comorbidities and once clinically ill, they are unlikely to be treated. In particular, veterinarians also reported an apparent association between diseases such as pneumonia and infectious kerato-conjunctivitis in herds following exposure to PI cattle, thus reducing herd welfare overall.

Veterinarians ($n = 12$) were aware that producers sometimes use "vampire vaccination" (collect blood from PI cattle to administer to BVDV naïve cattle to stimulate immunity). Veterinarians suggested that the motivation for the use of "vampire vaccination" was a perceived improvement of exposure (the number exposed can be controlled and is guaranteed) and a reduced welfare risk to PI cattle (as PI cattle are not required to live for longer than required for the blood collection). Two veterinarians suggested that the drivers for this activity were economic and practical benefits; other options such as commercial vaccination, are too expensive and ineffective. One veterinarian stated that if commercial vaccination was of a "high quality with high levels of long-lasting immunity, it would reduce the desire of producers to create their own cost-effective control measures." Some veterinarians ($n = 3$) expressed concern for this practice due to the risk of spreading other diseases due to inadequate hygiene and a lack of awareness of disease risk among producers.

When asked for additional comments, veterinarians indicated that the willingness of producers to implement control was believed to differ between beef and dairy producers, with dairy producers more likely to appreciate the benefits of eliminating BVDV compared with beef producers. Some veterinarians also believed that trading patterns and neighbouring farms make the prevention of exposure unfeasible, and the resulting exposures keep herd seroprevalence high.

Some veterinarians ($n = 3$) thought that producers' knowledge of BVDV, its production impacts and control measures was poor. Awareness of comorbidities in PI cattle was also believed to be low.

Approximately half of the veterinarians ($n = 21$) suggested that with veterinarian involvement, the management of BVDV on properties could be improved, and some veterinarians said that producer knowledge also needed improvement.

Additionally, there was a general opinion by veterinarians that the current available vaccine in Australia is too expensive and not sufficiently effective, with one veterinarian declaring that until alternative options become available "it is not fair to take away other practices" such as the use of PIs.

4. Discussion

This study highlighted that veterinarians' knowledge of herd-level BVDV prevalence—a key parameter for surveillance to determine whether control measures are effective—in their workplace region is limited. They appeared uncertain; in general, classifying their area as having a "low" or "high" herd-level prevalence, as well as estimating broad lower and upper limits around this parameter. This study further highlighted that recommendations by veterinarians for BVDV control do not always align with producers' preferred strategies, especially regarding the use of PI calves for deliberate exposure. However, although veterinarians generally do not support the use of deliberate exposure for BVDV control, some are willing to work with producers who use it. It also highlighted veterinarians' concern for the welfare of PI cattle, the use of a previously undocumented form of deliberate exposure which we term "vampire vaccination," and the risk of disease transmission (other than BVDV) between PI cattle and non-infected cattle.

Most veterinarians in this study believed that PI cattle have compromised welfare because they are clinically unhealthy and suffer early deaths. This was consistent with findings from previous studies which reported significant welfare implications due to ill-thrift, mucosal disease and predisposition to secondary diseases [22,36,37]. In the current study, veterinarians perceived that producer concern about the welfare of PI calves was low. This was also consistent with a previous study which found a lack of producer interest in welfare concerns associated with BVDV [38]. Authors found that unpredictable disease consequences and perceived costs of disease control influenced producer motivation, and that producers were more interested in production than animal welfare [37]. The current study also highlighted another welfare concern regarding the administration of blood collected from PI cattle to administer to BVDV naïve cattle as part of vampire vaccination. Veterinarians who were aware of this practice raised concerns about the risk of spreading diseases other than BVDV when using the vampire vaccination. Veterinarians believed that the use of this practice was driven by producers' perception that it was a cost-effective vaccination which provided life-long immunity. As such, vampire vaccination provided a cheaper alternative to the current commercial annual vaccination. Further investigation of vampire vaccination as part of BVDV control is required to determine incidence, the costs and benefits to producers, and the impact on the welfare of cattle exposed to this practice.

Veterinarians identified a range of enteric, respiratory, and systemic pathogen risks that could also be transmitted from PI to BVDV naïve cattle in both beef and dairy systems, as well as infectious kerato-conjunctivitis (pinkeye) and lice in beef cattle. Wide variation of within-herd prevalence of enteric and respiratory diseases in southern Australia (including the current study region) has been previously documented [38–41]. Therefore, the range of diseases and similar variation in veterinarians' estimations of prevalence of enteric and respiratory pathogens in the current study were expected. Although there have been studies of the health status of PI cattle and the presence of concurrent diseases in BVDV infected animals, there has been minimal research into the impact of secondary disease transmission from PI to BVDV naïve cattle and the subsequent effect on within-herd prevalence of disease. While difficult to quantify, this is worth investigation to understand these additional influences of introduction of PI cattle into BVDV naïve herds. It is possible that this is an underestimated impact of BVDV on herd health. Additionally, further studies are needed to determine the prevalence of BVDV within different regions and climate zones in Australia. Current literature identifies varied prevalence across Australia, without determining prevalence within a single climate zone or discerning between beef and dairy industries. Multiple other studies have cited a range of seroprevalences across Australia between 13–100% [9,10,42]. These studies involved different herd sizes across different Australian states, with likely differing herd management strategies that potentially contributed to the variation in prevalence [9,10,42].

Veterinarians are a crucial part of biosecurity at farm level through improving producer knowledge [29,43]. However, in this study, veterinarians were uncertain about the proportion of herds that were BVDV positive in their regions. Consequently, they were also unsure about the proportion of producers who used BVDV control and prevention methods, although the median estimate was consistent with a previous southern Australian study in which 36% of cattle producers implemented BVDV control [11]. However, this proportion might be influenced by concurrent control measures for another disease that are beneficial in the control of BVDV. Internationally, surveys of producers and veterinarians have indicated that insufficient knowledge is the most common reason for the absence of control protocols for BVDV [44]. Recent studies also indicated that Australian producers were considered to have a low knowledge of BVDV [11,17]. As comprehensive knowledge of a disease is needed for disease control at a national level, increased herd-level surveillance and education is essential for Australian BVDV control.

Most veterinarians in the current study did not support the use of PI calves for deliberate exposure to induce immunity. Instead, veterinarians usually recommended the use of vaccination and biosecurity (often in combination). This aligns with international standards, which recommend prevention programs that include development of herd immunity to BVDV [3,18,20]. Overall, little is known about deliberate exposure in Australia in terms of its incidence and efficacy in different herd types and environments. There are potential shortfalls in achieving BVDV disease control using deliberate exposure [15,23,45,46], such as incorrect timing, length of exposure and failure to ensure all susceptible animals seroconvert [15,22,45]. A previous survey of southern Australian producers found that deliberate exposure was less commonly used than vaccination, and was also generally inadequately managed when used [11]. In contrast, veterinarians in the current study reported that deliberate exposure was used relatively more commonly than the commercially available vaccination, especially on beef properties. Overall, this study highlighted that deliberate exposure is occurring without the recommendation of veterinarians and might have become a more popular option for BVDV control than commercial vaccination. This emphasises the need to investigate and assess drivers for this practice if the Australian cattle industry were to consider national control of BVDV.

Selection bias could have influenced the results of this study due to the targeting of participants who were members of cattle veterinary groups; those who responded to the survey might have been more likely to have a particular interest in BVDV control. In addition, we also acknowledge that veterinarians' knowledge of how clients employ measures to control BVDV might only reflect clients with close working relationships with their veterinarians, rather than producers who, for example, have small farms that require less veterinary input or only engage veterinary services for emergency reasons. Studies have shown the producers with good working relationships with veterinarians and prior knowledge are more likely to engage in discussion and follow advice [33,47,48]. Although sample size was small, the aim of this survey was to gain a range of responses from veterinarians, rather than a statistically significant consensus. For the purposes of BVDV control, it is important to appreciate and understand this range, because even a relatively small proportion of people with particular KAPs can influence control of a disease such as BVDV. The representation of a range of views, rather than majority opinions, are a valuable contribution to gaining an understanding of the challenges associated with BVDV control.

5. Conclusions

Veterinarians' recommendations generally acknowledge and reflect their concerns about the welfare associated with BVDV infection, but do not necessarily match producers' preferred strategies for BVDV control and management in their regions. To improve the control and management of BVDV, alignment of attitudes and practices is required. We suggest that this could be achieved by improving the knowledge of both veterinarians and producers about local BVDV prevalence to provide a baseline for surveillance and improve certainty about the impacts within their region. These include the direct economic impacts of BVDV control as well as indirect economic impacts and poor welfare in affected cattle. In particular, the drivers and impacts of the administration of blood from persistently infected cattle to BVDV naïve cattle that were documented in this study are worth further investigation. Finally, the differences in veterinarians recommended practices and those that they observe on farms likely represent differences in values between producers and veterinarians. A much greater understanding of how these values arise and their influence on BVDV control is needed.

Supplementary Materials: Figure S1: Count of veterinarians working on beef or dairy properties and the number of properties seen each week in a survey of veterinarians' knowledge, attitudes and practices associated with bovine viral diarrhoea virus management on farms in the temperate zone of south-east Australia in 2019. Figure S2: Counts of veterinarians in each age group in a survey of the knowledge, attitudes and practices associated with bovine viral diarrhoea virus management on farms in the temperate zone of south-east Australia in 2019. Figure S3: Barplot of the number of tests reported as being used by veterinarians to detect the presence of BVDV, in a survey of veterinarians' knowledge, attitudes and practices associated with BVDV management on properties in the temperate climate zone of south-east Australia in 2019. VNT = Virus neutralisation test, AGID = Agar Gel Immunodiffusion Assay, VI = viral isolation, IH = immunohistochemistry, PCR = Polymerase chain reaction, ELISA = enzyme-linked immunosorbent assay. Figure S4: Number of veterinarians reporting deliberate exposure to different stock types, in a survey of veterinarians' knowledge, attitudes and practices associated with BVDV management on farms in the temperate zone of south-east Australia in 2019. Figure S5: Boxplots of the estimated within herd prevalence of the grouped diseases, prevalence of the grouped diseased in BVDV persistently infected cattle (PI), and the proportion of producers testing for the grouped diseases on beef (left) and dairy (right) properties, in a survey of veterinarians' knowledge, attitudes and practices associated with BVDV management on farms in the temperate zone of south-east Australia in 2019. Other = lice and infectious bovine keratoconjunctivitis.

Author Contributions: Conceptualization, C.M., M.H.-J. and V.J.B.; Data curation, C.M.; Formal analysis, C.M., A.J.G., S.K. and V.J.B.; Investigation, C.M. and V.J.B.; Methodology, C.M., M.H.-J. and V.J.B.; Project administration, V.J.B.; Writing—original draft, C.M.; Writing—review and editing, C.M., A.J.G., S.K., M.H.-J. and V.J.B. All authors have read and agreed to the published version of the manuscript.

Acknowledgments: The authors thank the experts who contributed to the design of the survey and the study participants. We thank the Australian Veterinary Association (AVA) and the Australian and New Zealand College of Veterinary Scientists (ANZCVS) for distributing the survey. We also thank the Spatial Data Analysis Network, Charles Sturt University, for creating the survey and Cara Wilson for her help mapping data.

References

1. Richter, V.; Lebl, K.; Baumgartner, W.; Obritzhauser, W.; Käsbohrer, A.; Pinior, B. A systematic worldwide review of the direct monetary losses in cattle due to bovine viral diarrhoea virus infection. *Vet. J.* **2017**, *220*, 80–87. [CrossRef] [PubMed]
2. Lanyon, S.R.; Hill, F.I.; Reichel, M.P.; Brownlie, J. Bovine viral diarrhoea: Pathogenesis and diagnosis. *Vet. J.* **2014**, *199*, 201–209. [CrossRef] [PubMed]
3. Brownlie, J.; Clarke, M.C.; Howard, C.J.; Pocock, D.H. Pathogenesis and epidemiology of bovine virus diarrhoea virus infection of cattle. *Ann. Rech. Vet.* **1987**, *18*, 157–166. [PubMed]
4. Bruschke, C.J.; Haghparast, A.; Hoek, A.; Rutten, V.P.M.G.; Wentink, G.; Van Rijn, P.A.; Van Oirschot, J. The immune response of cattle, persistently infected with noncytopathic BVDV, after superinfection with antigenically semi-homologous cytopathic BVDV. *Vet. Immunol. Immunopathol.* **1998**, *62*, 37–50. [CrossRef]
5. Grooms, D.L. Reproductive consequences of infection with bovine viral diarrhea virus. *Vet. Clin. N. Am. Food Anim. Pract.* **2004**, *20*, 5–19. [CrossRef]
6. Lane, J.; Jubb, T.; Shephard, R.; Webb-Ware, J.; Fordyce, G. *Priority List of Endemic Diseases for the Red Meat Industries*; MLA Report B.AHE.0010: Sydney, Australia, 2015.
7. McGowan, M.; Holroyd, R. Reproductive inefficiencies and opportunities in dairy and beef cattle in Australia. *Proc. Aust. Soc. Anim. Prod.* **2008**, *27*, 1–9.
8. Burns, B.; Fordyce, G.; Holroyd, R. A review of factors that impact on the capacity of beef cattle females to conceive, maintain a pregnancy and wean a calf—Implications for reproductive efficiency in northern Australia. *Anim. Reprod. Sci.* **2010**, *122*, 1–22. [CrossRef]
9. Graham, D.; Clegg, T.A.; O'Sullivan, P.; More, S.J. Influence of the retention of PI calves identified in 2012 during the voluntary phase of the Irish national bovine viral diarrhoea virus (BVDV) eradication programme on herd-level outcomes in 2013. *Prev. Vet. Med.* **2015**, *120*, 298–305. [CrossRef]
10. Stott, A.W.; Humphry, R.; Gunn, G.; Higgins, I.M.; Hennessy, T.; O'Flaherty, J.; Graham, D.A. Predicted costs and benefits of eradicating BVDV from Ireland. *Ir. Vet. J.* **2012**, *65*, 12. [CrossRef]
11. Long, R. Knowledge, Attitudes and Management of Bovine Viral Diarrhoea Virus among Cattle Producers—Prevention, Control and Eradication. Honours Thesis, Charles Sturt University, Bathurst, Australia, 2019.

12. Saliki, J.T.; Dubovi, E.J. Laboratory diagnosis of bovine viral diarrhea virus infections. *Vet. Clin. N. Am. Food Anim. Pract.* **2004**, *20*, 69–83. [CrossRef]
13. Houe, H. Epidemiological features and economical importance of bovine virus diarrhoea virus (BVDV) infections. *Vet. Microbiol.* **1999**, *64*, 89–107. [CrossRef]
14. Brownlie, J. The pathogenesis of bovine virus. *Revne Sci. Tech. Int. Off. Epizoot.* **1990**, *9*, 43–59. [CrossRef]
15. Givens, M.D.; Newcomer, B.W. Perspective on BVDV control programs. *Anim. Health Res. Rev.* **2015**, *16*, 78–82. [CrossRef] [PubMed]
16. Reichel, M.P.; Lanyon, S.; Hill, F.I. Perspectives on Current Challenges and Opportunities for Bovine Viral Diarrhoea Virus Eradication in Australia and New Zealand. *Pathogens* **2018**, *7*, 14. [CrossRef] [PubMed]
17. Lanyon, S.; Anderson, M.; Reichel, M. Survey of farmer knowledge and attitudes to endemic disease management in South Australia, with a focus on bovine viral diarrhoea (bovine pestivirus). *Aust. Vet. J.* **2015**, *93*, 157–163. [CrossRef]
18. Lindberg, A.; Houe, H. Characteristics in the epidemiology of bovine viral diarrhea virus (BVDV) of relevance to control. *Prev. Vet. Med.* **2005**, *72*, 55–73. [CrossRef] [PubMed]
19. Smith, D.R. Epidemiologic tools for biosecurity and biocontainment. *Vet. Clin. N. Am. Food Anim. Pract.* **2002**, *18*, 157–175. [CrossRef]
20. Smith, D.R.D.; Grotelueschen, D.M. Biosecurity and biocontainment of bovine viral diarrhea virus. *Vet. Clin. N. Am. Food Anim. Pract.* **2004**, *20*, 131–149. [CrossRef]
21. Morton, J.M.; Phillips, N.; Taylor, L.; Gowan, M. Bovine viral diarrhoea virus in beef heifers in commercial herds in Australia: Mob-level seroprevalences and incidences of seroconversion, and vaccine efficacy. *Aust. Vet. J.* **2013**, *91*, 517–524. [CrossRef]
22. Evans, C.A.; Pinior, B.; Larska, M.; Graham, D.; Schweizer, M.; Guidarini, C.; DeCaro, N.; Ridpath, J.; Gates, M.C. Global knowledge gaps in the prevention and control of bovine viral diarrhoea (BVD) virus. *Transbound. Emerg. Dis.* **2018**, *66*, 640–652. [CrossRef]
23. Lindberg, A.; Alenius, S. Principles for eradication of bovine viral diarrhoea virus (BVDV) infections in cattle populations. *Vet. Microbiol.* **1999**, *64*, 197–222. [CrossRef]
24. PUBCRIS. Australian Pesticides and Veterinary Medicines Authority, Pestigard®, Product Number 53867. Available online: http://www.apvma.gov.au/ (accessed on 26 September 2019).
25. Ridpath, J.F.; Fulton, R.W.; Kirkland, P.D.; Neill, J.D. Prevalence and antigenic differences observed between Bovine viral diarrhea virus subgenotypes isolated from cattle in Australia and feedlots in the southwestern United States. *J. Vet. Diagn. Investig.* **2010**, *22*, 184–191. [CrossRef] [PubMed]
26. Henry, B.; Charmley, E.; Eckard, R.; Gaughan, J.B.; Hegarty, R. Livestock production in a changing climate: Adaptation and mitigation research in Australia. *Crop Pasture Sci.* **2012**, *63*, 191–202. [CrossRef]
27. Heffernan, C.; Misturelli, F.; Nielsen, L.; Gunn, G.J.; Yu, J. Analysis of Pan-European attitudes to the eradication and control of bovine viral diarrhoea. *Vet. Rec.* **2009**, *164*, 163–167. [CrossRef] [PubMed]
28. Ståhl, K.; Alenius, S. BVDV control and eradication in Europe—An update. *Jpn. J. Vet. Res.* **2012**, *60*, S31–S39.
29. Barrett, D.; More, S.J.; Graham, D.; O'Flaherty, J.; Doherty, M.L.; Gunn, H.M. Considerations on BVD eradication for the Irish livestock industry. *Ir. Vet. J.* **2011**, *64*, 12. [CrossRef] [PubMed]
30. Pinior, B.; Firth, C.L.; Richter, V.; Lebl, K.; Trauffler, M.; Dzieciol, M.; Hutter, S.E.; Burgstaller, J.; Obritzhauser, W.; Winter, P. A systematic review of financial and economic assessments of bovine viral diarrhea virus (BVDV) prevention and mitigation activities worldwide. *Prev. Vet. Med.* **2017**, *137*, 77–92. [CrossRef] [PubMed]
31. Hasler, B.; Howe, K.S.; Presi, P.; Stark, K. An economic model to evaluate the mitigation programme for bovine viral diarrhoea in Switzerland. *Prev. Vet. Med.* **2012**, *106*, 162–173. [CrossRef]
32. Valle, P.S.; Skjerve, E.; Martin, S.W.; Larssen, R.B.; Østerås, O.; Nyberg, O. Ten years of bovine virus diarrhoea virus (BVDV) control in Norway: A cost-benefit analysis. *Prev. Vet. Med.* **2005**, *72*, 189–207. [CrossRef]
33. Hernández-Jover, M.; Higgins, V.; Bryant, M.; Rast, L.; McShane, C. Biosecurity and the management of emergency animal disease among commercial beef producers in New South Wales and Queensland (Australia). *Prev. Vet. Med.* **2016**, *134*, 92–102. [CrossRef]
34. Australian Climate Averages—Climate Classifications. Available online: http://www.bom.gov.au/jsp/ncc/climate_averages/climate-classifications/index.jsp?maptype=kpn#maps (accessed on 25 September 2019).
35. R Core Team. *R: A Language and Environment for Statistical Computing*; R Foundation for Statistical Computing: Vienna, Austria, 2019; Volume Inclusive Pagination.

36. Brownlie, J.; Clarke, M.; Howard, C. Experimental production of fatal mucosal disease in cattle. *Vet. Rec.* **1984**, *114*, 535–536. [CrossRef] [PubMed]
37. Ridpath, J.F. The Contribution of Infections with Bovine Viral Diarrhea Viruses to Bovine Respiratory Disease. *Vet. Clin. N. Am. Food Anim. Pract.* **2010**, *26*, 335–348. [CrossRef] [PubMed]
38. Gunn, G.; Saatkamp, H.; Humphry, R.; Stott, A.W. Assessing economic and social pressure for the control of bovine viral diarrhoea virus. *Prev. Vet. Med.* **2005**, *72*, 149–162. [CrossRef]
39. Hay, K.; Barnes, T.; Morton, J.; Gravel, J.; Commins, M.; Horwood, P.F.; Ambrose, R.; Clements, A.; Mahony, T.J. Associations between exposure to viruses and bovine respiratory disease in Australian feedlot cattle. *Prev. Vet. Med.* **2016**, *127*, 121–133. [CrossRef] [PubMed]
40. Izzo, M.; Kirkland, P.; Mohler, V.; Perkins, N.; Gunn, A.A.; House, J. Prevalence of major enteric pathogens in Australian dairy calves with diarrhoea. *Aust. Vet. J.* **2011**, *89*, 167–173. [CrossRef] [PubMed]
41. Swiatek, D.; Palombo, E.A.; Lee, A.; Coventry, M.; Britz, M.; Kirkwood, C.D. Detection and analysis of bovine rotavirus strains circulating in Australian calves during 2004 and 2005. *Vet. Microbiol.* **2010**, *140*, 56–62. [CrossRef]
42. Taylor, L.; Black, P.; Pitt, D.; Mackenzie, A.; Johnson, S.; Rodwell, B. A seroepidemiological study of bovine pestivirus in Queensland beef and dairy herds conducted in 1994/95. *Aust. Vet. J.* **2006**, *84*, 163–168. [CrossRef]
43. Azbel-Jackson, L.; Heffernan, C.; Gunn, G.; Brownlie, J. Exploring the role of voluntary disease schemes on UK farmer bio-security behaviours: Findings from the Norfolk-Suffolk Bovine Viral Diarrhoea control scheme. *PLoS ONE* **2018**, *13*, e0179877. [CrossRef]
44. Pritchard, K.; Wapenaar, W.; Brennan, M.L. Cattle veterinarians' awareness and understanding of biosecurity. *Vet. Rec.* **2015**, *176*, 546. [CrossRef]
45. Fray, M.D.; Paton, D.J.; Alenius, S. The effects of bovine viral diarrhoea virus on cattle reproduction in relation to disease control. *Anim. Reprod. Sci.* **2000**, *60*, 615–627. [CrossRef]
46. Houe, H.; Meyling, A. Prevalence of bovine virus diarrhoea (BVD) in 19 Danish dairy herds and estimation of incidence of infection in early pregnancy. *Prev. Vet. Med.* **1991**, *11*, 9–16. [CrossRef]
47. Hernández-Jover, M.; Hayes, L.; Woodgate, R.; Rast, L.; Toribio, J.-A.L. Animal Health Management Practices Among Smallholder Livestock Producers in Australia and Their Contribution to the Surveillance System. *Front. Vet. Sci.* **2019**, *6*, 191. [CrossRef] [PubMed]
48. Ritter, C.; Jansen, J.; Roth, K.; Kastelic, J.P.; Adams, C.; Barkema, H.W. Dairy farmers' perceptions toward the implementation of on-farm Johne's disease prevention and control strategies. *J. Dairy Sci.* **2016**, *99*, 9114–9125. [CrossRef]

3

Circulation of Indigenous Bovine Respiratory Syncytial Virus Strains in Turkish Cattle: The First Isolation and Molecular Characterization

Zafer Yazici [1,*], Emre Ozan [2], Cuneyt Tamer [1], Bahadir Muftuoglu [2], Gerald Barry [3], Hanne Nur Kurucay [1], Ahmed Eisa Elhag [1,*], Abdurrahman Anil Cagirgan [4], Semra Gumusova [1] and Harun Albayrak [1]

1 Department of Veterinary Virology, Faculty of Veterinary Medicine, Ondokuz Mayis University, 55139 Samsun, Turkey; cuneyt_tamer@hotmail.com (C.T.); kurucayhannenur@gmail.com (H.N.K.); semragumusova@hotmail.com (S.G.); harunalbayrak55@msn.com (H.A.)
2 Department of Veterinary Experimental Animals, Faculty of Veterinary Medicine, Ondokuz Mayis University, 55139 Samsun, Turkey; emre.ozan@omu.edu.tr (E.O.); bahadirmuftuoglu@hotmail.com (B.M.)
3 Veterinary Science Centre, School of Veterinary Medicine, University College of Dublin, Dublin 4, Ireland; gerald.barry@ucd.ie
4 Bornova Veterinary Control Institute, Veterinary Control Institute Directorates, Ministry of Agriculture and Forestry, 35010 Izmir, Turkey; a.anilcagirgan@gmail.com
* Correspondence: zyazici@omu.edu.tr (Z.Y.); ahmedeisa_85@hotmail.com (A.E.E.)

Abstract: Bovine respiratory disease (BRD) is a huge economic burden on the livestock industries of countries worldwide. Bovine respiratory syncytial virus (BRSV) is one of the most important pathogens that contributes to BRD. In this study, we report the identification and first isolation, with molecular characterization, of a new BRSV strain from lung specimens of three beef cows in Turkey that died from respiratory distress. After the screening of lung tissues for BRD-associated viruses using a multiscreen antigen-ELISA, a BRSV antigen was detected. This was then confirmed by real-time RT-PCR specific for BRSV. Following confirmation, virus isolation was conducted in MDBK cell cultures and clear CPE, including syncytia compatible with BRSV, were detected. RT-nested PCR, using F gene-specific primers, was performed on the cultured isolates, and the products were sequenced and deposited to Genbank with accession numbers MT179304, MT024766, and MT0244767. Phylogenetic analysis of these sequences indicated that the cattle were infected with BRSV from subgroup III and were closely related to previously identified American and Turkish strains, but contained some amino acid and nucleotide differences. This research paves the way for further studies on the molecular characteristics of natural BRSV isolates, including full genome analysis and disease pathogenesis, and also contributes to the development of robust national strategies against this virus.

Keywords: BRSV; cattle; isolation; respiratory disorders; sequencing

1. Introduction

Bovine respiratory disease (BRD) is a term used to describe respiratory disease in cattle caused by single or a range of pathogens. It is a complex disease, with multiple viruses, bacteria, and parasites potentially involved [1,2]. BRD can negatively affect production and is therefore considered a major economic burden on the livestock industry worldwide [1,3]. Bovine respiratory syncytial virus (BRSV), also called *Bovine orthopneumovirus,* is an important pathogen of this complex [2,4,5]. BRSV belongs to the genus *Orthopneumovirus* of the family *Pneumoviridae* in the order *Mononegavirales* [6] and has a negative sense, single-stranded RNA genome. The non-segmented virus genome consists of 10 genes that encode 11 proteins: Two non-structural proteins (NS1 and NS2); a nucleocapsid (N) protein; a phosphoprotein (P); a matrix protein (M); glycoproteins SH, G (attachment), and F (fusion); M2-1 and M2-2 (control transcription and RNA replication); and RNA polymerase (L) [7,8].

Phylogenetic analysis based on both F and G proteins has led to a subdivision of BRSV into eight subgroups, denoted I–VIII [7,9–11]. These subgroups tend to separate geographically; subgroup I BRSV strains are typically isolated in the UK and Switzerland, whereas subgroup II normally includes strains from the Netherlands, Denmark, Belgium, France, and Japan [9,12]. The strains from the USA are commonly included in subgroup III, while some strains from the USA and other European countries fall into subgroup IV [7,9]. Finally subgroups V and VI include BRSV strains usually found in Belgium and France [9]. Subgroups VII and VIII are a recent addition and are predominantly seen in Europe, particularly in Italy and Croatia [7,10]. In addition, a putative new BRSV subgroup, tentatively named subgroup IX, has been proposed, in order to classify recent strains isolated from Brazil, which have mutations in the immunodominant region of the G protein [11].

BRSV predominantly infects cattle, although sheep and goats can also be infected [8,12]. The virus is mainly transmitted by direct contact and/or aerosols and both clinical and sub-clinical animals are capable of transmitting [7,13,14]. BRSV outbreaks can occur in all ages of animals, but young calves (particularly those between 2 weeks and 9 months old) are especially vulnerable [12,13].

The clinical manifestations of BRSV infections in cattle can vary from mildly symptomatic to fatal, and the outcome is multifactorial. The breed of cattle; the strain of virus; and the contribution of other viruses, bacteria, and parasites all play a role, alongside other factors, such as management practices and environments [5,14,15]. Although BRSV infection is rarely fatal, it can lead to upper and lower respiratory damage in young calves and is characterized by a fever, cough, decreased feed intake, increased respiratory rate, and nasal discharge [14,15].

There is limited information available about the seroprevalence of BRSV in Turkey and very few BRSV sequences from Turkish isolates have been submitted to GenBank [4,5]. Cases of BRD are plentiful in Turkey and some have been characterized, but major gaps in our understanding remain, thus limiting the ability to control it [3,16]. In this context, the aim of this study was to present both the first isolation of BRSV in Turkey and its molecular characterization, consisting of both sequencing and phylogenetic analysis.

2. Material and Methods

2.1. Samples

Between December 2018 and January 2019, a veterinarian in the Samsun province of Northern Turkey reported three cases of respiratory disease in beef cattle from the same farm. The cattle were unvaccinated against any BRD-associated viruses, including BRSV. The cattle died from severe respiratory disorders, including pneumonia. Lung tissue samples were taken post-mortem and sent to the Virology Department of The Faculty of Veterinary Medicine, Ondokuz Mayis University, for diagnosis. To differentiate the samples, they were labeled 34TR2018, 43TR2018, and 07TR2019, according to the animal they came from.

2.2. Virus Isolation

For cell culture isolation, approximately 1 g of lung tissue was placed in 5 mL of cold Minimal Essential Medium (MEM) containing 2% penicillin/streptomycin (Sigma-Aldrich, St. Louis, MO, USA), and then homogenized on ice for 1 min at 6000 rpm using a tissue homogenizer (Heidolph Ins., Schwabach, Germany). The homogenate was then centrifuged at 1500× g for 15 min and the supernatant was sterile-filtered (0.22 μm) and stored at −20 °C. For PCR, approximately 30 mg of lung tissue was homogenized with a Tissue-Lyser (Qiagen AG, Hilden, Germany) in 1.8 mL of MEM containing 2% penicillin/streptomycin. Obtained homogenates were clarified by centrifugation at 1500× g for 15 min and the supernatant was then sterile-filtered (0.22 μm) and stored at −20 °C.

MDBK cells were used for the virus isolation studies. Briefly, MDBK cells were cultivated at 37 °C with 5% CO_2 in Dulbecco's Modified Eagle's Medium (DMEM, Gibco, Paisley, UK) supplemented with 10% fetal calf serum (FCS, Sigma-Aldrich) and 1% penicillin/streptomycin (Sigma-Aldrich). Virus isolation from suspected samples was conducted by performing blind passages. Supernatants from tissue homogenates were inoculated onto MDBK monolayers at 37 °C for 60 min and then replaced with DMEM containing 2% FCS. Cells were maintained at 37 °C with 5% CO_2, and checked daily for cytopathic effects (CPE).

2.3. Antigen-ELISA for BRD-Associated Viruses

The lung tissues were tested using a commercially available multiscreen antigen-ELISA kit (Bio-X, Rochefort, Belgium, Cat. No: BIO K, 340/5). The kit has been reported to detect Bovine parainfluenza-3 (BPIV-3), Bovine viral diarrhea virus (BVDV), BRSV, and Bovine herpesvirus-1 (BHV-1), and was used according to the manufacturer's instructions.

2.4. Nucleic Acid Extraction and Amplification

We performed RNA extractions from homogenized lung tissue, as well as infected cell culture lysates, using a GeneJET RNA Purification Kit (Thermo Fisher Scientific, Vilnius, Lithuania), according to the manufacturer's instructions. The extracted RNA was eluted in 75 μL of elution buffer and kept at −80 °C.

For the real time RT-PCR analysis, the primers and the TaqMan probe targeted the N gene of BRSV and have been previously described by Boxus et al. [17]. For the RT-nested PCR, F gene-specific primers were used as previously described by Vilcek et al. [18]. For the first round of RT-nested PCR, we used B1 and B2A primers that amplify a 711 bp product. This was followed by B3 and B4A primers that amplify a 481 bp product. The sequence data of the primers and probe are given in Table 1.

Table 1. Information on the primers and probes used in the analysis.

Primers and Probe	Sequences (5′-3′)	Product Size(bp)	Ref.
F primer	GCAATGCTGCAGGACTAGGTATAAT	124	Boxus et al. [17]
R primer	ACACTGTAATTGATGACCCCATTCT		
Probe	FAM-ACCAAGACTTGTATGATGCTGCCAAAGCA-TAMRA		
B1	AATCAACATGCAGTGCAGTTAG	711	Vilcek et al. [18]
B2A	TTTGGTCATTCGTTATAGGCAT		
B3	GTGCAGTTAGTAGAGGTTATCTTAGT	481	
B4A	TAGTTCTTTAGATCAAGTACTTTGCT		

The real time RT-PCR was carried out using an iTaq™ Universal Probes One-Step Kit (Biorad, Hercules, CA, USA, Cat No: 1725140) on a CFX Connect real time PCR machine (Biorad). The real time RT-PCR reactions were carried out in a final volume of 25 μL containing 5 μL of RNA, 12.5 μL of 2X buffer, 320 nM of each primer, 160 nM of probe, 0.5 μL of RT enzyme, and 5 μL of RNAse-free water. The PCR conditions were as follows: 10 min at 50 °C for reverse transcription and 3 min at 95 °C, followed by 45 cycles at 95 °C for 7 s and 59 °C for 10 s.

The RT-nested PCR was carried out using the Qiagen Onestep RT-PCR kit (Qiagen, Cat No:210212). The first round of PCR was performed in a final volume of 50 μL consisting of 5 μL of RNA, 10 μL of 5X buffer, 400 nM of each primer, 1 μL of dNTP, 1 μL of RT enzyme, and 29 μL of RNAse-free water. The PCR conditions were as follows: 30 min at 50 °C for reverse transcription and 15 min at 95 °C, followed by 35 cycles at 95 °C for 45 s, 50 °C for 45 s, 72 °C for 60 s, and finally a cycle at 72 °C for 10 min. The second round of PCR was also carried out in a final volume of 50 μL containing 5 μL of the first round RT-PCR product, 10 μL of 5X buffer, 400 nM of each primer, 1 μL of dNTP, 1 μL of RT enzyme, and 29 μL of RNAse-free water. The cycling conditions employed for the second round of PCR were as follows: 1 min at 95 °C and 45 s at 95 °C, followed by 35 cycles at 50 °C for 45 s, 72 °C for 1 min, and finally a cycle at 72 °C for 10 min. Positive controls for both RT-PCR tests were provided by the virology laboratory of the Samsun Veterinary Control Institute, Turkey. For the nested PCR, all amplicons were visualized on 1% agarose gels.

2.5. Sequencing and Phylogenetic Analysis

PCR products were purified using a QIAquick PCR purification kit (Qiagen), according to the manufacturer's instructions and then Sanger sequenced by RefGen Biotechnology, Ankara, Turkey (http://www.refgen.com). The sequences were aligned using Bioedit, version 7.2.5, followed by BLAST analysis in GenBank databases [19]. For comparison, we selected seventeen representative isolate sequences from GenBank, including BRSV and human respiratory syncytial virus (HRSV) strains. The phylogenetic tree was constructed with the maximum likelihood method under the Tamura-3 parameter model using MEGA X (Molecular Evolutionary Genetics Analysis-MEGA, version 10.0.5) [20], and the bootstrap values were based on F gene nucleotide (nt) sequences. The tree was assessed using 1000 bootstrap replications. The sequences identified from animals 07TR2019, 34TR2018, and 43TR2018 were deposited in GenBank with the accession numbers MT179304, MT024766, and MT0244767, respectively.

3. Results

3.1. The Identification of Lung Tissue Samples Infected with BRSV

The first step of this study was the screening of all lung tissues for BRD-associated viruses using both the multiscreen antigen-ELISA and real time RT-PCR. All tissue samples were BRSV positive by ELISA, and negative for BVDV, BHV-1, and BPIV-3. The samples were also confirmed to be positive for BRSV by real time RT-PCR.

3.2. Virus Isolation

Lung homogenates from each animal, consisting of 43TR2018, 342TR2018, and 07TR2019, were added to MDBK cultures and incubated. Obvious CPE including syncytia were visible between 3- and 4-days post inoculation (Figure 1).

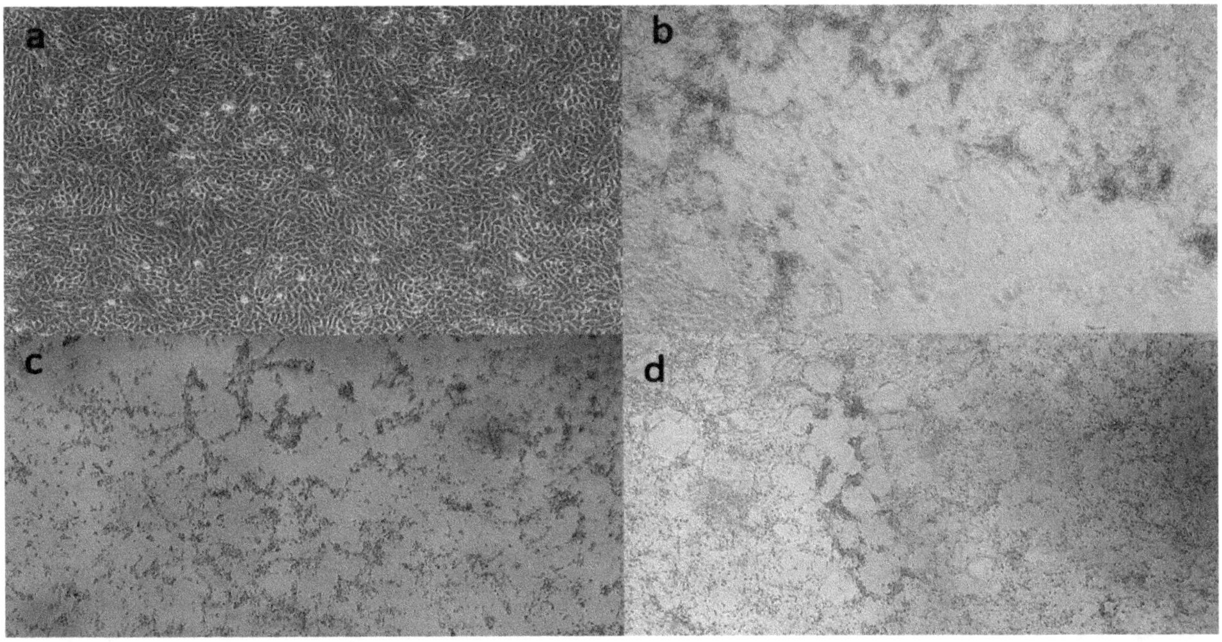

Figure 1. Photos of MDBK cells: (**a**) Cell control; (**b**,**c**) MDBK cells displaying cytopathic effects (CPE) and syncytia formation 72 h post-infection with isolates 43TR2018 and 34TR2018, respectively; (**d**) MDBK cells displaying limited CPE and syncytia foci 72 h post-infection with isolate 07TR2019.

3.3. *RT-Nested PCR*

Following virus propagation in culture, RNA was extracted from each of the infected MDBK cultures and nested PCR was performed. Based on this, 711 and 481 bp bands corresponding to the F gene were visible for 43TR2018 and 07TR2019, while only a 481 bp band, corresponding to the second round of PCR, was visible for isolate 34TR2018.

3.4. *Sequencing and Phylogenetic Analysis*

Following the RT-nested PCR, the 481 bp fragments were sequenced. As detailed in Table 2, the sequencing showed that the three isolates—MT179304, MT024766, and MT024767—had a 100% similarity to each other at the nucleotide (nt) level. Furthermore, the three isolates were found to be 99.49% and 99.22% identical to another Turkish strain—KY499619 [3]—at both nt and amino acid (aa) levels, respectively. The three isolates presented here were also 97.43% (nt) and 98.44% (aa) identical to the American reference strain KU159366.

As depicted in Figure 2, the phylogenetic analysis of the F gene revealed that our isolates—MT179304, MT024766, and MT024767—are in the same cluster in subgroup III, together with isolates KY499619 and KU159366, based on the nucleotide sequence.

Interestingly, however, there are some small amino acid differences that exist between these newly presented isolates and KY499619 and KU159366 (Table 3). Unlike the three isolates presented here, in isolate KU159366, a Threonine (T) at position 118 is an Alanine (A) and a Threonine (T) at position 173 is a Serine (S), while a Lysine (K) at position 176 is a Glutamic Acid (E) in isolate KY499619.

Table 2. Percentage of nucleotide and amino acid similarity between the isolates identified in this study (marked with *) and other bovine respiratory syncytial virus (BRSV) strains obtained from Genbank. NA: Not available.

			Amino Acid Similarities (%)												
	GenBank Number	**Strain Name and Country**	**NC038272**	**FJ543091**	**M82816**	**D00953**	**MG947594**	**KU159366**	**KY499619**	**MT179304***	**MT024766***	**MT024767***	**AF092942**	**AF124561**	**MF153477**
	NC038272	ATCC51908 NA		96.05	96.05	97.65	98.44	93.60	92.77	93.60	93.60	93.60	98.44	100.00	95.24
	FJ543091	BRSV-25-BR Brasil	96.14		98.44	95.24	96.05	89.38	88.51	89.38	89.38	89.38	94.42	96.05	91.09
	M82816	NA NA	96.14	99.49		95.24	96.05	90.24	89.38	90.24	90.24	90.24	94.42	96.05	91.93
	D00953	RB 93 NA	98.20	96.40	96.40		97.65	91.93	90.24	91.09	91.09	91.09	96.05	97.65	92.77
	MG947594	Lovsta 2016 Sweden	97.69	95.89	95.89	98.46		91.93	91.09	91.93	91.93	91.93	96.85	98.44	93.60
Nucleotide Similarities (%)	**KU159366**	USII/S1 USA	96.14	93.06	93.57	94.60	94.09		97.65	98.44	98.44	98.44	93.60	93.60	93.60
	KY499619	BRS/TR/Erz/2014 Turkey	95.63	93.06	93.57	94.09	93.57	97.43		99.22	99.22	99.22	92.77	92.77	92.77
	MT179304 *	07TR2019 Turkey	95.63	93.57	94.09	94.09	93.57	97.43	99.49		100.00	100.00	93.60	93.60	93.60
	MT024766 *	34TR2018 Turkey	95.63	93.57	94.09	94.09	93.57	97.43	99.49	100.00		100.00	93.60	93.60	93.60
	MT024767 *	43TR2018 Turkey	95.63	93.57	94.09	94.09	93.57	97.43	99.49	100.00	100.00		93.60	93.60	93.60
	AF092942	ATue51908 Germany	99.49	95.89	95.89	97.94	97.43	96.14	95.63	95.63	95.63	95.63		98.44	95.24
	AF124561	A2Gelfi France	99.49	95.63	95.63	97.69	97.17	95.63	95.12	95.12	95.12	95.12	98.97		95.24
	MF153477	BRSV-UnepJab-1 NA	96.66	93.06	93.06	95.12	94.60	94.86	94.34	94.34	94.34	94.34	96.66	96.14	

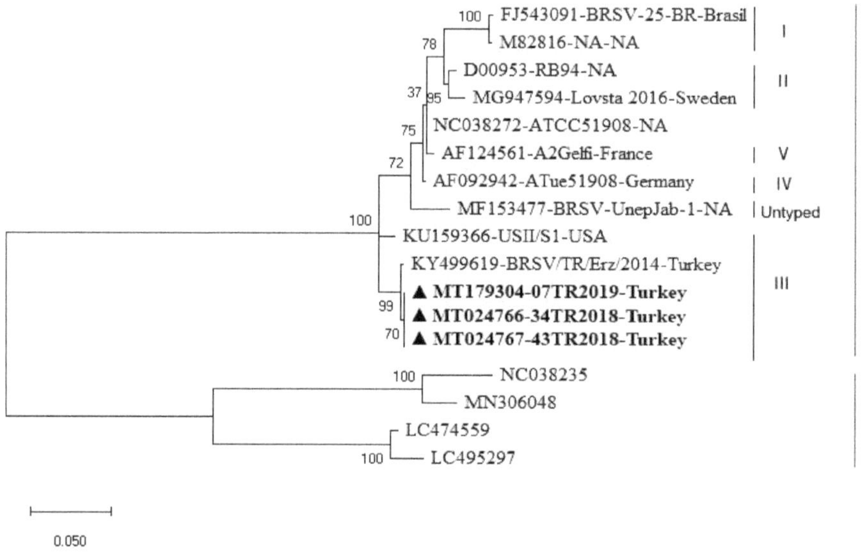

Figure 2. The phylogenetic analysis of the BRSV strains isolated in this study. The tree was constructed from a partial analysis of the BRSV F gene using the maximum likelihood method with MEGA X software. The robustness branching pattern was tested with 1000 bootstrap replications. According to the phylogenetic tree, the current strains were in subgroup III (marked in bold and with a ▲). The BRSV sequences were named using their GenBank accession number, strain name, and geographical origin. NA: Not available.

Table 3. Partial alignment of the F gene from the isolates identified in this study (marked with *), with a selection of strains from the different subgroups. NA: Not available.

Sub-Groups	GenBank Number	Strain Name	Amino Acid Positions of BRSV F Gene Sequence																			
			67	70	71	75	80	91	100	101	102	104	105	113	114	115	118	124	148	168	173	176
I	FJ543091	BRSV-25-BR	N	N	G	K	K	V	E	P	T	S	S	E	S	I	T	K	I	N	S	K
I	M82816	NA	.	.	.	.	.	A	.	.	.	.	.	.	.	.	.	.	.	K	.	.
II	D00953	RB 94	.	.	S	N	.	.	.	.	A	.	.	.	L	.	K	.	.	K	.	.
II	MG947594	Lovsta 2016	.	.	S	.	.	.	.	L	A	.	.	.	L	.	.	.	.	K	.	.
III	KU159366	USII/S1	D	K	S	.	.	T	V	.	A	F	N	.	L	M	A	R	.	K	.	.
III	KY499619	BRS/TR/Erz/2014	D	K	S	.	.	T	V	.	A	F	N	.	L	M	.	R	.	K	T	E
III	MT179304 *	07TR2019	D	K	S	.	.	T	V	.	A	F	N	.	L	M	.	R	.	K	T	.
III	MT024766 *	34TR2018	D	K	S	.	.	T	V	.	A	F	N	.	L	M	.	R	.	K	T	.
III	MT024767 *	43TR2018	D	K	S	.	.	T	V	.	A	F	N	.	L	M	.	R	.	K	T	.
IV	AF092942	ATue51908	.	K	S	.	.	.	.	.	A	F	.	.	L	.	.	.	V	K	.	.
V	AF124561	A2Gelfi	.	.	S	.	.	.	.	.	A	F	.	.	L	.	.	.	.	K	.	.
	NC038272	ATCC51908	.	.	S	.	.	.	.	.	A	F	.	.	L	.	.	.	.	K	.	.
Untyped	MF153477	BRSV-UnepJab-1	.	K	S	.	Q	I	.	.	A	F	.	G	L	T	.	R	.	K	.	.

4. Discussion

BRD is an economically important condition in the worldwide livestock industry that can be caused by a number of different viruses, bacteria, and parasites, individually or in combination [2,21]. The disease is typically caused by early virus infection, followed by bacterial secondary infection that can lead to lung damage and pneumonia-like illnesses [2,21]. Surprisingly, we have recently observed cattle with severe, sometimes fatal, BRD, associated with just single-pathogen infections, such as BRSV, BPIV3, or BHV-1 [3,5,22].

To investigate this and to understand potential changes in the viruses that may be causing an increased virulence, it is vital to be able to isolate and study the viruses in question. Previous studies in Turkey have mainly been diagnostic in nature, with limited phylogenetic analysis [4,5,23,24]. We present here, for the first time, the isolation and growth in culture of BRSV from infected cattle, phylogenetic analysis of the aforementioned isolates, and the identification of differences between them and previous isolates from Turkey and abroad. In this study, lung tissues from diseased animals were collected post-mortem and screened for the most common BRD-associated viruses, including BVDV, BHV-1, BPIV3, and BRSV, using commercially available ELISA kits, and only a BRSV antigen was found to be present [5]. No screening for bovine coronavirus or bacteria in the lung tissue was carried out, so the contribution from these pathogens to the disease state of the animals cannot be ruled out. Following a positive ELISA, lung homogenates were added to the cell culture and observed daily until CPE including syncytia and round apoptotic cells were visible. The isolation of BRSV in culture can be challenging because the virus is relatively labile and can struggle to grow in culture; however, this successful isolation now opens the door to extensive studies that would not have been possible otherwise [25–27].

The F gene of BRSV encodes a major structural protein that is commonly targeted by the adaptive immune response. It is a protein that is central to virus entry into cells, as well as being responsible for the fusion of infected cells with adjacent cells, resulting in the formation of large multinucleated syncytia [28]. Furthermore, the F gene is also a highly conserved region of the BRSV genome compared with the G gene [11]. The results of partial sequencing of the F gene of the current three isolates revealed that they were 100% identical to each other and were closely related to the sequence submitted (KY499619) from Turkey by Timurkan et al. [3]. We determined that the current strains—MT179304, MT024766, and MT024767—had a 99.49% nt and 99.22% aa similarity to the KY499619 strain. When compared to an international strain—KU159366—the isolates had a 97.43% nt and 98.44% aa similarity.

Phylogenetic analysis classified the isolates in subgroup III, similar to isolate KY499619, which was previously identified in Turkey and KU159366 from the USA. Considering the geographical location of Turkey, one could imagine a scenario where European strains would be readily imported into Turkey as globalization and international trade may hold potential risks for the spreading of diseases [29]; however, this does not seem to be the case for the outbreak on the farm in the present study. The amino acid change at position 118 is particularly interesting because that is the −2 position for an N-glycosylation sequence. The −2 position can have an influence on the efficiency of glycosylation of the local Asparagine [30]. Position 118 is also in the middle of the virokinin that is cleaved from the fusion protein of BRSV and is known to increase pulmonary inflammation during infection [31,32]. It is possible that this glycosylation efficiency may impact cleavage at the fusion protein furin cleavage sites, or that the amino acid change may impact the function of the virokinin itself. The second amino acid difference identified in the fusion protein compared to strain KY499619 is in the F2 subunit. Changes in this region could impact antibody recognition and may have consequences for vaccine development. All of these questions are areas for future exploration using the isolates in culture from this study.

Turkey has strong economic links to the USA and live animals are transported to Turkey from this region [33]. This is a possible source of the virus and illustrates the risks associated with globalized trade. Animals are known to harbor BRSV without symptoms, meaning the virus could easily be transported without detection [3], and constant introductions of new strains will increase the diversity of viruses in circulation, thus potentially complicating control efforts.

While the sample number is small in this study and from just one farm, it is a clear warning to the agricultural industry in Turkey that variant strains of BRSV exist in Turkey—variants that may have an increased virulence—and an increased molecular understanding of those variants is needed, along with better, more widespread surveillance and control strategies, in order to reduce the impact of this virus.

5. Conclusions

It is believed that BRSV is endemic in Turkey; however, minimal information is available on the prevalence of the virus, along with an understanding of the strains present. In order to successfully control infection, defining the target is essential. This study reports the identification and isolation of a new strain of BRSV that has not previously been identified in Turkey. It was associated with animals that died from respiratory distress and the strain shows amino acid differences in the Fusion protein (compared to the only other Turkish isolate) that are known to contribute to virulence. Importantly, the virus has been isolated in culture, which will allow further investigations into its virulence and the significance of those amino acid changes.

Author Contributions: Conceptualization, Z.Y., H.A., E.O., and G.B.; methodology, C.T., B.M., H.N.K., and A.E.E.; software, E.O., and B.M.; validation, Z.Y., E.O., and G.B.; formal analysis, E.O. and Z.Y.; investigation, C.T., B.M., H.N.K., and A.E.E.; writing—original draft preparation, Z.Y.; writing—review and editing, G.B., E.O., S.G., A.A.C., and A.E.E.; supervision, Z.Y. All authors have read and agreed to the published version of the manuscript.

References

1. Fulton, R.W. Bovine respiratory disease research (1983–2009). *Anim. Health. Res. Rev.* **2009**, *10*, 131–139. [CrossRef] [PubMed]
2. Headley, S.A.; Okano, W.; Balbo, L.C.; Marcasso, R.A.; Oliveira, T.E.; Alfieri, A.F.; NegriFilho, L.C.; Michelazzo, M.Z.; Rodrigues, S.C.; Baptista, A.L.; et al. Molecular survey of infectious agents associated with bovine respiratory disease in a beef cattle feedlot in southern Brazil. *J. Vet. Diagn. Invest.* **2018**, *30*, 249–251. [CrossRef] [PubMed]

3. Albayrak, H.; Yazici, Z.; Ozan, E.; Tamer, C.; Abd El Wahed, A.; Wehner, S.; Ulrich, K.; Weidmann, M. Characterisation of the First Bovine Parainfluenza Virus 3 Isolate Detected in Cattle in Turkey. *Vet. Sci.* **2019**, *6*, 56. [CrossRef] [PubMed]
4. Hacioglu, I.K.; Coskun, N.; Duran, S.; Sevinc, S.; Alkan, F. Phylogenetic Analysis of Bovine Respiratory Syncytial Virus from Calves with Respiratory Disorders. *Kafkas Univ. Vet. Fak. Derg.* **2019**, *25*, 251–256. [CrossRef]
5. Timurkan, M.O.; Aydin, H.; Sait, A. Identification and Molecular Characterisation of Bovine Parainfluenza Virus-3 and Bovine Respiratory Syncytial Virus-First Report from Turkey. *J. Vet. Res.* **2019**, *63*, 167–173. [CrossRef]
6. International Committee on Taxonomy of Viruses. 2019 Release. Available online: https://talk.ictvonline.org/ictv-reports/ictv_online_report/negative-sense-rna-viruses/mononegavirales/w/pneumoviridae/738/genus-orthopneumovirus/ (accessed on 3 September 2020).
7. Bertolotti, L.; Giammarioli, M.; Rosati, S. Genetic characterization of bovine respiratory syncytial virus strains isolated in Italy: Evidence for the circulation of new divergent clades. *J. Vet. Diagn. Invest.* **2018**, *30*, 300–304. [CrossRef]
8. Taylor, G.; Wyld, S.; Valarcher, J.F.; Guzman, E.; Thom, M.; Widdison, S.; Buchholz, U.J. Recombinant bovine respiratory syncytial virus with deletion of the SH gene induces increased apoptosis and pro-inflammatory cytokines in vitro, and is attenuated and induces protective immunity in calves. *J. Gen. Virol.* **2014**, *95*, 1244–1254. [CrossRef]
9. Valarcher, J.F.; Schelcher, H.B.; Bourhy, H. Evolution of Bovine Respiratory Syncytial Virus. *J. Virol.* **2000**, *74*, 10714–10728. [CrossRef]
10. Krešić, N.; Bedeković, T.; Brnić, D.; Šimić, I.; Lojkić, I.; Turk, N. Genetic analysis of bovine respiratory syncytial virus in Croatia. *Comp. Immunol. Microbiol. Infect. Dis.* **2018**, *58*, 52–57. [CrossRef]
11. Leme, R.A.; Agnol, A.M.D.; Balbo, L.C.; Pereria, F.L.; Possatti, F.; Alfieri, A.F.; Alfieri, A.A. Molecular characterization of Brazilian wild-type strains of Bovine respiratory syncytial virus reveals genetic diversity and putative subgroup of the virus. *Vet. Q.* **2020**, *40*, 83–96. [CrossRef]
12. Sarmiento-Silva, R.E.; Nakamura-Lopez, Y.; Vaughan, G. Epidemiology, Molecular Epidemiology and Evolution of Bovine Respiratory Syncytial Virus. *Viruses* **2012**, *4*, 3452–3467. [CrossRef] [PubMed]
13. Hoppe, I.B.A.L.; Medeiros, A.S.R.; Arns, C.W.; Samara, S.I. Bovine respiratory syncytial virus seroprevalence and risk factors in non-vaccinated dairy cattle herds in Brazil. *BMC Vet. Res.* **2018**, *14*, 208. [CrossRef] [PubMed]
14. Urban-Chmiel, R.; Wernicki, A.; Puchalski, A.; Dec, M.; Stęgierska, D.; Grooms, D.L.; Barbu, N.I. Detection of bovine respiratory syncytial virus infections in young dairy and beef cattle in Poland. *Vet. Q.* **2014**, *35*, 33–36. [CrossRef] [PubMed]
15. Baptista, A.L.; Rezende, A.L.; Fonseca, P.D.A.; Massi, R.P.; Nogueira, G.M.; Magalhães, L.Q.; Headley, S.A.; Menezes, G.L.; Alfieri, A.A.; Saut, J.P.E. Bovine respiratory disease complex associated mortality and morbidity rates in feedlot cattle from southeastern Brazil. *J. Infect. Dev. Ctries.* **2017**, *11*, 791–799. [CrossRef]
16. Yazici, Z.; Gumusova, S.; Tamer, C.; Muftuoglu, B.; Ozan, E.; Arslan, S.; Bas, O.; Elhag, A.E.; Albayrak, H. The first serological report for genotype C bovine parainfluenza 3 virus in ruminant species of mid-northern Turkey: Traces from the past. *Trop. Biomed.* **2019**, *36*, 803–809, Scopus EID: 2-s2.0-85073422601.
17. Boxus, M.; Letellier, C.; Kerkhofs, P. Real Time RT-PCR for the detection and quantitation of bovine respiratory syncytial virus. *J. Virol. Methods* **2005**, *125*, 125–130. [CrossRef]
18. Vilcek, S.; Elvander, M.; Ballagi-Pordány, A.; Belák, S. Development of nested PCR assays for detection of bovine respiratory syncytial virus in clinical samples. J. *Clin. Microbiol.* **1994**, *32*, 2225–2231. [CrossRef] [PubMed]
19. Hall, T. BioEdit: A user-friendly biological sequence alignment editor and analysis program for Windows 95/98/NT. *Nucleic Acids Symp. Ser.* **1999**, *41*, 95–98.
20. Kumar, S.; Stecher, G.; Li, M.; Knyaz, C.; Tamura, K. MEGA X: Molecular evolutionary genetics analysis across computing platforms. *Mol. Biol. Evol.* **2018**, *35*, 1547–1549. [CrossRef]
21. Kurcubic, V.; Dokovic, R.; Ilic, Z.; Petrovic, M. Etiopathogenesis and economic significance of bovine respiratory disease complex (BRD). *Acta Agric. Serb.* **2018**, *45*, 85–100. [CrossRef]

22. Albayrak, H.; Tamer, C.; Ozan, E.; Muftuoglu, B.; Kadi, H.; Dogan, F.; Cagirgan, A.A.; Elhag, A.E.; Akman, A.; Kurucay, H.N.; et al. Molecular identification and phylogeny of bovine herpesvirus-1 (BoHV-1) from cattle associated with respiratory disorders and death in Turkey. *Med. Weter.* **2020**, *76*, 358–361. [CrossRef]
23. Alkan, F.; Ozkul, A.; Bilge-Dagalp, S.; Yesilbag, K.; Oguzoglu, C.; Akca, Y.; Burgu, I. Virological and serological studies on the role of PI-3 virus, BRSV, BVDV, and BHV- 1 on respiratory infections of cattle. I. The detection of etiological agents by direct immunofluorescence technique. *DTW. Dtsch. Tierarztl. Wochenschr.* **2000**, *107*, 193–195. [PubMed]
24. Yesilbag, K.; Gungor, B. Seroprevalence of bovine respiratory viruses in North-Western Turkey. *Trop. Anim. Health Prod.* **2008**, *40*, 55–60. [CrossRef] [PubMed]
25. Almeida, R.S.; Domingues, H.G.; Coswig, L.T.; D'Arce, R.C.F.; Carvalho, R.F.; Arns, C.W. Detection of bovive respiratory syncytial virus in experimentally infected balb/c mice. *Vet. Res.* **2004**, *35*, 189–197. [CrossRef] [PubMed]
26. Santangelo, P.; Nitin, N.; LaConte, L.; Woolums, A.; Bao, G. Live-cell characterization and analysis of a clinical isolate of bovine respiratory syncytial virus, using molecular beacons. *J. Virol.* **2006**, *80*, 682–688. [CrossRef] [PubMed]
27. Bortolin Affonso, I.; de Souza, A.; Cavalheiro Martini, M.; Bianchi dos Santos, M.; Rosado Spilki, F.; Weis Arns, C.; Issa Samara, S. Detection of an untyped strain of bovine respiratory syncytial virus in a dairy herd. *Semin. Cienc. Agrar.* **2014**, *35*, 2539–2549. [CrossRef]
28. Valentova, V. The antigenic and genetic variability of bovine respiratory syncytial virus with emphasis on the G protein. *Vet. Med.* **2003**, *48*, 254–266. [CrossRef]
29. Dean, A.S.; Fournié, G.; Kulo, A.E.; Boukaya, G.A.; Schelling, E.; Bonfoh, B. Potential risk of regional disease spread in West Africa through cross-border cattle trade. *PLoS ONE* **2013**, *8*, e75570. [CrossRef]
30. Domingues, H.G.; Spilki, F.R.; Arns, C.W. Molecular detection and phylogenetic analysis of bovine respiratory syncytial virus (BRSV) in swabs and lung tissues of adult cattle. *Pesq. Vet. Bras.* **2011**, *31*, 961–966. [CrossRef]
31. Valarcher, J.F.; Furze, J.; Wyld, S.G.; Cook, R.; Zimmer, G.; Herrler, G.; Taylor, G. Bovine respiratory syncytial virus lacking the virokinin or with a mutation in furin cleavage site RA(R/K)R109 induces less pulmonary inflammation without impeding the induction of protective immunity in calves. *J. Gen. Virol.* **2006**, *87*, 1659–1667. [CrossRef]
32. Zimmer, G.; Rohn, M.; McGregor, G.P.; Schemann, M.; Conzelmann, K.K.; Herrler, G. Virokinin, a bioactive peptide of the tachykinin family, is released from the fusion protein of bovine respiratory syncytial virus. *J. Biol. Chem.* **2003**, *278*, 46854–46861. [CrossRef] [PubMed]
33. Okur-Gumusova, S.; Tamer, C.; Ozan, E.; Cavunt, A.; Kadi, H.; Muftuoglu, B.; Eisa Elhag, A.; Yazici, Z.; Albayrak, H. An investigation of the seroprevalence of crimean-congo hemorrhagic fever and lumpy skin disease in domesticated water buffaloes in Northern Turkey. *Trop. Biomed.* **2020**, *37*, 165–173, Scopus EID: 2-s2.0-85086915081.

4

Prolonged Detection of Bovine Viral Diarrhoea Virus Infection in the Semen of Bulls

Andrew J. Read, Sarah Gestier, Kate Parrish, Deborah S. Finlaison, Xingnian Gu, Tiffany W. O'Connor and Peter D. Kirkland *

Virology Laboratory, Elizabeth Macarthur Agriculture Institute, Woodbridge Road, Menangle, New South, Wales 2568, Australia; andrew.j.read@dpi.nsw.gov.au (A.J.R.); sarah.gestier@dpi.nsw.gov.au (S.G.); kate.parrish@dpi.nsw.gov.au (K.P.); deborah.finlaison@dpi.nsw.gov.au (D.S.F.); xingnian.gu@dpi.nsw.gov.au (X.G.); tiffany.o'connor@dpi.nsw.gov.au (T.W.O.)

* Correspondence: peter.kirkland@dpi.nsw.gov.au.

Abstract: Infection of bulls with bovine viral diarrhoea virus (BVDV) can result in the development of virus persistence, confined to the reproductive tract. These bulls develop a normal immune response with high neutralizing antibody titres. However, BVDV can be excreted in the semen for a prolonged period. Although relatively rare, in this study we describe six separate cases in bulls being prepared for admission to artificial breeding centres. Semen samples were tested in a pan-Pestivirus-reactive real-time PCR assay and viral RNA was detected in semen from five of the bulls for three to eight months after infection. In one bull, virus was detected at low levels for more than five years. This bull was found to have one small testis. When slaughtered, virus was only detected in the abnormal testis. The low levels of BVDV in the semen of these bulls were only intermittently detected by virus isolation in cell culture. This virus-contaminated semen presents a biosecurity risk and confirms the need to screen all batches of semen from bulls that have been previously infected with BVDV. The use of real-time PCR is recommended as the preferred laboratory assay for this purpose.

Keywords: bovine viral diarrhoea virus; Pestivirus; persistent testicular infection; prolonged testicular infection; bovine; testes; semen

---

1. Introduction

Pestiviruses are a group of viruses that belong to the family Flaviviridae and are of animal health and economic importance worldwide [1]. The taxonomy of the Pestivirus genus has been reorganised to 11 species based on nucleotide and deduced amino acid sequence relatedness, antigenic similarity and host of origin [2,3] Bovine viral diarrhoea virus type 1 (BVDV-1) has been taxonomically classified as *Pestivirus A*, and BVDV type 2 (BVDV-2) has been classified as *Pestivirus B*. These viruses are predominantly pathogens of cattle, though sheep, other ruminants and pigs may also become infected.

Transmission of BVDV occurs horizontally by direct and indirect contact between cattle, and vertically by transplacental infection of the foetus. The virus replicates in mucosal epithelium and associated lymphoid tissues. A viraemia follows with subsequent viral replication throughout the body. Post-natal transient infections are often subclinical, but can result in a range of clinical conditions including reproductive losses, immune suppression, respiratory disease and acute diarrhoea [4]. Periconceptional infections can result in conception failure and embryonic deaths. Gestational infections can result in foetal death, congenital abnormalities, or a calf that becomes persistently infected (PI) for life [4].

The detection of BVDV in the semen of bulls is well documented [5–10]. Contamination of semen can arise from three types of infection. Firstly, male calves exposed to BVDV in utero, before they become immunocompetent, are born PI and will shed virus from most organs including in the semen for life [11,12]. These calves are born immunotolerant to BVDV and are often weak, ill-thrifty and are frequently infertile. However, occasionally PI bulls may grow normally, have semen of normal quality and can even gain entry to an artificial breeding centre [13]. There is usually a high concentration of BVDV in the semen of PI bulls (10^4 to $10^{7.6}$ $TCID_{50}$/mL) [5,9,14]. Semen with high titres of virus can infect susceptible cows following insemination [15,16].

Secondly, post-pubertal bulls exposed to BVDV undergo a transient infection and may shed virus in semen for up to 14 days [9], or perhaps 28 days [17] following infection. Virus levels tend to be low ($10^{0.9}$ to $10^{1.8}$ $TCID_{50}$/mL) but can occasionally infect a susceptible female [9]. These bulls will eventually mount an immune response to the virus which prevents further shedding.

Thirdly, some post-pubertal bulls exposed to BVDV become acutely infected but develop a prolonged or perhaps persistent testicular infection. These bulls are not PI, become transiently infected and mount a normal antibody response. The virus is cleared systemically, yet the virus is excreted in semen for prolonged periods. For this study, we have defined this prolonged testicular infection as the detectable presence of BVDV RNA in semen more than 60 days from when the systemic infection occurred. Until recently, these prolonged testicular infections (PTI) were considered to be rare. The first case was reported in 1998 [18]. This bull was not viraemic and therefore not PI. Nevertheless, infectious BVDV was detected in his semen at a moderate level ($10^{3.3}$ $TCID_{50}$/mL) for the rest of his life.

PTIs were induced experimentally in 2003 by inoculating susceptible post-pubertal bulls with BVDV [14]. Following acute infection, the bulls appeared to mount a typical immune response with the cessation of detectable viraemia. BVDV RNA was detected in the semen of these bulls by reverse transcription-nested PCR for a prolonged period of time. Attempts to isolate BVDV from the semen of these bulls were unsuccessful in cell culture, however semen collected five months after inoculation established infection in a naïve calf when given intravenously. These results were replicated by the same research team [6]. While the aetiology of PTIs with BVDV is still poorly understood, administration of a live attenuated vaccine virus has also been shown to induce PTI [7].

The incidence of PTI is considered to be very low and few have been described [17–19], yet due to the economic significance of BVDV infection, the World Organization for Animal Health (OIE) recommends that semen from seropositive bulls be screened for the presence of BVDV [20]. Before entry to a semen collection centre, bulls are tested to demonstrate that they are not viraemic or PI. Bulls that give negative results are then held in isolation at least 28 days [21] to undertake pre-entry testing and to ensure that animals recently exposed to BVDV can be reliably identified by allowing time for seroconversion. Once admitted to the semen collection centre, semen collections from all bulls with neutralising antibodies to BVDV are tested by a real-time, reverse transcription PCR (qRT-PCR). Following the introduction of this requirement, we have identified six bulls that have exhibited prolonged or persistent testicular infection. The detailed investigation and subsequent longitudinal sampling of these bulls is described.

2. Materials and Methods

2.1. Specimens

Blood samples and commercially prepared, extended semen from six bulls were submitted to the Virology Laboratory at the Elizabeth Macarthur Agriculture Institute (EMAI), New South Wales, Australia by veterinarians from artificial breeding centres. These samples were tested to meet regulatory protocols for the export of semen, where the serological status of an animal is determined and, if seropositive, their semen was subjected to virus detection. Subsequent to testing of the initial samples from these bulls, both archival samples and prospective collections were requested.

Bull 2 was sent to an abattoir where the testes were collected and sent to EMAI. The testes were measured, weighed and dissected. Cut surfaces from various positions within the testes were swabbed using cotton tipped swabs which were placed into 3 mL of phosphate buffered gelatin saline (PBGS) and tested with a pan-Pestivirus-reactive qRT-PCR.

2.2. Serology

A virus neutralisation test [20,22] based on a non-cytopathogenic Australian reference strain of BVDV (Trangie, subtype 1c) [23,24] was used as the primary assay for the detection of anti-Pestivirus antibodies. In some instances, an agar gel immunodiffusion assay [22] had been used to test samples prior to the introduction of the international protocol for the screening of bulls entering semen collection centres.

2.3. Virus and Nucleic Acid Detection

Serum from each of the bulls was tested to determine if the bull was persistently infected with BVDV using a commercial antigen capture ELISA (IDEXX BVDV Ag/Serum Plus, IDEXX Laboratories, Liebefeld-Bern, Switzerland) run according to the manufacturer's instructions.

The detection of BVDV RNA was performed by qRT-PCR as described previously [25]. Briefly, total nucleic acid was extracted from semen samples with a magnetic particle handling system, using a volume of 25 μL of undiluted semen and 50 μL of semen diluted 1/4 in PBGS. An exogenous internal control was included in the extraction buffer for each sample. The qRT-PCR utilised pan-Pestivirus reactive primers and probe [26] run on an ABI 7500 thermocycler in standard mode for a total of 45 cycles. Cycling conditions were as specified by the Ag-Path master mix manufacturer (Ambion, Austin, TX, USA). The fluorescence threshold was set manually at 0.05 and background was automatically adjusted. qRT-PCR results were expressed as cycle threshold (Ct) values and classified as negative if no amplification was observed after 45 cycles.

Semen samples were processed [20] and virus isolation (VI) was conducted with primary bovine testis cells grown in Basal Medium Eagle (BME) with Hank's salts containing antibiotics and supplemented with serum from BVDV antibody- and virus-free donor animals. After primary culture, samples were passaged at weekly intervals for 2 additional sub-cultures and then screened for evidence of BVDV antigen by immunoperoxidase staining [22] using a mixture of anti-Pestivirus monoclonal antibodies (P1H11, P4G11, P1D8 and 2NB2) [27]. Virus isolation was attempted on the earliest available semen samples and then periodically throughout the sampling period when BVDV RNA had been detected by qRT-PCR.

2.4. Immunohistochemistry (IHC)

Sections (4 μm thickness) of formalin fixed testes from Bull 2 were cut, mounted on Superfrost Plus slides (Menzel Gläser, Thermo Fisher Scientific, Waltham, MA, USA) and oven-dried for 30 min. Sections were de-waxed in xylene and rehydrated in an ethanol series. Endogenous peroxides were then blocked with a 1.8% solution of peroxide in methanol for 20 min. Slides were washed briefly in distilled water followed by 2 × 5 min washes in phosphate buffered saline (PBS) with 0.05% Tween 20 (MP Biomedicals, Santa Ana, CA, USA). Antigens were unmasked at 37 °C for 15 min in undiluted Proteinase K (Dako, Agilent, Santa Clara, CA, USA). Sections were washed twice with distilled water and once with PBS/0.05% Tween 20 before being blocked for 1 h with 0.5% bovine serum albumin (Roche, Basel, Switzerland) and 1% normal goat serum in PBS. Following a rinse in PBS/0.05% Tween 20, 150 μL of mouse MAb 15C5 (IDEXX Laboratories, Westbrooke, ME, USA) at a 1/10 dilution was added to each section and incubated at room temperature (RT; approximately 25 °C) for 1 h. The sections were washed twice in PBS/0.05% Tween 20 and incubated in EnVision™ anti-mouse serum (Dako, Agilent, Santa Clara, CA, USA) at RT for 1 h. Following three PBS/0.05% Tween 20 washes, 200 μL Dakocytomation DAB+ (Dako, Agilent, Santa Clara, CA, USA) chromogenic solution was added to each section and developed for 10 min in the dark. Slides were rinsed with distilled water to stop the colour reaction, counterstained with Mayers haematoxylin, dehydrated and mounted with dibutylphthalate polystyrene xylene (DPX) mounting medium (Sigma-Aldrich, St. Louis, MO, USA).

3. Results

Bulls that enter semen collection centres are shown to not be viraemic for BVDV and neutralizing antibody titres are determined. A review of records held at EMAI indicated that during the period November 2012 to October 2019, 586 bulls were tested at EMAI for entry to artificial breeding centres. The majority of bulls in this group were *Bos taurus* breeds (95.9%), with *Bos taurus* × *Bos indicus* breeds (2.5%) and *Bos indicus* breeds (1.6%) making up the remainder. Neutralizing antibodies to BVDV were detected in 295 (50.3%) of these bulls at the time of screening. Semen samples from all bulls that had virus neutralizing antibodies to BVDV were tested by qRT-PCR.

Six bulls were identified to have PTIs because BVDV RNA was detected in semen more than 60 days after the first detection of infection. The 60-day limit provided sufficient time to elapse to exclude the possibility of residual RNA or virus from a recent acute infection being detected. All of these bulls gave negative results in the antigen ELISA, confirming that none was persistently infected. All bulls had high neutralizing antibody titres during the observation period. Live attenuated Pestivirus vaccines are not used in Australia and none of the bulls in this study had been vaccinated. Full details for the six infected bulls are described in Appendix A Tables A1–A6

Both beef (five) and dairy (one) bulls were involved, with ages at the time of first detection of virus infection ranging from 10 to 21 months (Table 1). BVDV RNA was detected in the semen of these bulls for periods ranging from 3 to 73 months after the latest date at which the bulls could have been infected. Due to the very low levels of RNA detected on many occasions, virus isolation was only attempted on a limited proportion of samples. BVDV was successfully isolated from 12.5% (4/32) of samples subjected to virus isolation.

Table 1. Summary of details for bulls studied.

Bull Number	Breed	Estimated Age at First Detection of Infection (Months) [a]	Estimated Duration of Shedding (Months) [b]	qRT-PCR Results in Semen (Ct)	Virus Isolation (Pos/Total Tested)
1	Main Anjou	21	3	32.8–35.8	0/6
2	Holstein	10	73	29.7–38.4	2/10
3	Angus	18	3	29.1–32.6	0/5
4	Angus	19	4	30.1–32.0	1/3
5	Angus	20	6	32.6–34.8	0/6
6	Wagyu	21	8	27.6–38.0	1/2 [c]

[a] Detection of seroconversion or detection of bovine viral diarrhoea virus (BVDV) RNA in semen, whichever occurred earlier. [b] Time between detection of infection and last detection of BVDV RNA in semen. [c] Virus isolation successful in the early phase of infection.

The data for Bull 2 (Table A2) provides an interesting insight into PTIs. BVDV was retrospectively detected in the semen of this bull over a period of more than five years. The first detection of BVDV RNA was in 2017 during the routine screening protocol for seropositive bulls. A review of the testing history for this bull indicated that it had been infected with BVDV prior to late January 2012. Fifteen batches of semen were available over a six-month period between April and October 2012. Interestingly, when this semen was tested in 2018, BVDV RNA was only detected in the last of these 15 samples (26 October 2012). After the detection of BVDV RNA in May 2017, 10 consecutive positive semen samples were identified in 2018, followed by two negative semen samples prior to this bull being sent to an abattoir. No semen was available for testing between October 2012 and May 2017.

Each of these bulls with a presumed PTI was clinically normal and without any physical abnormalities, with the exception of Bull 2. Soon after arriving at the artificial breeding centre, this bull had scrotal measurements recorded on two occasions, with a circumference of 31 cm on 20 February 2012 and 34 cm on 16 April 2012. These measurements were considered normal for a bull of his breed and age [28]. Six years later, Bull 2 was sent an abattoir in June 2018. The testes from this bull were forwarded to EMAI where they were measured, weighed and dissected. One testis was 20 cm long and weighed 720 g. The other was 16 cm long and weighed 431 g. Swabs were taken from freshly cut surfaces at various locations within each testis and qRT-PCR performed. The 16 swabs taken from the larger of the testes gave negative qRT-PCR results, while positive results were obtained from seven of the nine swabs taken from the smaller one. The highest levels of BVDV RNA (as indicated by the lowest Ct values) were found in swabs taken from the parenchyma of the testis (Figure 1). However, this result was not uniform across the testicle with one of the four parenchymal swabs yielding a very high Ct value (37.3). Lower levels of BVDV RNA were detected along the epididymis and no viral RNA was detected in the deferent duct or the rete testis (Figure 1). BVDV was isolated from the testicular parenchyma.

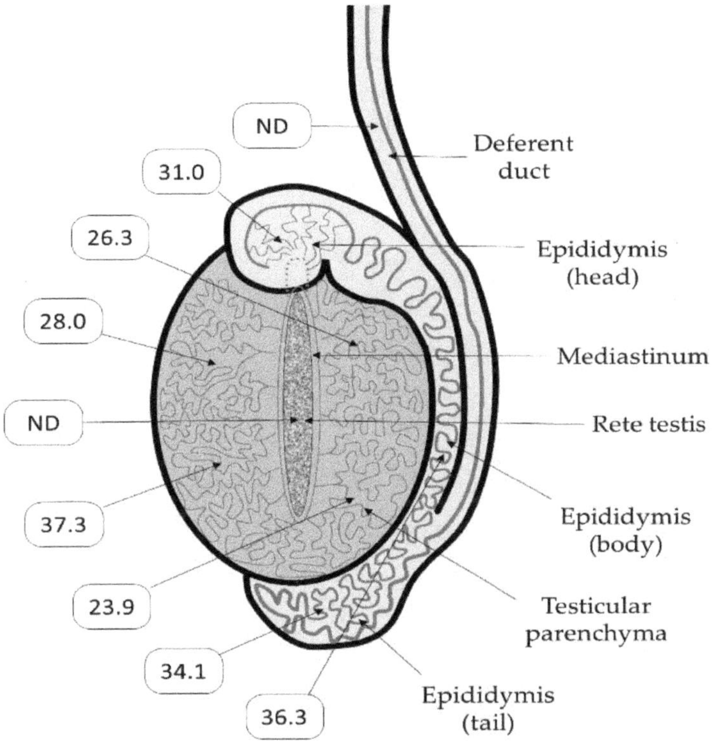

Figure 1. Schematic view of the affected testis of Bull 2. The numbers indicate the Ct values of swabs taken from the sites indicated by arrow heads. ND = BVDV RNA was not detected.

When examined microscopically, the abnormal testis from Bull 2 showed multifocal but locally extensive areas of seminiferous tubular atrophy (Figure 2A,C) characterised by reduced or absent germinal cell stages and aspermia. Affected tubules had either a reduced lumen diameter lined by a variably intact Sertoli cell layer or else were collapsed with complete or near total loss of Sertoli cells. Tubular atrophy was accompanied by moderate to marked tubular hyalinization and fibrosis and an increased prominence of Leydig cells. Immunohistochemical staining for BVDV antigen in these areas showed intense circumferential staining of the tubular luminal surface (Figures 2B and 3B). Within these tubules, there was also occasional staining of the subjacent thickened tubular wall mesenchyme and rarely within the cytoplasm of free intraluminal degenerative cells (Figure 3B). Adjacent to some areas of collapsed tubules were small clusters of less-affected tubules (Figure 2C) with low or no BVDV staining at the tubular luminal surface but containing numerous identifiable germinal cell stages which contained BVDV staining, including primary spermatocytes, round spermatids and elongate spermatids (Figure 3A). There was no evidence of inflammation associated with the affected tubules. Areas predominated by tubular lesions containing BVDV staining often intermingled with nearby histologically relatively normal tubules in which BVDV staining was not detected (Figure 2D). Representative sections of the epididymis were examined, found to be histologically unremarkable and BVDV IHC negative. The contralateral testicular tissue was histologically within normal limits (Figure 2E) and BVDV IHC negative (Figure 2F).

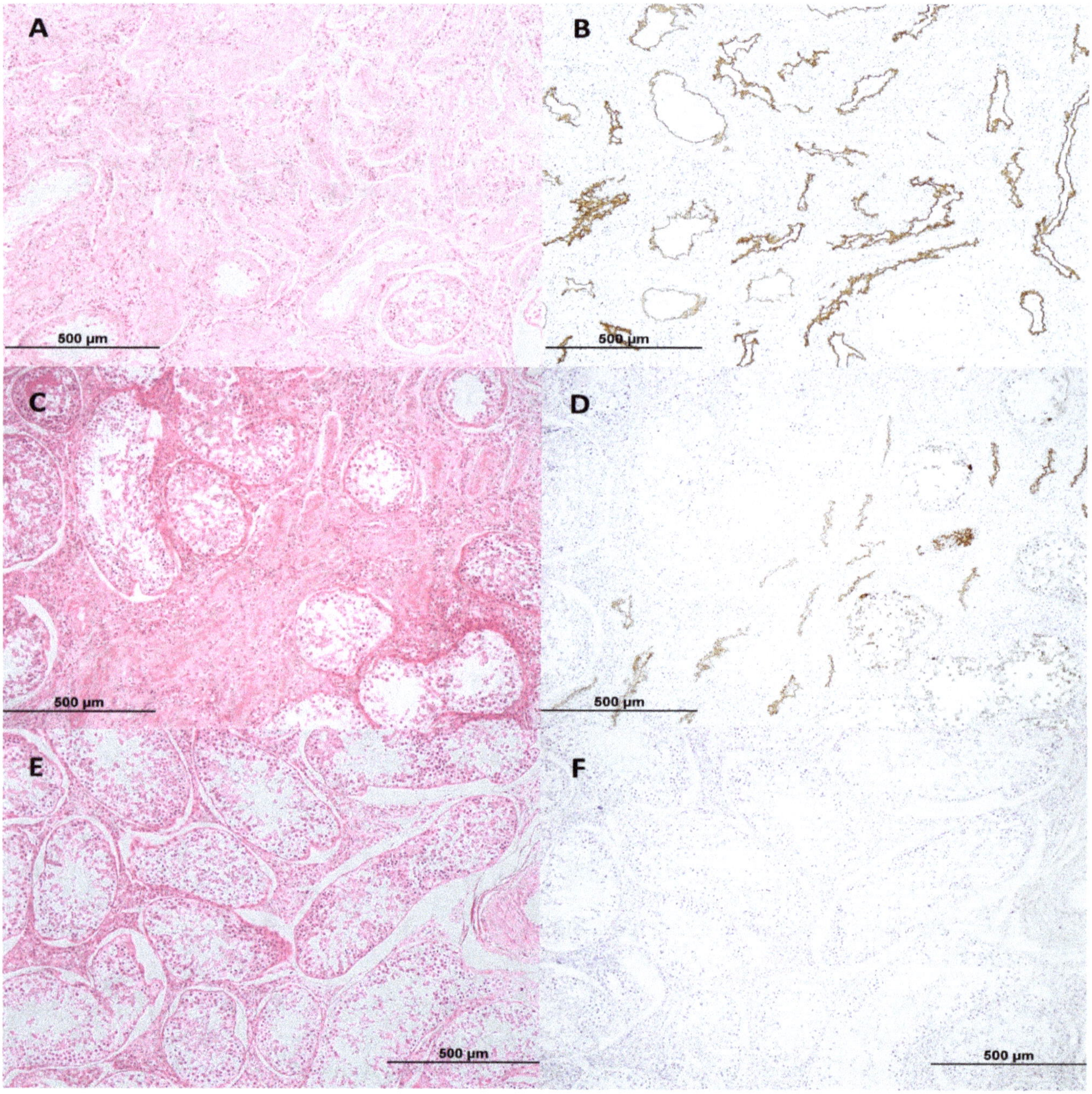

Figure 2. (**A**) Locally extensive areas of seminiferous tubular atrophy and fibrosis in a BVDV-infected bovine testicle. Many tubules are collapsed and shrunken with total loss of Sertoli cells, with a few tubules retaining some Sertoli cells but no germinal cells. The lower right quadrant contains a tubule with germinal cells. Haematoxylin and eosin (H&E) stain, 10×. (**B**) Non-serial section of A. Collapsed tubules have circumferential profiles of intense BVDV staining at the luminal surface. BVDV immunohistochemistry (IHC), 10×. (**C**) Collapsed seminiferous tubules intermingle with less-affected or relatively histologically normal tubules (lower right and upper left, respectively) in a BVDV-infected testicle. H&E stain, 10×. (**D**) Serial section of C; Collapsed tubules have intense BVDV staining while adjacent less-affected tubules (lower right) have BVDV staining within still-existing germinal cell stages and Sertoli cells. Histologically normal tubules (upper left) are BVDV antigen negative. BVDV IHC, 10×. (**E**) Histologically normal testicular tissue in the BVDV PCR negative contralateral testicle from Bull 2. H&E stain, 10×. (**F**) Serial section of E. The contralateral testicle is BVDV antigen negative. BVDV IHC, 10×.

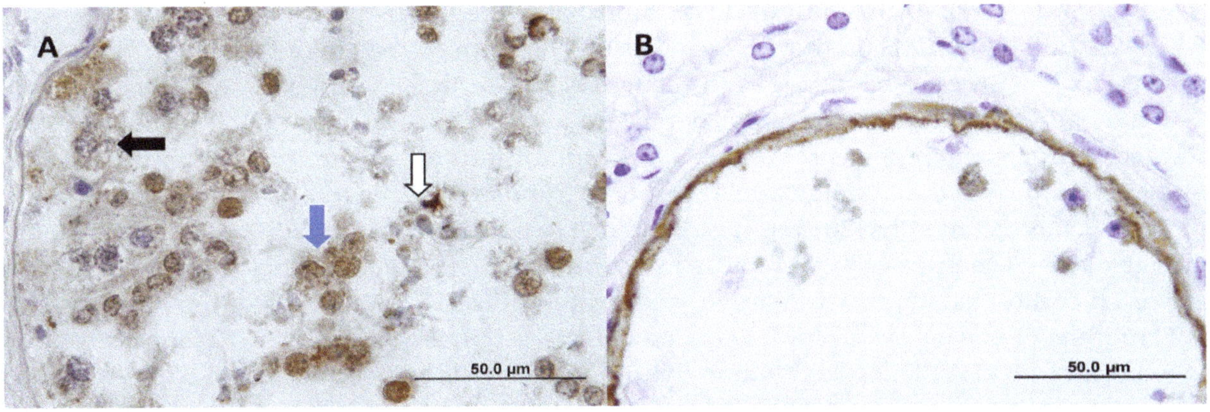

Figure 3. (**A**) A seminiferous tubule containing still-existing germinal cell stages in a BVDV-infected bovine testicle. BVDV staining is present in cells morphologically consistent with primary spermatocytes (black arrow), round spermatids (blue arrow) and elongated spermatids (white arrow). BVDV IHC, 100× (oil). (**B**) An atrophic seminiferous tubule in a BVDV-infected bovine testicle. The tubular luminal surface has intense BVDV staining which appears to occasionally extend into the superficial tubular mesenchyme and within degenerate free intraluminal cells. BVDV IHC, 100× (oil).

4. Discussion

International semen collection protocols and the associated health certification of donor bulls [21] are designed to ensure that bovine semen is free of contamination with BVDV. In addition to the exclusion of PI animals, measures are aimed at the exclusion of both transiently infected bulls and those with PTI. It was the adoption of these measures that resulted in the detection of the PTI bulls that are the subject of this report, and the detection of contaminated batches following retrospective testing. This study adds to the collective knowledge of prolonged or persistent testicular infection (PTI) in bulls through the identification and detailed investigation of six bulls. The longitudinal sampling, histopathology and IHC results have increased our understanding of the pathology and pathogenesis of PTI.

Studies of transiently infected bulls in the past have relied on virus isolation for the detection of BVDV in the semen. The use of qRT-PCR to detect BVDV in semen is recommended by the OIE [20], yet there is a lack of published literature on investigations of either transiently infected bulls or those with a PTI using qRT-PCR. It is not clear precisely how long BVDV RNA may be detected in semen following a transient infection. The possibility that some of these bulls were undergoing a transient infection when BVDV RNA was detected in the semen has to be considered due to the higher sensitivity of qRT-PCR, which may detect virus for a much longer time than virus isolation [26]. The date when Bull 5 was first infected can be estimated with the greatest precision due to the rising neutralizing antibody titre on the first two serum samples. Notably, the first semen sample to be tested gave a positive result and this sample was collected at least two months after the likely time of infection. Additionally, positive qRT-PCR results were obtained for semen samples for another two months. Therefore, it would seem unlikely that this RNA detection was the product of a transient infection. Similarly, with the exception of Bull 2, the other bulls were observed to shed viral RNA in semen for periods between three and eight months. Bull 2 shed virus for more than five years. Each of these bulls was likely to have experienced PTIs because the length of these shedding periods is in marked contrast to the 10 to 14 day periods reported for transiently infected bulls [9,10].

In 1998, Voges et al. described a post-pubertal bull that was shown to shed BVDV in semen over an 11-month period. This bull had a consistently high antibody titre against BVDV and yet was not viraemic and virus could not be detected in any organ apart from the testes. This bull was described as being in good health until his slaughter at 22 months of age. His growth rate and testicular development were unremarkable. Two other cases of PTI in bulls have been described in 2005 and 2014. [17,19]. In the latter report, a post-pubertal bull was also shown to be not PI. Infectious virus and viral RNA were detected in this bull up to 42 months of age. Virus was not detected for the last six months of this bull's life. IHC on this bull's testes at 48 months of age failed to detect viral antigen.

Voges et al. [18] proposed that for PTI to occur, BVDV infection should occur shortly before puberty, however, the pathogenesis of prolonged or persistent testicular infection is not clear. In cattle, puberty is evaluated on the basis of testicular growth and quantitative measures of sperm production [29]. Published estimates for the average age at puberty in bulls put this at approximately 10.5 months, ranging from 9.4 to 12.1 months [30–32]. It is of interest to note that five of the six bulls in our study were in the range of 17–21 months old when virus infection was first detected. The age at which three bulls seroconverted could be determined relatively accurately (Bulls 4, 5 and 6). These bulls were between 18 and 20 months of age when infection was first detected. Bull 2 was less than 10 months of age when he was exposed to BVDV. The age at which the other two bulls seroconverted to BVDV could not be accurately determined but their virus detection results indicate an upper age limit (18–21 months) at which infection may have occurred and is similar to the age at which the other three bulls became infected. The results of the three bulls whose age at infection could be estimated with some reliability challenges the notion that infection of PTI bulls only occurs at or around puberty.

The localization of BVDV in the reproductive tract of Bull 2 was different to what had been observed for transiently infected bulls. BVDV RNA was only detected in the smaller of the testes. Relatively high levels of RNA and antigen were detected in the parenchyma of this infected testis and BVDV was also isolated in cell culture. This is in contrast to what had been observed for transiently infected bulls, where virus was not isolated from the testicular parenchyma. In this bull, trace levels of BVDV RNA were also detected in the epididymis but, unlike observations of transiently infected bulls, no antigen was detected. Unfortunately, the accessory glands of Bull 2 were not examined, preventing further comparisons with the observations made in transiently infected bulls where virus was only isolated from the accessory glands.

The pathology and IHC staining of Bull 2 clearly demonstrated that the persistence of the BVDV infection was localized within the immune-privileged seminiferous tubule compartment. The bovine testis consists of two compartments, the peritubular compartment (Leydig cells and testicular macrophages) and the seminiferous tubule compartment (germ cells protected by Sertoli cells). The Sertoli cells span the basal to adluminal sections of the tubule and tight junctions between these cells form the blood–testes barrier [33]. This barrier protects developing germ cells from stimulating the adaptive immune system while allowing nutritional and structural support [34]. The peritubular compartment is exposed to the full immune response of the animal, while the seminiferous tubule compartment is in an immune-privileged site [35].

The pattern of pathology detected in this testis shows a continuum of tubular degenerative change correlating closely with a progression of BVDV staining, suggesting that the infection in this case was confined to seminiferous tubules and chronicity resulted in the eventual destruction of the normal tubule structure. It is also noteworthy that the concentration of BVDV RNA was not uniform across the testis. Within one area of the testicular parenchyma, the qRT-PCR gave a Ct value of 37.3. This result indicates that the level of BVDV RNA present was very close to the limit of detection for this assay. Yet, in the other areas of the testicular parenchyma tested, the Ct values ranged from 23.9 to 28.0. These values are typically seen in the semen of PI cattle. We speculate that the infection in PTI remains largely hidden from the immune system and manages to smoulder within the seminiferous tubules for a variable amount of time. The case of the bull from which the testes were collected at the abattoir supports this notion as there was a lack of interstitial or tubular inflammatory cellular infiltrates in response to the widespread presence of BVDV within the tubules, even in areas where BVDV tubule staining appears to extend superficially into the subjacent thickened peritubular mesenchyme of intensely stained tubules This latter observation may be a by-product of excessive antigen accumulation in these tubules, or perhaps the peritubular fibrosis assisted to shelter the infection from the peritubular compartment immune response. We speculate that the destruction of the tubules contributed to the small overall size of this testis. It was not possible to determine if the uninfected testis was ever infected, though no histological signs of past infection were detected. BVDV RNA was only detected in one of the early semen collections in 2012. It is not clear if BVDV RNA levels were too low to detect in these collections, or if there was deterioration in the RNA over the six years between when the RNA was shed and when it was tested by qRT-PCR. Additionally, the final two semen collections for this bull gave negative results in the qRT-PCR. Nevertheless, the ability to isolate virus from the testis of this bull 73 months after the initial infection demonstrates the capacity of the infection to persist in the testis for long periods.

The time course over which a PTI may be detected appears to range from a few months to many years. Eventually infection may be cleared, as appeared to occur in Bull 5 and as described by Newcomer et al., [17], or infection may remain persistent as demonstrated by Bull 2. Distinctions between persistent testicular infections and prolonged testicular infections have been proposed based on the ability to infect susceptible animals [17]. This distinction has not been applied to this series of bulls. BVDV was isolated from three of the six bulls (Bulls 2,4 and 6). Moreover, BVDV was isolated from the semen of Bull 2 on two occasions but was not isolated on eight. It is probable that differences between the ability to detect BVDV by qRT-PCR and by VI reflect shedding of the virus in semen, which in turn may vary between semen batches and progress of the infection.

Virus isolation has been considered the gold standard for BVDV detection when screening semen for the presence of BVDV-1. However, the results of the current investigations demonstrate the benefits of using qRT-PCR, which offers both higher analytical sensitivity and speed for the detection of BVDV infection. It is important that qRT-PCR assays employ broadly reactive pan-Pestivirus primers and probes to ensure that the potential genetic variability of all strains of Pestiviruses are reliably detected [20]. Many of the Ct values recorded for these positive bull semen samples were relatively high. The work of Hoffman et al. demonstrated that, for qRT-PCR assays, Ct values greater than 38 represent less than 10 genome copies per 5 μL of sample [26]. However, the volume of sample should not be overlooked because detection of 10 copies in a qRT-PCR assay represents approximately 1000 copies of RNA in a single 500 μL straw of semen. Parallel qRT-PCR and virus isolation experiments demonstrated that qRT-PCR had 100 to 1000 times greater sensitivity in contrast to the limit of detection for virus isolation methods. While qRT-PCR does not provide an indication of whether the sample contains infectious virus, a positive result in this assay does identify a batch as presenting a risk that infectious virus may be present. This risk is exemplified by experimental work [14] that demonstrated that, despite BVDV being detected by PCR, virus isolation attempts in cell culture with the semen of PTI bulls were unsuccessful. This same semen was capable of producing a systemic infection when injected into calves. Therefore, as recommended by the OIE [20], a reliable qRT-PCR should be the preferred diagnostic assay for BVDV detection for the screening of semen. Diagnostic laboratories are encouraged to undertake regular evaluation of any qRT-PCR assays that are being used to detect BVDV. This evaluation should involve comparison of published assays considering both the nucleic acid extraction and qRT-PCR components, using suitable samples from the country of origin, assessing the limit of detection and participating in proficiency testing.

With an increasing number of countries progressing towards freedom from BVDV, consideration may need to be given to screening of batches of stored semen. Most collections of semen from bulls that experience a PTI have very low levels of infectious virus and perhaps often at levels that would be lower than an infective dose following insemination. Nevertheless, this semen does present a biosecurity risk. Indeed, it had been shown that use of semen from the bull with the first recognized PTI was able to establish a systemic infection in an inseminated heifer [36], thereby confirming this risk. Contaminated semen can be used many years after collection and is often transported long distances internationally. These factors, combined with the potential for exposure of a large number of breeding females to a single batch of semen, increase the potential for the introduction of BVDV into free herds and countries, or potentially the introduction of other species of Pestivirus (such as BVDV-2 and Hobi-like Pestiviruses) into countries where these viruses are absent and where appropriately protective vaccines are not used.

In conclusion, although prolonged or persistent testicular infections are a relatively rare event, the findings of this study emphasize the recommendations [20] for all batches of semen from seropositive bulls to be screened to exclude the possibility of BVDV. Further, it is recommended that this screening is more effectively carried out by qRT-PCR rather than by virus isolation methods.

Author Contributions: Conceptualization, A.J.R. and P.D.K.; methodology and investigation, A.J.R., S.G., K.P., D.S.F., X.G., T.W.O. and P.D.K.; data curation, A.J.R.; writing—Original draft preparation, A.J.R., S.G. and P.D.K.; writing—Review and editing, A.J.R., S.G., K.P., D.S.F., X.G., T.W.O. and P.D.K. All authors have read and agreed to the published version of the manuscript.

Acknowledgments: We acknowledge contributions of Megan Beca, Pennie Harkness, Steve Williams and Reon Holmes for supplying additional information about the bulls and providing additional samples. We are indebted to the staff of the Virology Laboratory at EMAI for their invaluable assistance during the testing of the samples described in this study and to the technical staff of the EMAI pathology laboratory for preparation of the tissue sections. Roger Cook provided helpful comments on the histological findings.

Appendix A

Table A1. Serological and virological test results for Bull 1.

Sample Date	Sample Type	Age (Months)	qRT-PCR (Ct)	Virus Isolation	Antigen ELISA	VNT (Titre)
28/08/2012	Serum	21			Negative	512
22/10/2012	Serum	23		Negative		≥512
12/11/2012	Extended semen	23	Positive (35.4)	Negative		
23/11/2012	Extended semen	24	Positive (35.4)	Negative		
26/11/2012	Extended semen	24	Positive (35.8)	Negative		
28/11/2012	Extended semen	24	Positive (32.8)	Negative		
30/11/2012	Extended semen	24	Positive (35.5)	Negative		
6/12/2012	Serum	24				≥512

Breed: Maine-Anjou. Date of birth: December 2010. Time of infection: prior to 28 August 2012. VNT—virus neutralisation titre.

Table A2. Serological and virological test results for Bull 2.

Sample Date	Sample Type	Age (Months)	qRT-PCR (Ct)	Virus Isolation	Antigen ELISA	AGID	VNT (Titre)
23/01/2012	Serum	10			Negative	3	
13/03/2012	Serum	12			Negative	2	
17/04/2012	Extended semen	13	Negative [a]	Negative			
17/04/2012	Extended semen	15	Negative [a]				
19/06/2012	Extended semen	15	Negative [a]				
29/06/2012	Extended semen	16	Negative [a]				
20/07/2012	Extended semen	17	Negative [a]				
8/08/2012	Extended semen	17	Negative [a]				
20/08/2012	Extended semen	17	Negative [a]				
24/08/2012	Extended semen	17	Negative [a]				
31/08/2012	Extended semen	18	Negative [a]				
4/09/2012	Extended semen	18	Negative [a]				
7/09/2012	Extended semen	18	Negative [a]				
11/09/2012	Extended semen	18	Negative [a]				
21/09/2012	Extended semen	18	Negative [a]				
28/09/2012	Extended semen	19	Negative [a]				
26/10/2012	Extended semen	20	Positive (36.5) [a]				
13/11/2012	Serum	26			Negative	>3	
7/05/2013	Serum	38			Negative	3	
5/05/2014	Serum	50			Negative	3	
4/05/2015	Serum	62			Negative	3	
2/05/2016	Serum	74			Negative		≥512
1/05/2017	Extended semen	82	Positive (29.7)	Positive			
18/01/2018	Extended semen	82	Positive (32.6)	Negative			
23/01/2018	Extended semen	82	Positive (32.4)	Negative			
25/01/2018	Extended semen	83	Positive (30.9)	Positive			

Table A2. *Cont.*

Sample Date	Sample Type	Age (Months)	qRT-PCR (Ct)	Virus Isolation	Antigen ELISA	AGID	VNT (Titre)
1/02/2018	Extended semen	83	Positive (35.9)	Negative			
6/02/2018	Extended semen	83	Positive (32.5)	Negative			
8/02/2018	Serum	83			Negative		
12/02/2018	Extended semen	83	Positive (33.3)	Negative			
13/02/2018	Extended semen	83	Positive (34.4)	Negative			
15/02/2018	Extended semen	83	Positive (31.58)	Negative			
16/02/2018	Extended semen	83	Positive (38.46)				
20/02/2018	Extended semen	83	Positive (36.82)				
22/02/2018	Extended semen	83	Negative				
27/02/2018	Extended semen	84	Negative				

Breed: Holstein. Date of birth: March 2011. Time of infection: prior to 23 January 2012. [a] Tested in 2018. AGID—agar gel immunodiffusion assay

Table A3. Serological and virological test results for Bull 3.

Sample Date	Sample Type	Age (Months)	qRT-PCR (Ct)	Virus Isolation	Antigen ELISA	VNT(Titre)
20/02/2013	Serum	15			Negative	
22/05/2013	Extended semen	18	Positive (29.2)			
24/05/2013	Extended semen	18	Positive (29.7)	Negative		
28/05/2013	Extended semen	18	Positive (29.3)	Negative		
30/05/2013	Extended semen	18	Positive (29.1)			
3/06/2013	Extended semen	18	Positive (32.6)			
7/06/2013	Extended semen	18	Positive (30.0)			
10/06/2013	Serum	18		Negative		≥512
12/06/2013	Extended semen	18	Positive (31.0)			
14/06/2013	Extended semen	19	Positive (30.5)			
18/06/2013	Extended semen	19	Positive (29.5)			
20/06/2013	Extended semen	19	Positive (30.0)			
24/06/2013	Extended semen	19	Positive (30.4)			
26/06/2013	Extended semen	19	Positive (30.5)			
3/07/2013	Extended semen	19	Positive (30.5)			
8/07/2013	Extended semen	19	Positive (32.0)			
12/07/2013	Extended semen	19	Positive (31.0)			
12/07/2013	Extended semen	19	Positive (30.5)	Negative		
16/07/2013	Extended semen	20	Positive (30.4)			
18/07/2013	Extended semen	20	Positive (31.4)			
23/07/2013	Extended semen	20	Positive (32.2)			
15/08/2013	Extended semen	21	Positive (30.7)	Negative		

Breed: Angus. Date of birth: December 2011. Time of infection: prior to 22 May 2013.

Table A4. Serological and virological test results for Bull 4.

Sample Date	Sample Type	Age (Months)	qRT-PCR (Ct)	Virus Isolation	Antigen ELISA	AGID	VNT (Titre)
3/09/2013	Serum	18			Negative	Negative	
8/10/2013	Serum	19			Negative	>3	
22/10/2013	Extended semen	20	Positive (31.7)	Positive			
24/10/2013	Extended semen	20	Positive (32.0)	Negative			
16/12/2013	Seminal fluid	22	Positive (30.2)	Negative			
16/02/2014 [a]	Extended semen	24	Positive (30.1)				
16/02/2014 [a]	Serum	24					≥512

Breed: Angus. Date of birth: March 2012. Time of infection: between late August and September 2013. [a] Slaughtered immediately after this collection.

Table A5. Serological and virological test results for Bull 5.

Sample Date	Sample Type	Age (Months)	qRT-PCR (Ct)	Virus Isolation	Antigen ELISA	VNT(Titre)
31/03/2014	Serum	20			Negative	4
12/05/2014	Serum	21		Negative		256
15/05/2014	Extended semen	21	Positive (32.6)			
24/05/2014	Neat semen	22	Positive (34.2)	Negative		
11/06/2014	Extended semen	22	Positive (34.8)	Negative		
2/07/2014	Neat semen	23	Positive (34.1)	Negative		
17/07/2014	Extended semen	23	Positive (33.9)	Negative		
20/02/2015	Serum	31			Negative	≥512
8/04/2015	Extended semen	32	Negative			
20/04/2015	Serum	32		Negative		≥512
22/04/2015	Extended semen	33	Negative			
27/04/2015	Extended semen	33	Negative			
14/05/2015	Extended semen	33	Negative			
19/05/2015	Extended semen	33	Negative			
21/05/2015	Extended semen	34	Negative			
25/05/2015	Extended semen	34	Negative			
28/05/2015	Extended semen	34	Negative			
2/06/2015	Extended semen	34	Negative			
4/06/2015	Extended semen	34	Negative			
8/06/2015	Extended semen	34	Negative			
12/06/2015	Extended semen	34	Negative			
16/06/2015	Extended semen	34	Negative			
28/06/2015	Extended semen	35	Negative			
18/07/2015	Extended semen	35	Negative			
17/08/2015	Extended semen	36	Negative			
21/08/2015	Extended semen	37	Negative			
24/08/2015	Extended semen	37	Negative			
31/08/2015	Extended semen	38	Negative			
6/02/2017	Serum	54			Negative	512
3/04/2017	Serum	56				128
1/05/2017	Extended semen	57	Negative			
4/05/2017	Extended semen	57	Negative			

Breed: Angus. Date of birth: August 2012. Time of infection: probably infected mid-March 2014.

Table A6. Serological and virological test results for Bull 6.

Sample Date	Sample Type	Age (Months)	qRT-PCR (Ct)	Virus Isolation	Antigen ELISA	VNT
14/12/2018	Extended semen	15	Negative			
6/04/2019 [a]	Serum	19			Negative	
21/05/2019	Extended semen	20	Positive (27.6)	Positive		
1/09/2019	Serum	24			Negative	>512
24/09/2019	Serum	24				>512
17/10/2019	Extended semen	25	Positive (38.0)	Negative		
22/11/2019	Extended semen	26	Positive (36.4)			
8/01/2020	Extended semen	28	Positive (36.2)			
23/01/2020	Extended semen	28	Negative			

Breed: Wagyu. Date of birth: September 2017. Time of infection: estimated infected between mid-April and mid-May 2019. [a] A BVDV antibody ELISA was performed on serum taken on 6 April 2019 with negative results (data not shown).

References

1. Richter, V.; Lebl, K.; Baumgartner, W.; Obritzhauser, W.; Kasbohrer, A.; Pinior, B. A systematic worldwide review of the direct monetary losses in cattle due to bovine viral diarrhoea virus infection. *Vet. J.* **2017**, *220*, 80–87. [CrossRef] [PubMed]
2. Smith, D.B.; Meyers, G.; Bukh, J.; Gould, E.A.; Monath, T.; Scott Muerhoff, A.; Pletnev, A.; Rico-Hesse, R.; Stapleton, J.T.; Simmonds, P.; et al. Proposed revision to the taxonomy of the genus Pestivirus, family Flaviviridae. *J. Gen. Virol.* **2017**, *98*, 2106–2112. [CrossRef] [PubMed]

3. Walker, P.J.; Siddell, S.G.; Lefkowitz, E.J.; Mushegian, A.R.; Dempsey, D.M.; Dutilh, B.E.; Harrach, B.; Harrison, R.L.; Hendrickson, R.C.; Junglen, S.; et al. Changes to virus taxonomy and the International Code of Virus Classification and Nomenclature ratified by the International Committee on Taxonomy of Viruses. *Arch. Virol.* **2019**, *164*, 2417–2429. [CrossRef] [PubMed]
4. Walz, P.H.; Grooms, D.L.; Passler, T.; Ridpath, J.F.; Tremblay, R.; Step, D.L.; Callan, R.J.; Givens, M.D.; American College of Veterinary Internal, M. Control of bovine viral diarrhea virus in ruminants. *J. Vet. Intern. Med.* **2010**, *24*, 476–486. [CrossRef] [PubMed]
5. Bielanski, A.; Dubuc, C.; Hare, W.C.D. Failure to Remove Bovine Diarrhea Virus (BVDV) from Bull Semen by Swim up and other Separatory Sperm Techniques Associated with in vitro Fertilization. *Reprod. Domest. Anim.* **1992**, *27*, 303–306. [CrossRef]
6. Givens, M.D.; Riddell, K.P.; Edmondson, M.A.; Walz, P.H.; Gard, J.A.; Zhang, Y.; Galik, P.K.; Brodersen, B.W.; Carson, R.L.; Stringfellow, D.A. Epidemiology of prolonged testicular infections with bovine viral diarrhea virus. *Vet. Microbiol.* **2009**, *139*, 42–51. [CrossRef] [PubMed]
7. Givens, M.D.; Riddell, K.P.; Walz, P.H.; Rhoades, J.; Harland, R.; Zhang, Y.; Galik, P.K.; Brodersen, B.W.; Cochran, A.M.; Brock, K.V.; et al. Noncytopathic bovine viral diarrhea virus can persist in testicular tissue after vaccination of peri-pubertal bulls but prevents subsequent infection. *Vaccine* **2007**, *25*, 867–876. [CrossRef]
8. Kirkland, P.D.; McGowan, M.R.; Mackintosh, S.G.; Moyle, A. Insemination of cattle with semen from a bull transiently infected with pestivirus. *Vet. Rec.* **1997**, *140*, 124–127. [CrossRef]
9. Kirkland, P.D.; Richards, S.G.; Rothwell, J.T.; Stanley, D.F. Replication of bovine viral diarrhoea virus in the bovine reproductive tract and excretion of virus in semen during acute and chronic infections. *Vet. Rec.* **1991**, *128*, 587–590. [CrossRef]
10. Whitmore, H.L.; Gustafsson, B.K.; Havareshti, P.; Duchateau, A.B.; Mather, E.C. Inoculation of bulls with bovine virus diarrhea virus: Excretion of virus in semen and effects on semen quality. *Theriogenology* **1978**, *9*, 153–163. [CrossRef]
11. McClurkin, A.W.; Coria, M.F.; Cutlip, R.C. Reproductive performance of apparently healthy cattle persistently infected with bovine viral diarrhea virus. *J. Am. Vet. Med. Assoc.* **1979**, *174*, 1116–1119. [PubMed]
12. Barlow, R.M.; Nettleton, P.F.; Gardiner, A.C.; Greig, A.; Campbell, J.R.; Bonn, J.M. Persistent bovine virus diarrhoea virus infection in a bull. *Vet. Rec.* **1986**, *118*, 321–324. [CrossRef] [PubMed]
13. Howard, T.H.; Bean, B.; Hillman, R.; Monke, D.R. Surveillance for persistent bovine viral diarrhea virus infection in four artificial insemination centers. *J. Am. Vet. Med. Assoc.* **1990**, *196*, 1951–1955. [PubMed]
14. Givens, M.D.; Heath, A.M.; Brock, K.V.; Brodersen, B.W.; Carson, R.L.; Stringfellow, D.A. Detection of bovine viral diarrhea virus in semen obtained after inoculation of seronegative postpubertal bulls. *Am. J. Vet. Res.* **2003**, *64*, 428–434. [CrossRef] [PubMed]
15. Kirkland, P.; Mackintosh, S.; Moyle, A. The outcome of widespread use of semen from a bull persistently infected with pestivirus. *Vet. Rec.* **1994**, *135*, 527–529. [CrossRef] [PubMed]
16. Meyling, A.; Jensen, A.M. Transmission of bovine virus diarrhoea virus (BVDV) by artificial insemination (AI) with semen from a persistently-infected bull. *Vet. Microbiol.* **1988**, *17*, 97–105. [CrossRef]
17. Newcomer, B.W.; Toohey-Kurth, K.; Zhang, Y.; Brodersen, B.W.; Marley, M.S.; Joiner, K.S.; Zhang, Y.; Galik, P.K.; Riddell, K.P.; Givens, M.D. Laboratory diagnosis and transmissibility of bovine viral diarrhea virus from a bull with a persistent testicular infection. *Vet. Microbiol.* **2014**, *170*, 246–257. [CrossRef] [PubMed]
18. Voges, H.; Horner, G.W.; Rowe, S.; Wellenberg, G.J. Persistent bovine pestivirus infection localized in the testes of an immuno-competent, non-viraemic bull. *Vet. Microbiol.* **1998**, *61*, 165–175. [CrossRef]
19. Dunser, M.; Altmann, M.; Dengg, J.; Eichinger, M.; Loitsch, A.; Revilla-Fernandez, S.; Schweighardt, H. Localised persistent infection of the genital tract with bovine viral diarrhoea virus in an immunocompetent bull. *Wien. Tierarztl. Mon.* **2005**, *92*, 227–232.
20. International Office of Epizootics (OIE). Chapter 3.4.7. Bovine viral diarrhoea. In *Manual of Diagnostic Tests and Vaccines for Terrestrial Animals*; Office international des épizooties: Paris, France, 2019; pp. 1075–1096.
21. International Office of Epizootics (OIE). Chapter 4.7. Collection and processing of bovine, small ruminant and porcine semen. In *Terrestrial Animal Health Code*; Office international des épizooties: Paris, France, 2019.
22. Kirkland, P.D.; MacKintosh, S.G. Ruminant Pestivirus Infections. In *Australia and New Zealand Standard Diagnostic Procedures*; Department of Agriculture, Australian Government: Canberra, Australia, 2006; pp. 1–30.

23. Mahony, T.J.; McCarthy, F.M.; Gravel, J.L.; Corney, B.; Young, P.L.; Vilcek, S. Genetic analysis of bovine viral diarrhoea viruses from Australia. *Vet. Microbiol.* **2005**, *106*, 1–6. [CrossRef]
24. Gong, Y.; Trowbridge, R.; Macnaughton, T.B.; Westaway, E.G.; Shannon, A.D.; Gowans, E.J. Characterization of RNA synthesis during a one-step growth curve and of the replication mechanism of bovine viral diarrhoea virus. *J. Gen. Virol.* **1996**, *77 Pt 11*, 2729–2736. [CrossRef]
25. Gu, X.; Davis, R.J.; Walsh, S.J.; Melville, L.F.; Kirkland, P.D. Longitudinal study of the detection of Bluetongue virus in bull semen and comparison of real-time polymerase chain reaction assays. *J. Vet. Diagn. Investig.* **2014**, *26*, 18–26. [CrossRef] [PubMed]
26. Hoffmann, B.; Depner, K.; Schirrmeier, H.; Beer, M. A universal heterologous internal control system for duplex real-time RT-PCR assays used in a detection system for pestiviruses. *J. Virol. Methods* **2006**, *136*, 200–209. [CrossRef] [PubMed]
27. Brown, L.M.; Papa, R.A.; Frost, M.J.; Mackintosh, S.G.; Gu, X.; Dixon, R.J.; Shannon, A.D. A single amino acid is critical for the expression of B-cell epitopes on the helicase domain of the pestivirus NS3 protein. *Virus Res.* **2002**, *84*, 111–124. [CrossRef]
28. Hueston, W.D.; Monke, D.R.; Milburn, R.J. Scrotal circumference measurements on young Holstein bulls. *J. Am. Vet. Med. Assoc.* **1988**, *192*, 766–768.
29. Wolf, F.R.; Almquist, J.O.; Hale, E.B. Prepuberal Behavior and Puberal Characteristics of Beef Bulls on High Nutrient Allowance. *J. Anim. Sci.* **1965**, *24*, 761–765. [CrossRef] [PubMed]
30. Brito, L.F.; Barth, A.D.; Rawlings, N.C.; Wilde, R.E.; Crews, D.H., Jr.; Mir, P.S.; Kastelic, J.P. Effect of nutrition during calfhood and peripubertal period on serum metabolic hormones, gonadotropins and testosterone concentrations, and on sexual development in bulls. *Domest. Anim. Endocrinol.* **2007**, *33*, 1–18. [CrossRef] [PubMed]
31. Dance, A.; Thundathil, J.; Wilde, R.; Blondin, P.; Kastelic, J. Enhanced early-life nutrition promotes hormone production and reproductive development in Holstein bulls. *J. Dairy Sci.* **2015**, *98*, 987–998. [CrossRef]
32. Harstine, B.R.; Maquivar, M.; Helser, L.A.; Utt, M.D.; Premanandan, C.; DeJarnette, J.M.; Day, M.L. Effects of dietary energy on sexual maturation and sperm production in Holstein bulls. *J. Anim. Sci.* **2015**, *93*, 2759–2766. [CrossRef]
33. Fawcett, D.W.; Leak, L.V.; Heidger, P.M., Jr. Electron microscopic observations on the structural components of the blood-testis barrier. *J. Reprod Fertil Suppl.* **1970**, *10*, 105–122.
34. Mital, P.; Hinton, B.T.; Dufour, J.M. The blood-testis and blood-epididymis barriers are more than just their tight junctions. *Biol. Reprod.* **2011**, *84*, 851–858. [CrossRef] [PubMed]
35. Setchell, B.P.; Pollanen, P.; Zupp, J.L. Development of the blood-testis barrier and changes in vascular permeability at puberty in rats. *Int. J.* **1988**, *11*, 225–233. [CrossRef] [PubMed]
36. Niskanen, R.; Alenius, S.; Belak, K.; Baule, C.; Belak, S.; Voges, H.; Gustafsson, H. Insemination of susceptible heifers with semen from a non-viraemic bull with persistent bovine virus diarrhoea virus infection localized in the testes. *Reprod. Domest. Anim.* **2002**, *37*, 171–175. [CrossRef] [PubMed]

5

Clinical and Serological Evaluation of LINDA Virus Infections in Post-Weaning Piglets

Alexandra Kiesler [1,†], Kerstin Seitz [1,†], Lukas Schwarz [2,†], Katharina Buczolich [1], Helga Petznek [1], Elena Sassu [2], Sophie Dürlinger [2], Sandra Högler [3], Andrea Klang [3], Christiane Riedel [1], Hann-Wei Chen [1], Marlene Mötz [1], Peter Kirkland [4], Herbert Weissenböck [3], Andrea Ladinig [2], Till Rümenapf [1] and Benjamin Lamp [1,*,‡]

1 Institute of Virology, Department for Pathobiology, University of Veterinary Medicine, Veterinaerplatz 1, 1210 Vienna, Austria; Alexandra.Kiesler@vetmeduni.ac.at (A.K.); Kerstin.Seitz@vetmeduni.ac.at (K.S.); katharina.buczolich@gmx.net (K.B.); Helga.Petznek@vetmeduni.ac.at (H.P.); Christiane.Riedel@vetmeduni.ac.at (C.R.); Hann-Wei.Chen@vetmeduni.ac.at (H.-W.C.); Marlene.Moetz@vetmeduni.ac.at (M.M.); Till.Ruemenapf@vetmeduni.ac.at (T.R.)

2 Department for Farm Animals and Veterinary Public Health, University Clinic for Swine, University of Veterinary Medicine, Veterinaerplatz 1, 1210 Vienna, Austria; Lukas.Schwarz@vetmeduni.ac.at (L.S.); Elena.Sassu@vetmeduni.ac.at (E.S.); Sophie.Duerlinger@vetmeduni.ac.at (S.D.); Andrea.Ladinig@vetmeduni.ac.at (A.L.)

3 Institute of Pathology and Forensic Veterinary Medicine, Department of Pathobiology, University of Veterinary Medicine, Veterinaerplatz 1, 1210 Vienna, Austria; Sandra.Hoegler@vetmeduni.ac.at (S.H.); Andrea.Klang@vetmeduni.ac.at (A.K.); Herbert.Weissenboeck@vetmeduni.ac.at (H.W.)

4 Virology Laboratory, Elizabeth Macarthur Agriculture Institute, Woodbridge Rd, Menangle, New South Wales 2568, Australia; Peter.Kirkland@dpi.nsw.gov.au

* Correspondence: Benjamin.J.Lamp@vetmed.uni-giessen.de.

† These authors contributed equally to the work.

‡ Current affiliation: Institute of Virology, Faculty of Veterinary Medicine, Justus-Liebig-Universität, Schubertstrasse 81, 35392 Giessen, Germany; Benjamin.J.Lamp@vetmed.uni-giessen.de.

Abstract: The novel pestivirus species known as lateral-shaking inducing neuro-degenerative agent (LINDA) virus emerged in 2015 in a piglet-producing farm in Austria. Affected piglets showed strong congenital tremor as a result of severe lesions in the central nervous system. Here, we report the results of a controlled animal infection experiment. Post-weaning piglets were infected with LINDA to determine the susceptibility of pigs, the clinical consequences of infection and the humoral immune response against LINDA. No clinically overt disease signs were observed in the piglets. Viremia was hardly detectable, but LINDA was present in the spleen and several lymphatic organs until the end of the experiment on day 28 post-infection. Oronasal virus shedding together with the infection of one sentinel animal provided additional evidence for the successful replication and spread of LINDA in the piglets. Starting on day 14 post-infection, all infected animals showed a strong humoral immune response with high titers of neutralizing antibodies against LINDA. No cross-neutralizing activity of these sera with other pestiviral species was observed. According to these data, following postnatal infection, LINDA is a rather benign virus that can be controlled by the pig's immune system. However, further studies are needed to investigate the effects of LINDA on the fetus after intrauterine infection.

Keywords: Linda virus; serological profile; virus neutralization assay; virus pathogenicity; humoral immune response

1. Introduction

The genus *Pestivirus* within the family Flaviviridae currently comprises 11 different species—recently termed *Pestivirus A–K* [1]. In addition to the long known classical swine fever virus (CSFV, *Pestivirus C*), a number of other pestivirus species have been identified in the porcine host in recent years, such as border disease virus (BDV, *Pestivirus D*), bovine viral diarrhea virus (BVDV-1, *Pestivirus A*), Bungowannah virus (BUNGO, *Pestivirus F*), and atypical porcine pestivirus (APPV, *Pestivirus K*) [1–5]. In 2015, we detected a yet unknown pestivirus species in a piglet-producing farm in Austria, which was termed lateral-shaking inducing neuro-degenerative agent (LINDA) virus [6]. Since the nucleotide sequence of LINDA shows a significant divergence of over 30% compared to the accepted pestivirus species, we proposed it as the new species *Pestivirus L* [1,6].

Pestiviruses are small enveloped viruses with a positive-sense, single-stranded, non-segmented RNA genome with a length of about 12 to 13 kilobases (kb) [7]. The genome consists of one large open reading frame (ORF), flanked by 5′- and 3′-non-coding regions [7]. This single ORF encodes a hypothetical polyprotein, that is co- and post-translationally processed into non-structural and structural proteins by viral and cellular proteases [8]. The three structural glycoproteins, termed E^{rns}, E1 and E2, and the nucleocapsid protein named Core are generated by cellular proteases [9,10]. The generation of the non-structural proteins N^{pro}, p7, NS2, NS3, NS4A, NS4B, NS5A and NS5B is very complex. Multiple processing steps mediated by autoproteases (N^{pro} and NS2) and the major NS3/4A protease yield partially processed precursors, mature proteins and enzymatically active protein fragments [8,11–13]. The presence of the autoprotease N^{pro} and the envelope glycoprotein E^{rns} are recognized as characteristic of the genus *Pestivirus* [1,7]. Since the corresponding proteins have been found in the genome of LINDA, it can undoubtedly be classified in the genus *Pestivirus* [6].

CSFV is listed by the World Organization for Animal Health (OIE) as an economically important pig pathogen [14]. The clinical signs of classical swine fever (CSF) vary significantly depending on the virulence of the virus strain as well as the age and susceptibility of the infected pigs. CSF is usually characterized by fever, skin lesions, convulsions and, especially in young animals, death within a few days [15]. BUNGO emerged on a pig farm in Australia in 2003, causing an increased rate of stillbirths, mummification and sudden deaths of piglets [2,16]. Experimental studies were conducted to investigate the pathogenicity of BUNGO in weaner pigs and porcine fetuses under laboratory conditions. Despite the low pathogenicity of the virus in weaned piglets, a long-lasting viremia, efficient virus shedding and rapid seroconversion were detected [17]. In contrast, a multifocal non-suppurative myocarditis with myonecrosis was observed following direct fetal exposure to BUNGO mimicking intrauterine infection [18]. APPVs were discovered in the United States in 2015 by next-generation sequencing [4], and subsequently detected in many countries around the world [19–23]. A close correlation between intrauterine APPV infections and the occurrence of congenital tremor (CT) type A-II in newborn piglets was reported [24]. The simultaneous detection of nucleic acids of APPV and hypomyelination in the central nervous system of these piglets implied a causative role of APPV for the appearance of the so-called shaking piglet syndrome [20]. This causal relationship is further supported by the birth of shaking piglets after inoculation of pregnant sows with APPV-containing material [24].

LINDA was discovered during the investigation of an outbreak of CT in a piglet-producing farm. We identified the agent, isolated the virus, sequenced its genome and established a RT-PCR assay as well as serological reagents for its detection [6]. Since then, LINDA has not been found in any other farm in Austria or elsewhere in the world [25]. To gain a deeper insight into the biology of this virus, we infected weaned piglets with LINDA under controlled experimental conditions. The aim of this small-scale animal experiment was the determination of susceptibility, pathogenicity and virulence of LINDA in the immunocompetent porcine host. Sera from the experimentally infected piglets were further used to characterize the humoral immune response against LINDA and to study the induction of cross-neutralizing antibodies against other pestiviruses.

2. Materials and Methods

2.1. Cells and Viruses

SK-6 cells [26] and MDBK cells (ATCC® CCL-22™) [27] were grown in Dulbecco's modified Eagle's medium (DMEM) supplemented with 10% fetal bovine serum (FCS, Bio and Sell GmbH, Feucht, Germany; negatively tested for the presence of pestiviruses), 100 U/mL penicillin and 100 μg/mL streptomycin. All cells were maintained at 37 °C and 5% CO_2. Cell culture-derived LINDA was used for the experiments. After initial cell culture isolation from a clinical case (passage 1, P1), a primary LINDA stock was generated containing a 50% tissue culture infectious dose ($TCID_{50}$) of 1.1×10^7 (P2, GenBank® KY436034) [6]. The virus was titrated in an endpoint dilution assay and supernatant from a single focus was harvested (P3) to ensure freedom from other pathogens. A master stock (P4) was prepared and characterized by RT-PCR and subsequent Sanger sequencing. In direct comparison with the consensus sequence of the original isolate no mutations were detected. All LINDA infection doses used for animal inoculations were recovered from the master stock and thus represent cell culture passage 5 of LINDA. BVDV-1a strain NADL and BVDV-1b strain NCP7 were obtained from E. Dubovi (Cornell University College of Veterinary Medicine, Ithaca, NY) [28]. CSFV 2.3 Alfort-Tübingen [29], BDV-1 X818 [30], BVDV-2 strain 890 [31], and BVDV-3 (unpublished strain isolated from FCS, South American origin) were obtained from the virus collection of the Institute of Virology in Giessen (Justus-Liebig-University, Giessen, Germany). Pestivirus strain Giraffe-1 [32] was a gift from D. J. Paton, Animal Health and Veterinary Laboratory Agency (AHVLA, Weybridge, United Kingdom). BUNGO was obtained from stocks of the Elizabeth Macarthur Agricultural Institute (Department of Primary Industries, Menangle, New South Wales, Australia) [2].

2.2. Virus Infection and Titration

Infections of MDBK and SK-6 cells with various strains of the different pestivirus species were performed with the indicated multiplicity of infection (MOI). Virus stocks for the experiments were generated using 10-cm cell culture dishes infected with a MOI of 0.1. At 72 h post-infection, the cell culture supernatant was harvested, filtered through a 0.45 μm cellulose filter (Sartorius, Göttingen, Germany), aliquoted and stored at −80 °C until use. The $TCID_{50}$ of viral supernatants was determined in three replicates by an end-point dilution assay (EPDA). The virus titer was calculated using the Spearman-Kaerber algorithm [33]. Re-isolation of LINDA was performed using SK-6 cells and fresh sample material.

2.3. RT-PCR Detection

RNA was extracted from serum and tissue samples, saliva, feces, cultured cells or virus cell culture supernatant using the QIAamp Viral RNA Mini Kit and the RNeasy Mini Kit (Qiagen, Hilden, Germany) according to the manufacturer's instructions. RNA was eluted in 60 μL RNase free distilled water and directly used for RT-PCR or stored at –80 °C for subsequent analysis. RT-PCR was carried out using the OneTaq One-Step RT-PCR Kit (NEB, Ipswich, USA) or the One Step RT-PCR Kit (Qiagen) using the oligonucleotides PPF 5′-GTKATHCAATACCCTGARGC-3′ and PPR 5′-GGRTTCCAGGARTACATCA-3′ [6]. PCR amplicons were subjected to gel electrophoresis and purified with the peqGOLD Gel Extraction Kit (Peqlab, Erlangen, Germany), if needed.

2.4. Calibration-Curve-Estimated Copy Number of LINDA Genome Equivalents

For the quantification of virus excretion, viremia and virus loads of organ homogenates, qRT-PCRs were performed on an ABI 7500 cycler (Applied Biosystems, Foster City, USA) using the LINDA and BUNGO specific primers LVqRTfor196 (5′-CACTGGWAAGGATCACCCACT-3′) and LVqRTrev351 (5′-AATYACAACGGATAWTMTTTATACTGG-3′) and the FAM/TAMRA labeled probe, LVqRTprobe322 (5′-Fam-ATAGGATGCCGGCGGATGCCCTGT-TamRa -3′). For the generation of a calibration curve, a T-vector plasmid fragment harboring the cDNA target sequence was produced using EcoRI digest, gel-purified and spectrophotometrically quantified. The copy number of recombinant plasmid fragment was calculated following the formula: N (molecules per μL) = (C

(DNA concentration in μg/μL) / K (fragment size in bp)) $\times$ 185.5 $\times$ 10^{13}. The factor results from the weight of the genome-equivalent ssDNA molecules (330 daltons per base), the volume projection factors and the Avogadro constant (6.02 $\times$ 10^{23} mol^{-1}). In order to obtain a standard curve, a ten-fold dilution series of the DNA control was included in the qRT-PCR setup [34]. Cycling conditions were 50 °C for 10 min, 95 °C for 1 min and 40 cycles of 95 °C for 10 sec, 60 °C for 1 min (amplification and fluorescence detection step). Semi-quantitative copy number estimation was calculated by 7500 System SDS Software (Applied Biosystems) based on the calibration curve. The amplification of the dsDNA standard does not include reverse transcription, which is why minor deviations may occur between RNA samples and dsDNA standard amplification depending on the efficiency of the cDNA synthesis. The qRT-PCR assay presented here is linear up to 10 copies of the dsDNA template per reaction (Ct value of 38). Since 10 copies per reaction were included as the lowest template amount in the standard series, this value represents the limit of quantification and our lower assay cutoff. The genome equivalents of 1.0 μL of purified RNA were converted to copies per 1 mL liquid sample, 1 g tissue sample or copies per swab using appropriate projection factors. The samples from the animal experiment were measured once due to high numbers and limited financial resources. However, the qRT-PCR data were validated by virus isolation experiments carried out in parallel with all samples obtained during the experiment.

2.5. Virus Neutralization Assay

All virus neutralization assays (VNA) were prepared in triplicate in 96-well microtiter plates. Viruses used in the VNA were diluted in DMEM without FCS from stock solutions generating a final titer of 100 to 300 $TCID_{50}$ per 0.1 mL. Initial two-fold dilution series of the serum samples were prepared with DMEM without FCS generating a final serum dilution of 1:256 in the last wells. Highly reactive sera were further diluted in five-fold series to a final serum dilution of 1:$10^{5.6}$ in the last wells. 100 μL of each serum dilution were mixed with 100 μL of the respective virus solution containing between 100 to 300 $TCID_{50}$. After the virus was added, the VNA was incubated for 2 h at 37 °C in 5% CO_2. One hundred microliters of this virus/serum mixtures were added to 96-well flat bottom plates containing confluent cell monolayers and incubated for 48 h at 37 °C in 5% CO_2. Viral infections were detected by indirect immunofluorescence using murine monoclonal antibodies (MAbs) as indicated below. Back titration of each virus solution was performed in parallel. Defined positive and negative sera against the respective virus or groups were used as controls. The titers obtained from the VNAs were calculated using the Spearman-Kaerber algorithm and reported as the reciprocal of the serum dilution that inhibited infection of 50% of the cells (neutralization dose 50%, ND_{50}).

2.6. Indirect Immunofluorescence Assay and Antibodies

The immunofluorescence assays were performed as previously described [8]. Briefly, the cells were fixed with 4% paraformaldehyde for 20 min at 4 °C, permeabilized with 1% (vol/vol) Triton-X 100 (Merck, Darmstadt, Germany) in PBS and stained with the mouse MAb 6A5 [35] and A18 [36]. The monoclonal antibody 6A5 was used to detect the E2 molecule of BVDV-1, BVDV-2, BVDV-3, BDV, BUNGO, giraffe pestivirus and LINDA infections. CSFV E2 was detected by MAb A18. Goat anti-mouse IgG conjugated with Cy3 (Dianova, Hamburg, Germany) was used as a secondary antibody. A porcine BUNGO antiserum (748-09.10-1) collected from a naturally infected sow, which had produced an abnormal litter, was kindly provided by the Elizabeth Macarthur Agricultural Institute.

2.7. Animal Experiment

The animal experiment was approved by the ethics committee of the University of Veterinary Medicine, Vienna and the Federal Ministry of Science, Research and Economy according to the §§ 26ff. of the Austrian Animal Experiments Act from 2012 (Permission code: BMWF-68.205/0130-WF/V/3b/2017, permission date: 07.07.2017). Post-weaning crossbreed piglets (*Sus scrofa domestica*) were used for the study of LINDA pathogenesis and virulence in immunocompetent hosts. The pigs came from the breeding farm Medau of the University of Veterinary Medicine, Vienna. The entire herd of the farm was negative tested for swine pathogenic influenza A viruses (IAV; H3N2, H1N1, H1N2 and H1N1pan) and porcine reproductive and respiratory syndrome viruses (PRRSV). The mother sows of the experimental animals were vaccinated against parvovirus and erysipelas during lactation according to the manufacturer's instructions (Parvoruvac; Merial GmbH, Hallbergmoos, Germany). The piglets themselves were protected on day 21 with a combined vaccination against *Mycoplasma hyopneumoniae* and porcine circovirus-2 (Circoflex and Mycoflex; both from Boehringer Ingelheim Vetmedica GmbH, Ingelheim, Germany). No further special diagnostic tests were carried out as there were neither pathological nor clinical signs of disease in these piglets.

A week prior to the beginning of the trial (study days –7 to –1) 21 weaned piglets in the 13th week of life were housed in a biological safety unit (BSL-2) for adaptation. At the beginning of the animal experiment, six piglets were housed separately in order to later serve as sentinel animals. The remaining piglets were divided into three groups of five animals each and housed in separate units. One group was not infected and served as a negative control, one group was inoculated intramuscularly (i.m.) with 1×10^7 $TCID_{50}$ LINDA and the last group was infected intranasally (i.n.) with 1×10^7 $TCID_{50}$ LINDA (study day 0). One day after infection (study day 1), three sentinel animals were added to each of the infection-groups. A daily clinical score was determined for each individual animal. The general condition, behavior, body temperature, feed intake and weight gain of all animals were assessed and measured after the infection over a period of 28 days. Particular attention was paid to the occurrence of signs of disease. Each animal was assigned a daily clinical score, which included individual values for behavior, feed intake, dyspnea, ocular and nasal discharge, coughing and diarrhea in the range from 0 (physiological) to 3 (severe clinical symptoms) according to an established evaluation scheme of the University Clinic for Swine of the University of Veterinary Medicine, Vienna [37]. While the body temperature of all animals was also monitored daily, the body weight was assessed at the time point of arrival and on study days 0–7, 9, 14, 21 and 28. Blood and fecal samples as well as nasal and oral swabs were taken on the study days 0, 3, 5, 7, 14, 21 and 28/29. Urine samples (spontaneous urine samples or collected via cystocentesis) were obtained on study day 3 from most animals. All animals were euthanized with T61 (5.0 mg/mL tetracaine hydrochloride, 50 mg/mL mebezonium iodide and 200 mg/mL embutramide; 1 mL/10 kg) on study day 28 or 29 under general anesthesia (1.3 mg/kg azaperone and 10 mg/kg ketamine hydrochloride). During necropsy, organ samples were taken for molecular and pathohistological analysis. In particular, the LINDA RNA loads were analyzed in samples taken from the kidney, bladder, cerebellum, cerebrum, spinal cord, dorsal root ganglia, thymus, spleen, tonsils, lymph nodes (Lnn. inguinales, mesenteriales and mandibularis), parotid and sublingual glands, heart, lung, liver and intestinal segments from all animals.

2.8. Pathological Examinations

Tissue samples of the brain and spinal cord, dorsal root ganglia, liver, spleen, kidney, urinary bladder, thymus, spleen, tonsils, inguinal lymph node and mandibular gland were taken from all animals for histological examination. Additional samples of the coeliac ganglion, sciatic nerve, mesenteric and mandibular lymph nodes and parotid gland were included from the experimentally infected animals and sentinels. Five coronary sections of the brain were taken at the levels of telencephalon, diencephalon, cerebellum, mesencephalon and metencephalon. Transversal sections of the spinal cord were taken from cervical, thoracic and lumbar regions. The organ samples were fixed in 10% neutral buffered formalin, embedded in paraffin wax, sectioned at 2 μm and stained with hematoxylin and eosin (HE).

3. Results

3.1. Pathogenicity and Virulence of LINDA in Weaned Piglets

The animal experiment was performed with weaned piglets to investigate the clinical effects of LINDA infection in the immunocompetent host. The animals of all three groups (infected intranasally, intramuscularly or mock), including the sentinel animals, showed normal physiological parameters and good general condition throughout the 28-day infection period. Neither the individually examined clinical values nor the additive clinical score showed major pathological changes in individual animals or significant changes between the different groups (Figure 1). Mild ocular and nasal discharge and cough were observed early after infection (study days 0 to 7) in most animals of both LINDA infected groups. However, these changes were also observed in sentinel animals of these groups that did not show seroconversion to LINDA (n.i. sent., described below). Mild fever (maximum rectal temperature of 40.7 °C) occurred in all i.m. infected animals within the first three days after inoculation. The single sentinel animal that later seroconverted showed an elevated body temperature and mild diarrhea. No differences were found between the groups in necropsy and histological examination. Gross examination revealed alveolar emphysema of the lung in animals of all the groups. Alveolar edema and pulmonary hyperemia were detected in some animals of all groups. Macroscopically, the central nervous system of all animals appeared normal. However, in the histological examination the majority of the animals from all groups ($n = 17$) showed mild, oligofocal, randomly distributed perivascular, mononuclear infiltrations and some glial nodules in the brain and/or spinal cord. A slight follicular hyperplasia of the spleen was observed in one sentinel animal of the i.n. and i.m. group. Stomach lesions such as ulcerations, hyperkeratinization or follicular hyperplasia were found in almost all animals. Mild, predominantly mononuclear, sometimes suppurating, interstitial nephritis or cortical infarction were found in many animals ($n = 13$) including animals from the non-infected control group. An interstitial lymphocytic infiltration of the mandibular gland was evident in one sentinel animal each of intranasally and intramuscularly infected group. An abscess was observed in the snout of an intranasally infected animal. The initial body weight of each animal was defined as 100% and the relative weight gain for each piglet and the average weight gain of the groups were calculated for each study day. The non-infected control group showed a slightly higher weight gain compared to the infected groups and the sentinel animals. However, the differences in weight gain between the experimental groups were neither pronounced nor statistically significant (Figure 2).

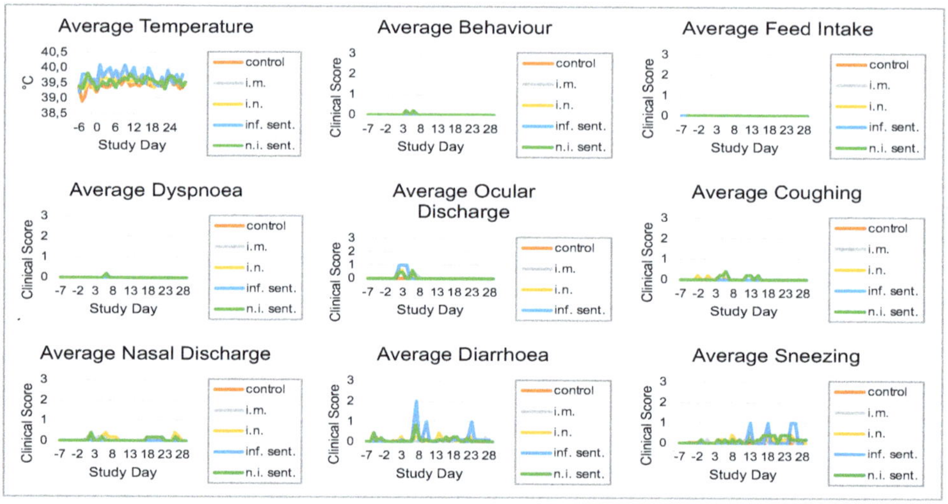

Figure 1. Pathogenicity of lateral-shaking inducing neuro-degenerative agent (LINDA) in immunocompetent piglets. A total of 21 piglets were divided in five groups: five negative control, five intramuscularly (i.m.) infected and five intranasally (i.n.) infected animals as well as three sentinel animals for the i.m. and three sentinel animals for the i.n. group. The animals from the i.m. and i.n. infection groups were inoculated with LINDA (1×10^7 $TCID_{50}$/mL) on study day 0. Body temperature, behavior, feed intake, dyspnea, ocular discharge, coughing, nasal discharge, diarrhea and sneezing were assessed daily and symptoms were classified by a scoring system with scores from 0 (physiological) to 3 (severe clinical symptoms). The mean of gathered parameters was calculated for the control, i.m. infected, i.n. infected, infected sentinel (inf. sent.) and non-infected sentinel (n.i. sent.) animals. No severe LINDA virus associated clinical signs were observed comparing infected and non-infected animals. However, mild fever and other signs of disease were seen in some infected animals, such as the infected sentinel animal within the i.m. group.

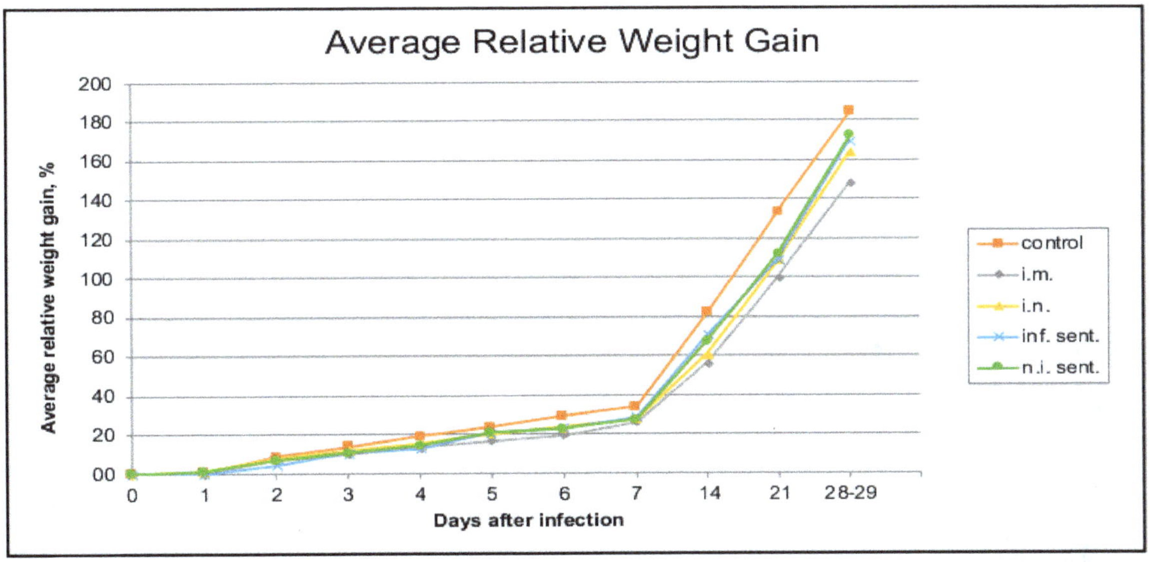

Figure 2. Average relative daily weight gain. Piglets were weighed on study days 0–7, 14, 21 and 28/29. The initial body weight was set as 100% value and relative weight gain was calculated for every individual at the indicated time-points. The mean value was calculated for every trial group. Infected groups show a slightly reduced weight gain compared to the negative control group after 7 days post-infection. However, the absolute differences between the groups were not significant.

3.2. Replication of LINDA in the Immunocompetent Porcine Host

Before the beginning of the experiment, blood samples of all animals were taken and tested for the presence of LINDA RNA and LINDA neutralizing antibodies. Serum samples were taken on study days 0, 3, 7, 14 and 28/29 of the experiment and analyzed in a LINDA-specific qRT-PCR assay as well as in virus isolation studies. No infectious LINDA or viral RNA were detected in the mock infected group at any time of the experiment. Most i.m. infected and all i.n. infected animals did not show a detectable viremia after LINDA inoculation. We observed a low level of viremia in two i.m. infected animals (5.0×10^5 GE/mL for animal 8 i.m. and 5.5×10^5 for animal 9 i.m. on study day 7) and a higher level in one sentinel animal of this group (2.3×10^7 GE/mL on study day 14, Figure 3). LINDA could be isolated from each of these qRT-PCR positive serum samples. Virus shedding was assessed using oral and nasal swabs as well as fecal and urine samples. Most of these samples gave negative results in the LINDA virus-specific qRT-PCR and virus isolation experiments. The oral swabs of one of the viremic piglets from the i.m. group (study day 7) and the oral and nasal swabs from three animals of the i.n. group gave signals below assay cutoff in the qRT-PCR assay (study days 3, 7 and/or 14). The RNA loads in these swabs were very low and cell culture virus isolation was not successful. An additional conventional RT-PCR was performed on the questionable samples as described before [6]. The amplification of LINDA-specific RT-PCR products was verified by nucleotide sequencing (Figure S1). LINDA RNA was not detectable in the fecal samples obtained on study days 3, 7 and 14 from the experimentally infected animals. However, the viremic sentinel animal (number 11) from the i.m. infected group showed substantial LINDA RNA loads in the feces (1.31×10^5 GE/g on study day 14) that also allowed successful virus isolation. All urine samples gave negative results in qRT-PCR and virus isolation. Multiple organs were sampled during necropsy on days 28/29 post-infection. Most organ samples gave negative results for the presence of LINDA RNA in the qRT-PCR. However, LINDA genomes were detectable in several lymphoid organs, such as the inguinal lymph nodes ($n = 4$), spleen ($n = 2$) and tonsils ($n = 4$) of animals of the i.m. infected group reaching values between 4.0×10^3 and 2.3×10^6 GE/g. LINDA RNA was also found in the infected sentinel animal of the i.m. group (animal 11) in the inguinal lymph nodes and spleen. Interestingly, the virus was detectable in the tonsils of all i.n. infected animals ($n = 5$), but only found in the inguinal lymph node of one of these animals ($n = 1$, Figure 3).

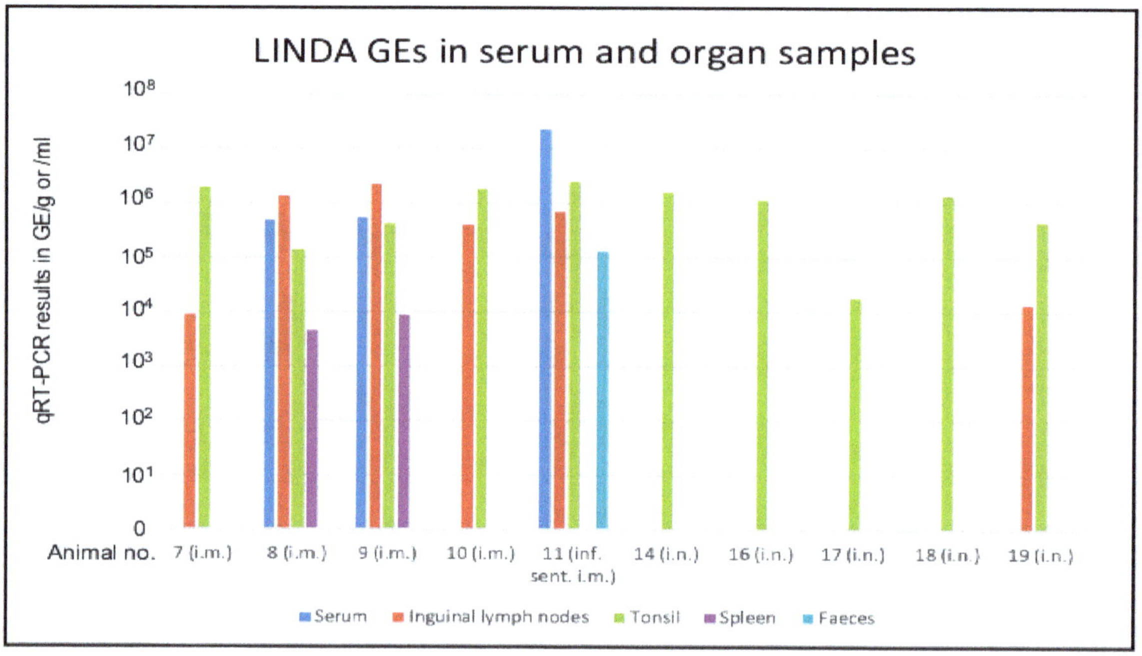

Figure 3. qRT-PCR results of the animal experiment. Multiple samples were analyzed for the presence of LINDA RNA before, during and after the experimental infection of piglets with LINDA. Blood and fecal samples as well as nasal and oral swabs were taken on study days 0, 3, 5, 7, 14, 21 and 28/29. Fecal samples were collected on study days 3, 7 and 14, while urine samples were only taken from most animals on day 3. Kidney, bladder, cerebellum, cerebrum, spinal cord, dorsal root ganglia, thymus, spleen, tonsils, different lymph nodes (Lnn. inguinales, mesenteriales and mandibularis), parotid and sublingual glands, heart, lung, liver and intestinal segments were sampled from all animals during necropsy on days 28/29. Most samples gave negative results for LINDA RNA. Only two i.m. infected animals showed detectable LINDA RNA loads in serum samples taken on study day 7 and one sentinel animal of the i.m. group on day 14. These serum samples also allowed the re-isolation of LINDA. Viral RNA was not detectable in urine samples and only detected in one fecal sample (animal 11, i.m. group, infected sentinel). However, the RNA of LINDA was detected in multiple samples from lymphoid organs demonstrating the presence of LINDA in the experimentally infected animals as well as in the infected sentinel animal until the end of the experiment.

3.3. Humoral Immune Response against LINDA

All serum samples obtained before, during and at the end of the experiment were tested for LINDA-specific antibodies using a LINDA virus neutralization assay (Figure 4). No virus neutralizing activity was measured in the serum samples taken before the start of the experiment ($ND_{50} < 1/2$, below limit of detection). Sera from the mock infected group and sera from the LINDA RNA negative sentinel animals showed no virus neutralizing activity at the end of the trial. A gradual onset of humoral immune responses was observed in all infected animals (i.m. and i.n.) between days 7 and 14 post-infection, reaching peak values of up to 1/8,640 ND_{50}/mL. A comparably strong reactivity of 1/1,028 was also seen in the serum sample of the i.m. infected animal 6, in which no LINDA RNA replication was detected throughout the experiment. Interestingly, the development of the humoral immune response was delayed to study day 21 in the LINDA infected sentinel animal 11.

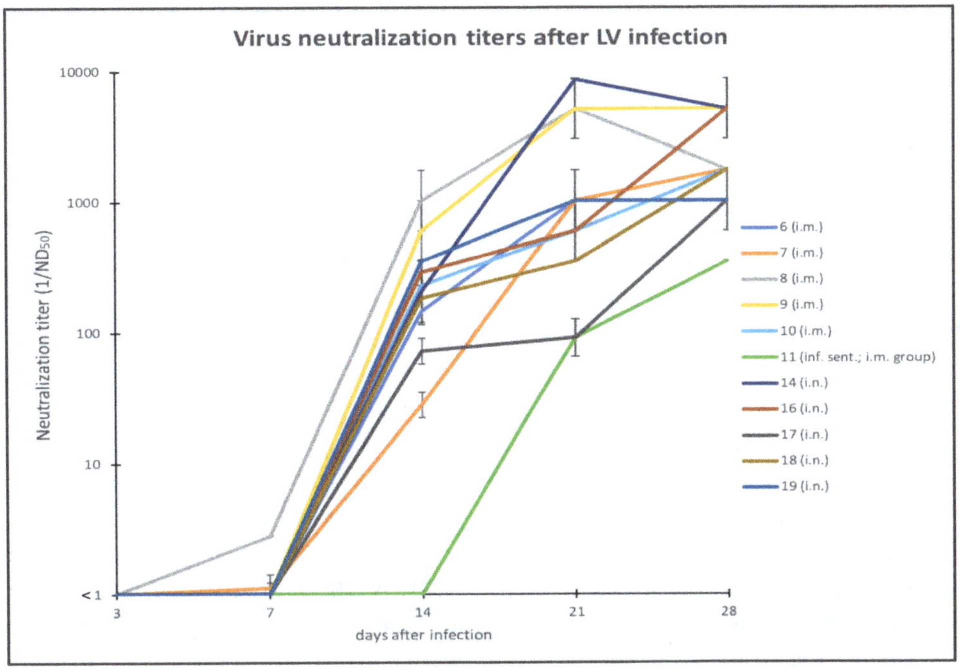

Figure 4. Virus neutralization activities of LINDA immune sera. The serum samples taken on study days 0, 3, 7, 14, 21 and 28/29 were tested in VNAs against LINDA. All VNAs were performed in triplicate and ND_{50} was calculated using the Spearman-Kaerber algorithm. The reciprocal ND_{50} value is presented for each serum sample including error bars for positive and negative standard deviation. All $1/ND_{50}$ values were less than 1 until study day 7, when the first weak neutralizing activities were measured in single animals. Significant neutralizing activities ($ND_{50} > 1:10$) were detected in all infected animals starting on day 14. Note the later onset of humoral immune response in the infected sentinel animal from the i.m. group on day 21.

3.4. Cross Neutralization of LINDA-Immune Sera with Other Pestivirus Species

To assess antigenic relations to other pestiviruses, we characterized the LINDA-immune sera from study days 28/29 for their cross-neutralizing activities against multiple pestiviral strains. In particular, we performed VNAs with the pestivirus species BVDV-1a (strain NADL), BVDV-1b (strain NCP7), BVDV-2 (strain 890), CSFV 2.3 (strain Alfort-Tübingen), BDV-1 (strain X818), pestivirus giraffe (strain giraffe 1), BUNGO and an unpublished BVDV-3 strain. We found no neutralizing activity of the LINDA-immune sera ($ND_{50} < 1/2$) against any of these viruses. Additionally, we tested a porcine BUNGO convalescence serum (748-09.10-1), initially obtained for immunodetection of BUNGO infections of cultured cells. This antiserum efficiently neutralized BUNGO (BUNGO ND_{50} 1/3200) as well as LINDA in our VNAs (LINDA ND_{50} 1/1,600) but had no effect on the infection of BVDV-1, BVDV-2 and CSFV (all $ND_{50} < 1/2$).

4. Discussion

The aim of this study was to investigate the pathogenicity of LINDA during post-natal infections and to characterize the humoral immune response against LINDA in order to obtain important basic data for sero-surveillance studies. Therefore, a small-scale animal experiment was set up using LINDA infections in post-weaning piglets. In this experiment, we found no evidence of severe acute disease in weaners caused by LINDA infection. Only mild clinical signs, such as mild fever, nasal discharge and mild changes in fecal consistency, were observed in single animals without significant influence on the growth rates of these piglets. Inflammatory infiltrates and glial nodules occurred in the brain and/or spinal cord of animals from all groups including the control group. Hence, these lesions were not associated with LINDA infection and were consequently interpreted as non-specific experimental background. Other findings of necropsy could be interpreted as random findings or might represent stress-related diseases, such as the typical gastric lesions. However, productive LINDA infections were observed in all animals, which were experimentally inoculated with 1×10^7 $TCID_{50}$, regardless of the infection route used. LINDA virus excretion was detected using qRT-PCR in oronasal fluids of some infected animals and excretion via feces was documented for a single animal. Viremia was hardly detectable in the serum of most animals, while all except one experimentally infected animal (animal 6 i.m.) showed a long-lasting presence of the virus in the tonsils and/or lymphatic organs. Unfortunately, no peripheral mononuclear blood cells (PBMCs) were preserved from the experiment that could have been used for a potentially more sensitive virus detection in the blood [38]. Therefore, future studies, also including pregnant sows, will investigate whether LINDA virus is associated with PBMCs and whether the analysis of isolated PBMCs allows a more sensitive diagnosis. The infection of one sentinel animal in the i.m. group confirmed that infectious loads of virus were secreted in this simulated acute infection scenario. When we consider the positive detection of LINDA in serum, nasal secretions and feces of some infected animals, blood contacts or oronasal uptake of the pathogen may be considered as possible pathways of infection as also demonstrated by the successful artificial i.m. and i.n. infection. Since the minimum infection dose of LINDA for piglets is unknown, it is up to future studies to clarify the natural routes of infection. The clinical data are in accordance with clinical and epidemiological data about other pestiviruses, such as BVDV, BDV or CSFV, showing that mononuclear cells and lymphoid organs are the primary targets of pestivirus infections [39,40]. Most pestiviruses are well-adapted to their host species and the acute infection of immunocompetent animals usually leads to mild to subclinical disease with limited virus replication [41,42]. Severe pestiviral disease, such as abortion, malformation or neurological disorders, is mostly a consequence of intrauterine infections and responsible for the high economic losses following pestiviral infections [43]. This circumstance also explains the differences in the clinical picture between the animal experiment with immunocompetent piglets presented here and the LINDA virus outbreak in a piglet breeding farm from which LINDA virus was originally isolated [6]. Similar results were obtained in infection studies with BUNGO in weaner piglets, where few clinical signs, a short phase of viremia (3 to 10 days post-inoculation) and low levels of virus excretion were observed [17]. We conclude that LINDA is not only the closest genetic relative of Bungowannah virus but also shows similar pathogenicity in pigs. The results of our post-natal experimental infection demonstrate that the clinical picture of BUNGO and LINDA in immunocompetent animals is distinct from symptoms of piglets affected by CSFV strains of high and moderate virulence but might be similar to low virulence CSFV strains [44]. Future studies evaluating LINDA infections of the unborn fetus will be necessary to assess the potential hazard of LINDA [18,45].

The acute infection of piglets with LINDA led to the development of a strong humoral immunity starting at about seven days post-infection (Figure 4). Despite high titers of neutralizing antibodies, viral RNA persisted in the tonsils and lymphoid organs as has also been shown for other pestiviruses. This phenomenon has been described for several pestiviruses and studied in detail for BVDV pointing to a potential risk of virus transmission from convalescent animals [46]. We used the generated LINDA-antisera to evaluate antigenic cross-reactivity between LINDA and other pestiviruses. Unfortunately, we could not include APPV in these tests, because no APPV strain was available that showed the necessary infectivity in the cell culture [19]. Our VNA data clearly demonstrate that antibodies from acute LINDA infections do not provide protection against infections with classical pestiviruses. Therefore, a serological interference with established VNAs for CSFV diagnosis is unlikely. However, further studies are needed to evaluate possible false positive reactions in serological CSFV tests using a larger sample size of LINDA-antisera as well as highly reactive immune sera obtained from sows infected during pregnancy with viremic, persistently infected piglets. Our data support the hypothesis that LINDA forms an independent species (*Pestivirus L*) within the genus *Pestivirus* with a highly divergent antigenic profile. Interestingly, the high titer BUNGO-antiserum showed a strong cross-neutralization activity in VNA against LINDA, while low to absent neutralization profiles of BUNGO-antisera against other pestiviruses were observed in previous studies [47]. This result is puzzling, because it is in conflict with the results obtained with the LINDA-antisera. A possible explanation could be that the species BUNGO and LINDA form an antigenic group within the genus *Pestivirus*, sharing conserved antigenic motifs important for virus neutralization. Again, future studies may answer this question by analyzing a larger sample size of BUNGO- and LINDA-antisera in cross-protection VNAs and, even more importantly, in controlled animal experiments.

5. Patents

The authors B.L., L.S. and T.R. are inventors on a patent on Linda pestivirus (PCT/EP2017/084453; Isolation of a novel pestivirus causing congenital tremor).

Author Contributions: Conceptualization, K.S., L.S. and B.L.; Data curation, A.K. (Alexandra Kiesler), H.P., S.D, H.-W.C. and B.L.; Formal analysis, A.K. (Alexandra Kiesler), K.S., L.S., K.B. and B.L.; Funding acquisition, T.R. and B.L.; Investigation, A.K. (Alexandra Kiesler), K.S., L.S., K.B., H.P., E.S., S.D., S.H., A.K. (Andrea Klang), C.R., H.-W.C., M.M., P.K., H.W., A.L., T.R. and B.L.; Methodology, K.S., L.S., K.B., H.P., E.S., S.D., S.H., A.K. (Alexandra Kiesler), C.R., H.-W.C., M.M. and T.R.; Project administration, B.L.; Resources, P.K., H.W., A.L., T.R. and B.L.; Supervision, H.W., A.L. and B.L.; Validation, A.K. (Alexandra Kiesler), L.S., H.P. and B.L.; Visualization, A.K. (Alexandra Kiesler) and B.L.; Writing—original draft, A.K. (Alexandra Kiesler), T.R. and B.L.; Writing—review and editing, A.K. (Alexandra Kiesler), L.S., T.R. and B.L.

Acknowledgments: The authors acknowledge Markus Cihar who was responsible for animal care and supporting during sampling. The authors thank Boehringer Ingelheim Vetmedica GmbH (Binger Strasse 173, 55216 Ingelheim am Rhein, Germany) for their financial support (Contract number: 396806) and Eric Vaughn (Boehringer Ingelheim Animal Health USA Inc., 2412 S Loop Dr, Ames, IA, United States) for valuable scientific discussions.

References

1. Smith, D.B.; Meyers, G.; Bukh, J.; Gould, E.A.; Monath, T.; Scott Muerhoff, A.; Pletnev, A.; Rico-Hesse, R.; Stapleton, J.T.; Simmonds, P.; et al. Proposed revision to the taxonomy of the genus Pestivirus, family Flaviviridae. *J. Gen. Virol* **2017**, *98*, 2106–2112. [CrossRef] [PubMed]
2. Kirkland, P.D.; Frost, M.J.; Finlaison, D.S.; King, K.R.; Ridpath, J.F.; Gu, X. Identification of a novel virus in pigs–Bungowannah virus: A possible new species of pestivirus. *Virus Res.* **2007**, *129*. [CrossRef] [PubMed]
3. Nagai, M.; Aoki, H.; Sakoda, Y.; Kozasa, T.; Tominaga-Teshima, K.; Mine, J.; Abe, Y.; Tamura, T.; Kobayashi, T.; Nishine, K.; et al. Molecular, biological, and antigenic characterization of a Border disease virus isolated from a pig during classical swine fever surveillance in Japan. *J. Vet. Diagn. Invest.* **2014**, *26*, 547–552. [CrossRef] [PubMed]
4. Hause, B.M.; Collin, E.A.; Peddireddi, L.; Yuan, F.; Chen, Z.; Hesse, R.A.; Gauger, P.C.; Clement, T.; Fang, Y.; Anderson, G. Discovery of a novel putative atypical porcine pestivirus in pigs in the USA. *J. Gen. Virol* **2015**, *96*, 2994–2998. [CrossRef]
5. Deng, Y.; Sun, C.Q.; Cao, S.J.; Lin, T.; Yuan, S.S.; Zhang, H.B.; Zhai, S.L.; Huang, L.; Shan, T.L.; Zheng, H.; et al. High prevalence of bovine viral diarrhea virus 1 in Chinese swine herds. *Vet. Microbiol* **2012**, *159*, 490–493. [CrossRef]
6. Lamp, B.; Schwarz, L.; Hogler, S.; Riedel, C.; Sinn, L.; Rebel-Bauder, B.; Weissenbock, H.; Ladinig, A.; Rumenapf, T. Novel Pestivirus Species in Pigs, Austria, 2015. *Emerg Infect. Dis* **2017**, *23*, 1176–1179. [CrossRef]
7. Simmonds, P.; Becher, P.; Bukh, J.; Gould, E.A.; Meyers, G.; Monath, T.; Muerhoff, S.; Pletnev, A.; Rico-Hesse, R.; Smith, D.B.; et al. ICTV Virus Taxonomy Profile: Flaviviridae. *J. Gen. Virol* **2017**, *98*, 2–3. [CrossRef]
8. Lamp, B.; Riedel, C.; Roman-Sosa, G.; Heimann, M.; Jacobi, S.; Becher, P.; Thiel, H.J.; Rumenapf, T. Biosynthesis of classical swine fever virus nonstructural proteins. *J. Virol.* **2011**, *85*, 3607–3620. [CrossRef]
9. Rümenapf, T.; Unger, G.; Strauss, J.H.; Thiel, H.J. Processing of the envelope glycoproteins of pestiviruses. *J. Virol.* **1993**, *67*, 3288–3294.
10. Stark, R.; Meyers, G.; Rümenapf, T.; Thiel, H.J. Processing of pestivirus polyprotein: Cleavage site between autoprotease and nucleocapsid protein of classical swine fever virus. *J. Virol.* **1993**, *67*, 7088–7095.

11. Lamp, B.; Riedel, C.; Wentz, E.; Tortorici, M.A.; Rumenapf, T. Autocatalytic cleavage within classical swine fever virus NS3 leads to a functional separation of protease and helicase. *J. Virol.* **2013**, *87*. [CrossRef] [PubMed]
12. Lackner, T.; Muller, A.; Pankraz, A.; Becher, P.; Thiel, H.J.; Gorbalenya, A.E.; Tautz, N. Temporal modulation of an autoprotease is crucial for replication and pathogenicity of an RNA virus. *J. Virol.* **2004**, *78*, 10765–10775. [CrossRef] [PubMed]
13. Tautz, N.; Elbers, K.; Stoll, D.; Meyers, G.; Thiel, H.J. Serine protease of pestiviruses: Determination of cleavage sites. *J. Virol.* **1997**, *71*, 5415–5422. [PubMed]
14. Inch, C. World Animal Health. *Can. Vet. J.* **2006**, *47*, 790–791.
15. Lohse, L.; Nielsen, J.; Uttenthal, A. Early pathogenesis of classical swine fever virus (CSFV) strains in Danish pigs. *Vet. Microbiol.* **2012**, *159*, 327–336. [CrossRef]
16. Kirkland, P.D.; Read, A.J.; Frost, M.J.; Finlaison, D.S. Bungowannah virus–a probable new species of pestivirus–what have we found in the last 10 years? *Anim. Health. Res. Rev.* **2015**, *16*, 60–63. [CrossRef]
17. Finlaison, D.S.; King, K.R.; Gabor, M.; Kirkland, P.D. An experimental study of Bungowannah virus infection in weaner aged pigs. *Vet. Microbiol.* **2012**, *160*, 245–250. [CrossRef]
18. Finlaison, D.S.; Cook, R.W.; Srivastava, M.; Frost, M.J.; King, K.R.; Kirkland, P.D. Experimental infections of the porcine foetus with Bungowannah virus, a novel pestivirus. *Vet. Microbiol.* **2010**, *144*, 32–40. [CrossRef]
19. Schwarz, L.; Riedel, C.; Högler, S.; Sinn, L.J.; Voglmayr, T.; Wöchtl, B.; Dinhopl, N.; Rebel-Bauder, B.; Weissenböck, H.; Ladinig, A.; et al. Congenital infection with atypical porcine pestivirus (APPV) is associated with disease and viral persistence. *Vet. Res.* **2017**, *48*, 1. [CrossRef]
20. Postel, A.; Hansmann, F.; Baechlein, C.; Fischer, N.; Alawi, M.; Grundhoff, A.; Derking, S.; Tenhundfeld, J.; Pfankuche, V.M.; Herder, V.; et al. Presence of atypical porcine pestivirus (APPV) genomes in newborn piglets correlates with congenital tremor. *Sci. Rep.* **2016**, *6*, 27735. [CrossRef]
21. Pan, S.; Yan, Y.; Shi, K.; Wang, M.; Mou, C.; Chen, Z. Molecular characterization of two novel atypical porcine pestivirus (APPV) strains from piglets with congenital tremor in China. *Transbound. Emerg. Dis.* **2019**, *66*, 35–42. [CrossRef] [PubMed]
22. Beer, M.; Wernike, K.; Drager, C.; Hoper, D.; Pohlmann, A.; Bergermann, C.; Schroder, C.; Klinkhammer, S.; Blome, S.; Hoffmann, B. High prevalence of highly variable atypical porcine pestiviruses found in Germany. *Transboun. Emerg. Dis.* **2016**. [CrossRef] [PubMed]
23. de Groof, A.; Deijs, M.; Guelen, L.; van Grinsven, L.; van Os-Galdos, L.; Vogels, W.; Derks, C.; Cruijsen, T.; Geurts, V.; Vrijenhoek, M.; et al. Atypical Porcine Pestivirus: A Possible Cause of Congenital Tremor Type A-II in Newborn Piglets. *Viruses* **2016**, *8*, 271. [CrossRef] [PubMed]
24. Arruda, B.L.; Arruda, P.H.; Magstadt, D.R.; Schwartz, K.J.; Dohlman, T.; Schleining, J.A.; Patterson, A.R.; Visek, C.A.; Victoria, J.G. Identification of a divergent lineage porcine pestivirus in nursing piglets with congenital tremors and reproduction of disease following experimental inoculation. *PLoS ONE* **2016**, *11*, e0150104. [CrossRef] [PubMed]
25. Cagatay, G.N.; Antos, A.; Meyer, D.; Maistrelli, C.; Keuling, O.; Becher, P.; Postel, A. Frequent infection of wild boar with atypical porcine pestivirus (APPV). *Transbound. Emerg. Dis.* **2018**, *65*, 1087–1093. [CrossRef] [PubMed]
26. Kasza, L.; Shadduck, J.A.; Christofinis, G.J. Establishment, viral susceptibility and biological characteristics of a swine kidney cell line SK-6. *Res. Vet. Sci.* **1972**, *13*, 46–51. [CrossRef]
27. Madin, S.H.; Darby, N.B., Jr. Established kidney cell lines of normal adult bovine and ovine origin. *Proc. Soc. Exp. Biol. Med.* **1958**, *98*, 574–576. [CrossRef]
28. Corapi, W.V.; Donis, R.O.; Dubovi, E.J. Monoclonal antibody analyses of cytopathic and noncytopathic viruses from fatal bovine viral diarrhea virus infections. *J. Virol.* **1988**, *62*, 2823–2827.
29. Meyers, G.; Rumenapf, T.; Thiel, H.J. Molecular cloning and nucleotide sequence of the genome of hog cholera virus. *Virology* **1989**, *171*, 555–567. [CrossRef]
30. Becher, P.; Shannon, A.D.; Tautz, N.; Thiel, H.J. Molecular characterization of border disease virus, a pestivirus from sheep. *Virology* **1994**, *198*, 542–551. [CrossRef]
31. Ridpath, J.F.; Bolin, S.R. The genomic sequence of a virulent bovine viral diarrhea virus (BVDV) from the type 2 genotype: Detection of a large genomic insertion in a noncytopathic BVDV. *Virology* **1995**, *212*, 39–46. [CrossRef] [PubMed]

32. Schmeiser, S.; Mast, J.; Thiel, H.J.; Konig, M. Morphogenesis of pestiviruses: New insights from ultrastructural studies of strain Giraffe-1. *J. Virol.* **2014**, *88*, 2717–2724. [CrossRef] [PubMed]
33. Hierholzer, J.C.; Killington, R.A. 2 - Virus isolation and quantitation. In *Virology Methods Manual*; Mahy, B.W.J., Kangro, H.O., Eds.; Academic Press: London, UK, 1996; Volume 1, pp. 25–46.
34. Sanders, R.; Mason, D.J.; Foy, C.A.; Huggett, J.F. Considerations for accurate gene expression measurement by reverse transcription quantitative PCR when analysing clinical samples. *Anal. Bioanal. Chem.* **2014**, *406*, 6471–6483. [CrossRef] [PubMed]
35. Gilmartin, A.A.; Lamp, B.; Rumenapf, T.; Persson, M.A.; Rey, F.A.; Krey, T. High-level secretion of recombinant monomeric murine and human single-chain Fv antibodies from Drosophila S2 cells. *Protein Eng. Des. Sel.* **2012**, *25*, 59–66. [CrossRef]
36. Weiland, E.; Ahl, R.; Stark, R.; Weiland, F.; Thiel, H.J. A second envelope glycoprotein mediates neutralization of a pestivirus, hog cholera virus. *J. Virol.* **1992**, *66*, 3677–3682.
37. Sinn, L.J.; Zieglowski, L.; Koinig, H.; Lamp, B.; Jansko, B.; Mosslacher, G.; Riedel, C.; Hennig-Pauka, I.; Rumenapf, T. Characterization of two Austrian porcine reproductive and respiratory syndrome virus (PRRSV) field isolates reveals relationship to East Asian strains. *Vet. Res.* **2016**, *47*, 17. [CrossRef] [PubMed]
38. Summerfield, A.; Hofmann, M.A.; McCullough, K.C. Low density blood granulocytic cells induced during classical swine fever are targets for virus infection. *Vet. Immunol. Immunopathol.* **1998**, *63*, 289–301. [CrossRef]
39. Karikalan, M.; Rajukumar, K.; Mishra, N.; Kumar, M.; Kalaiyarasu, S.; Rajesh, K.; Gavade, V.; Behera, S.P.; Dubey, S.C. Distribution pattern of bovine viral diarrhoea virus type 1 genome in lymphoid tissues of experimentally infected sheep. *Vet. Res. Commun.* **2016**, *40*, 55–61. [CrossRef]
40. Ridpath, J.F.; Falkenberg, S.M.; Bauermann, F.V.; VanderLey, B.L.; Do, Y.; Flores, E.F.; Rodman, D.M.; Neill, J.D. Comparison of acute infection of calves exposed to a high-virulence or low-virulence bovine viral diarrhea virus or a HoBi-like virus. *Am. J. Vet. Res.* **2013**, *74*, 438–442. [CrossRef]
41. Lanyon, S.R.; Hill, F.I.; Reichel, M.P.; Brownlie, J. Bovine viral diarrhoea: Pathogenesis and diagnosis. *Vet. J.* **2014**, *199*, 201–209. [CrossRef] [PubMed]
42. Strong, R.; La Rocca, S.A.; Paton, D.; Bensaude, E.; Sandvik, T.; Davis, L.; Turner, J.; Drew, T.; Raue, R.; Vangeel, I.; et al. Viral Dose and Immunosuppression Modulate the Progression of Acute BVDV-1 Infection in Calves: Evidence of Long Term Persistence after Intra-Nasal Infection. *PLoS ONE* **2015**, *10*, e0124689. [CrossRef] [PubMed]
43. Bielefeldt-Ohmann, H.; Tolnay, A.E.; Reisenhauer, C.E.; Hansen, T.R.; Smirnova, N.; Van Campen, H. Transplacental infection with non-cytopathic bovine viral diarrhoea virus types 1b and 2: Viral spread and molecular neuropathology. *J. Comp. Pathol.* **2008**, *138*, 72–85. [CrossRef] [PubMed]
44. Tarradas, J.; de la Torre, M.E.; Rosell, R.; Perez, L.J.; Pujols, J.; Munoz, M.; Munoz, I.; Munoz, S.; Abad, X.; Domingo, M.; et al. The impact of CSFV on the immune response to control infection. *Virus Res.* **2014**, *185*, 82–91. [CrossRef] [PubMed]
45. Passler, T.; Riddell, K.P.; Edmondson, M.A.; Chamorro, M.F.; Neill, J.D.; Brodersen, B.W.; Walz, H.L.; Galik, P.K.; Zhang, Y.; Walz, P.H. Experimental infection of pregnant goats with bovine viral diarrhea virus (BVDV) 1 or 2. *Vet. Res.* **2014**, *45*, 38. [CrossRef] [PubMed]
46. Collins, M.E.; Heaney, J.; Thomas, C.J.; Brownlie, J. Infectivity of pestivirus following persistence of acute infection. *Vet. Microbiol.* **2009**, *138*, 289–296. [CrossRef]
47. Kirkland, P.D.; Frost, M.J.; King, K.R.; Finlaison, D.S.; Hornitzky, C.L.; Gu, X.; Richter, M.; Reimann, I.; Dauber, M.; Schirrmeier, H.; et al. Genetic and antigenic characterization of Bungowannah virus, a novel pestivirus. *Vet. Microbiol.* **2015**, *178*, 252–259. [CrossRef]

6

The Outcome of Porcine Foetal Infection with Bungowannah Virus is Dependent on the Stage of Gestation at which Infection Occurs: Clinical Signs and Gross Pathology

Deborah S. Finlaison * and Peter D. Kirkland

Virology Laboratory, New South Wales Department of Primary Industries, Elizabeth Macarthur Agricultural Institute, Menangle, NSW 2568, Australia; peter.kirkland@dpi.nsw.gov.au
* Correspondence: deborah.finlaison@dpi.nsw.gov.au

Abstract: Bungowannah virus is a novel pestivirus identified from a disease outbreak in a piggery in Australia in June 2003. The aim of this study was to determine whether infection of pregnant pigs with Bungowannah virus induces the clinical signs and gross pathology observed during the initial outbreak and how this correlates with the time of infection. Twenty-four pregnant pigs were infected at one of four stages of gestation (approximately 35, 55, 75 or 90 days). The number of progeny born alive, stillborn or mummified, and signs of disease were recorded. Some surviving piglets were euthanased at weaning and others at ages up to 11 months. All piglets were subjected to a detailed necropsy. The greatest effects were observed following infection at 35 or 90 days of gestation. Infection at 35 days resulted in a significant reduction in the number of pigs born alive and an increased number of mummified foetuses (18%) and preweaning mortalities (70%). Preweaning losses were higher following infection at 90 days of gestation (29%) and were associated with sudden death and cardiorespiratory signs. Stunting occurred in chronically and persistently infected animals. This study reproduced the clinical signs and gross pathology of the porcine myocarditis syndrome and characterised the association between the time of infection and the clinical outcome.

Keywords: Bungowannah virus; foetus; pestivirus; porcine

---

1. Introduction

Bungowannah virus is a novel pestivirus identified from an outbreak of a disease in a piggery in New South Wales, Australia, in June 2003 [1]. It is genetically distinct from the other recognised pestiviruses of pigs, namely, classical swine fever virus (CSFV) and atypical porcine pestivirus (APPV) [2,3], with its closest genetic relationship to the recently identified Linda virus [4]. The disease was referred to as the porcine myocarditis syndrome, or PMC, because histological changes in the first affected animals consisted almost exclusively of multifocal, non-suppurative myocarditis, with myonecrosis observed in some cases. The outbreak initially presented as sudden death in 2–3-week-old weaning-age pigs, but soon after the onset, there was a marked increase in the birth of stillborn foetuses and a slight increase in the occurrence of mummified pigs [1]. Cumulative losses in some weeks exceeded 50% of pigs born, and it is estimated that as many as 50,000 pigs died in the initial outbreak. Due to the reproductive effects and disease becoming apparent almost exclusively in the first 2–3 weeks of life, it was presumed to be predominantly the consequence of in utero infection. This hypothesis was supported by the detection of elevated serum immunoglobulin G levels in up to 50% of stillborn pigs, and by the absence of disease in pigs after the immediate postweaning period or in sows farrowing affected litters [1].

The pestiviruses are well-recognised reproductive pathogens with the outcome of infection being dependent on a number of factors, including the stage of gestation that the infection occurs in relation to organogenesis and the development of immune competence [5–12]. CSFV has historically been the main pestivirus recognised to infect pigs (although infections with bovine viral diarrhoea virus (BVDV) and border disease virus (BDV) have been identified), and low virulence strains of CSFV may cause in utero infection and reproductive losses in the absence of disease in the rest of the herd [13–18].

Subsequent to the discovery of Bungowannah virus, two more pestiviral infections of pigs have been described: APPV [3] and Linda virus [4]. Both viruses have been associated with congenital tremors in piglets [4,10,19].

While there is strong epidemiological, virological [20] and preliminary experimental [21] evidence that Bungowannah virus is the causative agent of the PMC syndrome, the disease has not been reproduced experimentally. In an accompanying report [22], we described the virological and serological characteristics following the successful infection of the porcine foetus at four different stages of gestation. Regardless of the stage of gestation at which infection occurred, Bungowannah virus was detected in the serum/body fluid and excretions of infected pigs at birth and this was unrelated to the presence or absence of a precolostral Bungowannah virus-specific antibody in these animals. Persistent infections, as described for other pestiviruses, were observed following infection of the dam at 35 days of gestation, as was a chronic infection state where animals that had been presumed to be persistently infected (PI) following infection of the dam at 55 days later seroconverted. Viraemia, virus detection in tissues and viral shedding cleared more rapidly the later in gestation that infection occurred.

The aim of the current study was to determine whether infection of pregnant pigs with Bungowannah virus at different stages of gestation induces the clinical signs and gross pathology of PMC in the progeny that were observed during the initial outbreak. An in-depth description of the histopathological findings will be reported separately.

2. Materials and Methods

2.1. Study Design

Twenty-four pregnant pigs (22 gilts and two parity-1 sows) with known joining dates were obtained from a piggery known to be free of Bungowannah virus. Full details of the management of these pigs are described in a companion paper [22]. Pregnancy was confirmed using an ultrasound examination prior to selection for the study. The pigs were challenged intranasally at approximately 35 (34–36), 55 (55–58), 75 (72–76) or 90 (90–92) days of gestation ($n = 6$ per group—referred to as D35, D55, D75 and D90; Table 1). These time-points were selected as they were similar to those used in a previous study where foetuses were directly inoculated [21] and they span the gestational age at which the pig foetus is considered to become immunocompetent (70 days). All pregnancies were allowed to proceed to 113 days of gestation; then, all pigs were induced to farrow on day 114 to optimise the collection of blood from piglets prior to suckling.

Table 1. Summary of challenge details and reproductive outcomes following the inoculation of pregnant pigs with Bungowannah virus.

Group [1]	Sow Number (Litter ID)	Day of Gestation at Challenge	Day of Farrowing	Born Alive	Stillborn/AutolySing (%)	Mummified (%)	Total Litter Size	Preweaning Losses (%)	Number Weaned	Comments
D35	4558 (15)	34	112	8	1 (7%)	5 (36%)	14	8 (100%)	0	
D35	4536 (17)	34	114	7	6 (46%)	0 (0%)	13	2 (29%)	5	
D35	4540 (12)	35	111	7	3 (25%)	2 (17%)	12	7 (100%)	0	
D35	4596 (16)	35	114	4	4 (40%)	2 (20%)	10	3 (75%)	1	
D35	4570 (14)	36	114	9	0 (0%)	2 (18%)	11	4 (44%)	5	
Mean				**7.0**	**24%**	**18%**	**12**	**70%**	**2.2**	
D55	4261 (10)	55	114	11	1 (8%)	0 (0%)	12	2 (18%)	9	
D55	325 (11)	55	114	13	2 (13%)	0 (0%)	15	3 (23%)	10	Parity 1; pig 11-15 not infected
D55	4409 (8)	56	114	6	2 (25%)	0 (0%)	8	0 (0%)	6	
D55	4268 (7)	58	114	11	0 (0%)	0 (0%)	11	2 (18%)	6	3 piglets savaged
Mean				**10.3**	**12%**	**0%**	**11.5**	**15%**	**7.8**	
D75	4294 (3)	73	114	11	0	0	11	3 (27%)	8	
D75	4300 (4)	73	114	7	1	2	10	0 (0%)	7	
D75	4486 (5)	73	114	10	1	0	11	0 (0%)	0 [2]	10 piglets savaged/poor milk production
D75	4279 (1)	76	110	11	3	0	14	0 (0%)	0 [2]	11 piglets savaged
D75	4281 (2)	76	114	7	5	0	12	0 (0%)	7	
Mean				**9.2**	**16%**	**4%**	**11.6**	**5%**	**7.3**	
D90	739 (18)	90	111	6	3	1	10	1 (17%)	1	4 piglets savaged
D90	735 (22)	90	113	9	2	0	11	5 (56%)	4	
D90	738 (23)	90	114	10	1	0	11	0 (0%)	10	
D90	736 (20)	91	112	9	3	0	12	2 (22%)	7	
D90	2622 (21)	91	114	10	0	0	10	4 (40%)	6	
D90	2623 (19)	92	113	8	0	0	8	3 (38%)	5	
Mean				**8.7**	**14%**	**2%**	**10.3**	**29%**	**5.5**	
D35	35 (13)	36	114	13	3	1	17	1 (8%)	12	NI [3]; Parity 1
D55	4260 (9)	56	114	11	2	2	15	4 (38%)	6	NI; 1 death due to accident
D75	4292 (6)	72	114	10	0	0	10	1 (10%)	9	NI
Mean				**11.3**	**10%**	**6%**	**14.0**	**18%**	**9**	

[1] One sow from the D55 group did not farrow and has been excluded from the table. [2] Excluded from mean. [3] Litter not infected.

At birth, all pigs were weighed, their crown–rump lengths recorded, individually identified with ear tags and had their litter identity recorded. They were given an iron supplement intramuscularly between 2 and 4 days of age.

Farrowing outcomes, including the number of progeny born alive, stillborn or mummified, were recorded for each litter. Signs of disease observed throughout the study were documented.

Pigs from infected litters were weaned when they were 21–25 days old. As the presence of Bungowannah virus could still be detected at weaning in several challenge groups, as many pigs as the secure containment facilities could hold were weaned and retained until at least 8 weeks old. Selected pigs from D35 and D55 were kept in the study for a longer period to monitor clinical signs and virological and serological parameters [22]. Throughout the study, pigs that were moribund, not feeding or did not appear to be viable were euthanased.

Pigs from the three litters that did not become infected with Bungowannah virus (on the basis that the virus could not be detected in serum or body fluid for any of the pigs in the litter in a real-time reverse-transcription polymerase chain reaction (qRT-PCR) assay and negative precolostral serology results) were kept as control pigs until 14 to 21 days old, at which time they were euthanased. Because of the logistical considerations associated with the management of breeding sows in a secure containment facility, no mock-inoculated treatment group was included.

Individual pig IDs have been retained in the text where relevant to facilitate comparison between histopathology and virology and serology findings described in related manuscripts [22]. The first number relates to the litter ID and the second relates to the animal ID within the litter (generally in order of birth), e.g., 8-01 indicates the first pig to be born in litter 8.

All piglets were subjected to a detailed necropsy.

The animal studies were approved by the Animal Ethics Committee of the Elizabeth Macarthur Agricultural Institute, AEC Reference No. M09/02 (6 March 2009).

2.2. Inoculum

The pregnant pigs were challenged with a total of 5.3–5.8 $\log_{10}$ $TCID_{50}$ of Bungowannah virus in 5 mL of phosphate-buffered gelatin saline (2.5 mL per nostril), with the exception of litter 11, where the sow only received approximately 3.8 $\log_{10}$ $TCID_{50}$ of the virus. This inoculum was prepared as previously described [22,23].

2.3. Statistics

The confounding effect of treatment due to the separate cohorts was considered. The proportions of live, stillborn, mummified (of total born), weaned and lost/died pigs were analysed using a generalised linear model (GLM) as quasi-binomial (allowing for additional variation between sows). Each model included the time of challenge as a fixed effect. For the crown–rump length and birth weight data, a mixed model was fitted, with the time of challenge as a fixed effect, as well as random sow effects.

All calculations were performed with the R statistical software [24] using the glm function to fit the GLM model or the ASReml-R library [25] to fit the mixed models for length and weight.

3. Results

All 24 pigs challenged became infected. One pig from D55 failed to farrow and was not pregnant. As previously reported, the foetuses of 20/23 (87%) of the infected dams became infected with Bungowannah virus, as determined by the detection of Bungowannah virus nucleic acid using qRT-PCR in serum or body fluid at birth [22]. Within the 20 infected litters, 226 pigs (including stillborn and mummified foetuses) were born, of which, 225 had been infected in utero [22]. As all infected pigs were viraemic at birth, where individual animals are mentioned, reference is only made to their precolostral antibody level at birth. Three litters (n = 42 pigs) were uninfected at birth (as determined by negative qRT-PCR and precolostral serology results) and remained uninfected for the duration they remained in the study (14–21 days).

There were no significant differences in the crown–rump length ($p = 0.594$) and birth weight ($p = 0.180$) of pigs in the four treatment groups and uninfected litters.

3.1. *Incidence of Stillbirths, Preweaning Deaths and Mummified Pigs*

The day of gestation that the pregnant animals were challenged and their reproductive outcomes, including preweaning losses are summarised in Table 1. The greatest effects of infection were observed in the litters of dams infected at 35 or 90 days of gestation. While the use of cohorts confounded results, significant differences were associated with the time of challenge for the proportion born alive (of total) ($p = 0.029$) and proportion mummified ($p = 0.008$), where these values are lower and higher for the D35 group, respectively. For live-born pigs, there were significant differences between challenge groups in the proportion of preweaning losses ($p = 0.004$). The preweaning losses were significantly higher for D35 (there was also a numerically higher mean for D90 compared with D55 and D75; however, this was not statistically significant).

3.2. *Clinical Signs*

Table 2 summarises the reproductive effects, the likelihood of development of persistent infections and the most common clinical signs and necropsy findings observed in the progeny of sows following in utero infection with Bungowannah virus at different stages of gestation.

Table 2. Summary of the reproductive effects, and most common clinical signs and necropsy findings following in utero infection with Bungowannah virus.

			Clinical Signs		Necropsy Findings	
Day of Gestation at Challenge	Reproductive Effects [1]	Persistent Infections? [2]	Preweaning	Postweaning	Preweaning	Postweaning
35 days	Born alive ↓↓↓ Stillbirths ↑↑ Mummified foetuses ↑↑↑ Preweaning deaths ↑↑↑	Yes (>90%)	Purpura, subcutaneous oedema, absence of facial whiskers, weak-born pigs that did not suckle, neurological signs—abnormal behaviour	Stunting, pallor due to anaemia, conjunctivitis, subcutaneous facial skin mass, leukopaenia, thrombocytopaenia, purplish discolouration of the snout and ears, ecchymoses in the skin of the hind-quarter	Purpura, subcutaneous oedema, white foci in the cerebrum, orange/mottled liver, fibrinous adhesions in pleural and abdominal cavities (older animals)	Blood clots and serosanguinous fluid in abdomen/thoracic cavities, petechiae, red/haemorrhagic lymph nodes, ulcerated tonsils, facial mass
55 days	Stillbirths ↑	At birth, 18% were seronegative to Bungowannah virus and apparently persistently infected. The 3 seronegative animals retained postweaning later seroconverted	Melaena, pallor, ataxia	Stunting of apparently persistently infected pigs, occasional diarrhoea	Occasional fibrinous adhesions in thoracic and abdominal cavities	No significant findings
75 days	Stillbirths ↑	No	No disease observed	No disease observed	No significant findings	No significant findings
90 days	Stillbirths ↑ Preweaning deaths ↑↑	No	Sudden death, tachypnoea and dyspnoea	No disease observed	Cardiomegally, liver enlargement, fibrin tags in the thoracic and/or abdominal cavities, blood clots in abdominal cavity, pericardial/thoracic effusions, red/haemorrhagic mesenteric and/or inguinal lymph nodes	No significant findings

[1] ↑—mild increase, ↑↑—moderate increase, ↑↑↑—marked increase, ↓↓↓—marked decrease. [2] [22].

3.2.1. Group D35

The exposure of the pregnant animals at around 35 days of gestation resulted in a high percentage of infected pigs that were seronegative (96%) and presumably persistently infected at birth [22]. Clinically, a high proportion of stillborn (24%) and mummified pigs (18%) and a very high level of preweaning mortalities (70%) resulted (Table 1). The live-born pigs in these litters were often very weak, had difficulties moving from the rear of the sow after birth and some showed a limited ability to suckle. Many died soon after birth or were overlain, presumably as a consequence of their weakness or were euthanased due to their inability to feed. Additional abnormalities observed at birth in both stillborn and live-born pigs included purpura extending over the skin (n = 15) (Figure 1a,b) and/or subcutaneous oedema, particularly extending over the head, neck and ventral abdomen (n = 9) (Figure 1c). Pigs born with subcutaneous oedema had poor viability. All nine died soon after birth, were weak and were overlain or were euthanased on humane grounds within 3 days of birth. Mild subcutaneous oedema was noted in an additional two pigs at necropsy at 3 and 11 days of age. Of the four pigs with purpura that survived to be weaned, the purpura resolved with age and three of the four appeared to grow normally until weaning, although two developed conjunctivitis at approximately 3 weeks of age. They subsequently died or were euthanased when 26, 34, 35 and 57 days old. Several pigs exhibited neurological signs at birth, including walking into walls (14-04) and screaming, due to an inability to find the udder despite being able to suckle (most of litter 12). One pig (14-04) also developed haemorrhagic diarrhoea in the first week of life that resolved following antibiotic treatment. Three pigs developed diarrhoea in the first week of life, two of which were cross-fostered from their original mother due to milk supply issues, presumably due to poor udder stimulation from weak piglets and were ultimately euthanased (12-02, 12-05) by 2 weeks of age, and a third that had diarrhoea for 3–4 days that resolved following antibiotic treatment and then died suddenly 6 days later (16-02). One 2-week-old pig was euthanased as it failed to grow.

From the five infected litters, eleven pigs survived to weaning and were monitored until approximately 11 weeks old. Of these 11 pigs, nine were considered PI with Bungowannah virus based on ongoing viraemia and shedding of the virus throughout the study until death or euthanasia and negative precolostral serology at birth (14-01, 14-02, 14-04, 14-07, 14-09, 16-07, 17-01, 17-03, 17-04) [22]. The PI pigs grew poorly compared to their two cohorts (17-02, 17-06), which were not PI, based on their precolostral seropositive status at birth [22]. The PI pigs became stunted from soon after weaning (Figure 1d) and exhibited generalised skin pallor from 7 weeks of age. The first pig (17-03) was euthanased within 4 days of weaning after the sudden onset of recumbency; mouth breathing with a small amount of purulent nasal discharge; and purplish skin discolouration of the snout, ears, ventral abdomen and hind quarters (Figure 1e,f). Conjunctivitis was an ongoing problem in two pigs (17-01, 17-04). In addition, three pigs developed firm subcutaneous masses under their eyes between 5 and 9 weeks of age, which forced the lower eyelid dorsally, leaving them unable to open the affected eye (16-07, 17-01, 17-04) (Figure 1g); another developed an erosive lip lesion that resolved following antibiotic treatment at 6 weeks old (14-09). Investigation of the pallor diagnosed anaemia and only the PI pigs were affected. When sampled at 8 weeks old, the packed cell volume of the five affected animals ranged from 8% to 21% (reference interval for weaner pigs 26–41%; [26]). The low levels of circulating reticulocytes (0–0.4%) (corrected reticulocyte percentages <1%) and the normal mean corpuscular volume indicated that the anaemias were non-regenerative and normocytic. In addition, three animals were leukopaenic [26] and three were thrombocytopaenic. While one PI pig survived to 75 days of age (14-01), the remaining PI pigs that did not succumb to other problems were ultimately euthanased due to severe anaemia.

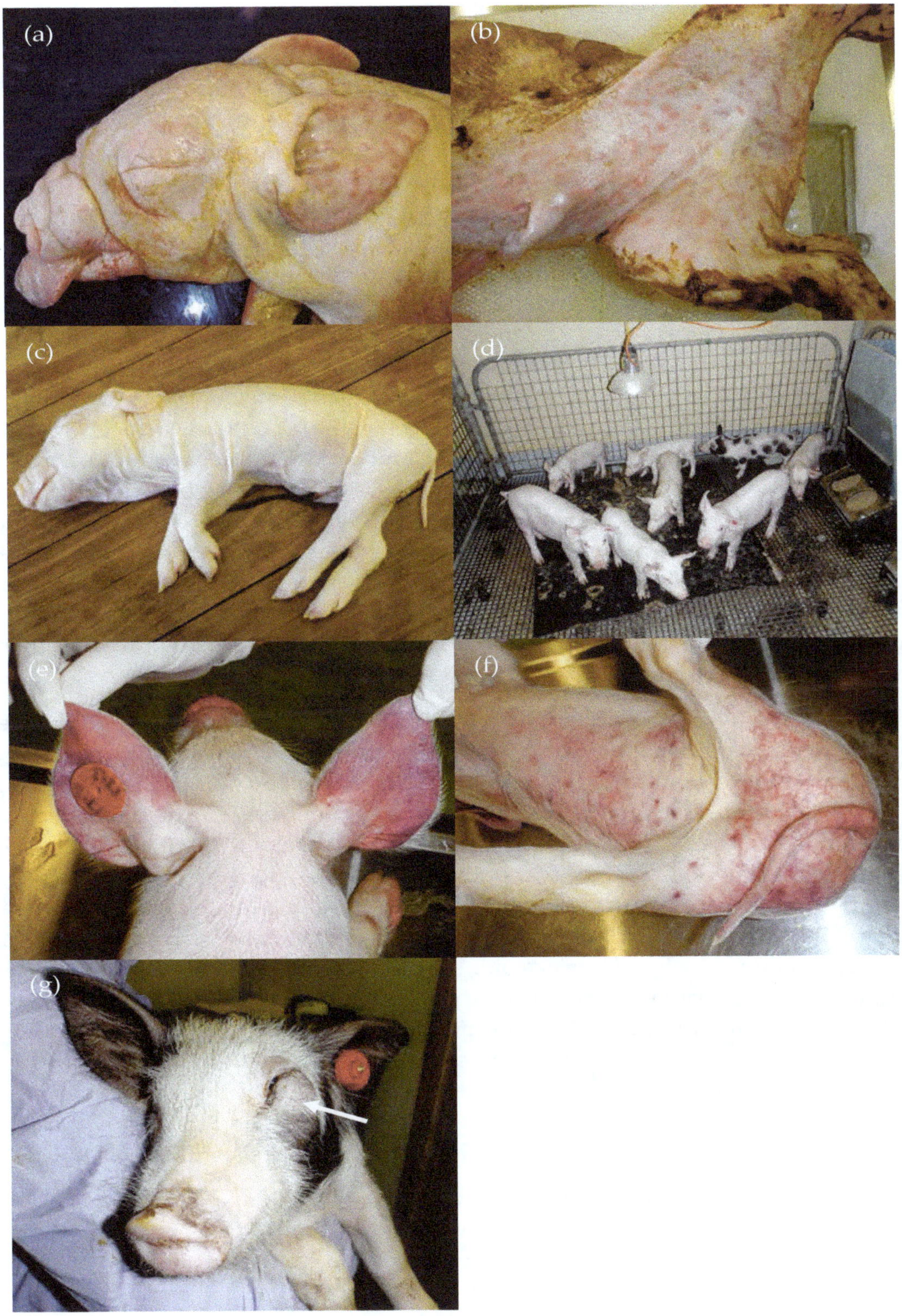

Figure 1. Clinical signs observed in D35 pigs: (**a**) purpura, subcutaneous oedema and absence of facial whiskers (12-09, stillborn); (**b**) purpura (17-11, stillborn); (**c**) subcutaneous oedema—most evident ventrally (12-10, 1 day old); (**d**) remaining pigs at 7 weeks of age with stunting of 6 smaller pigs compared with the 2 larger, non-PI pigs; (**e**) 26-day-old pig with purplish discolouration of the ears and snout (17-03); (**f**) same pig as (e) with purplish discolouration ventrally and on hind-quarters; and (**g**) 16-07 (62 days old) with mass under left eye, resulting in closure of the eyelids (arrow).

3.2.2. Group D55

There were no clear reproductive effects observed following infection at approximately 55 days gestation (Table 1), with 82% of the infected pigs being seropositive at birth. Two of the stillborn pigs that were seronegative [22] exhibited mild subcutaneous oedema, although the significance is unclear as they were also moderately autolysed. In the immediate postnatal period (first 2 days of life), deaths were attributed to savaging ($n = 3$), overlay ($n = 3$) and runts ($n = 1$). Commencing at about one week after birth, in two litters, four pigs had dark faeces on a rectal swab that was consistent with melaena, suggesting upper gastrointestinal tract bleeding (7-10, 7-11, 10-04, 10-12) and one pig passed bloody liquid at the time of sampling (10-10) (the precolostral antibody titres for 10-04 and 10-10 were 10 and 80 respectively; the three other pigs had suckled prior to the initial sampling). Melaena was detected again on a rectal swab at 14 days of age in one of these pigs (7-11). This pig exhibited pallor, grew poorly compared to its littermates and was euthanased when it failed to gain weight and was unable to compete for food. Another pig (10-12) also grew poorly after melaena was detected at 6 days of age and was euthanased rather than weaned. The third pig (10-04) with melaena grew normally until 13 days old but then grew little in the following week, and at 20 days old, it exhibited pallor and mild jaundice. It was weaned at 28 days, and at this time, it was still growing poorly and exhibiting mild hind limb ataxia. At 19 days old, one pig (7-06; precolostral antibody titre of 1280) was pyrexic (40.7 °C), mildly ataxic with a slight tremor and showed retarded growth compared to its littermates. Despite antibiotic treatment, it was still pyrexic (40.2 °C) 2 days later and continued to exhibit neurological signs, including poor balance with a wide base stance; there was no obvious head tilt or nystagmus. It was noticed that one pig from litter 8 (8-01; seronegative at birth) appeared weaker than the other pigs in its litter in the first couple of days of life and was sometimes slow to move to the teat to feed.

In litters 7 ($n = 4$), 8 ($n = 3$, including 8-01 and 8-05) and 10 ($n = 5$, including 10-01), the pigs with the highest viral loads in serum and oropharyngeal secretions at 2 weeks of age, as well as all pigs surviving to weaning age from litter 11 ($n = 10$), were weaned to clarify whether the ongoing viraemia was due to a persistent infection, given that the dams were infected prior to the expected timing of foetal immunocompetence [22]. All weaned pigs were raised until at least 10 weeks old. Disease was not observed during this period, with the exception of occasional diarrhoea, and at 6.5 and 8 weeks of age, 10-04 had two episodes of pyrexia and lethargy, which responded well to antibiotic treatment on both occasions. The most dramatic clinical difference was the variation in size of the littermates from litter 8 (Figure 2) and litter 10 when 11 weeks old. Across both of these litters, five pigs were live born and seronegative for Bungowannah virus antibody [22]. The two small pigs (Figure 2; 8-01 and 8-05) appeared to be PI on the basis of qRT-PCR results and the absence of antibodies against Bungowannah virus at birth and were markedly stunted compared to their non-PI littermates (seropositive at birth). When 6 to 7 months old, Bungowannah virus RNA could no longer be detected in the serum of these stunted animals; they concurrently developed high antibody titres and their growth rate improved markedly and they are described here as chronically rather than persistently infected [22].

One of the stunted pigs was reared until 6 months of age (10-01), and another two until 11 months of age (8-01 and 8-05). At approximately 3.5 months old, 8-01 and 10-01 experienced an episode of diarrhoea due to a *Salmonella* infection, but otherwise, no disease was observed. At 189 days of age, pig 10-01 weighed 105 kg; at 11 months of age, 8-01 and 8-05 weighed 183 and 153 kg respectively.

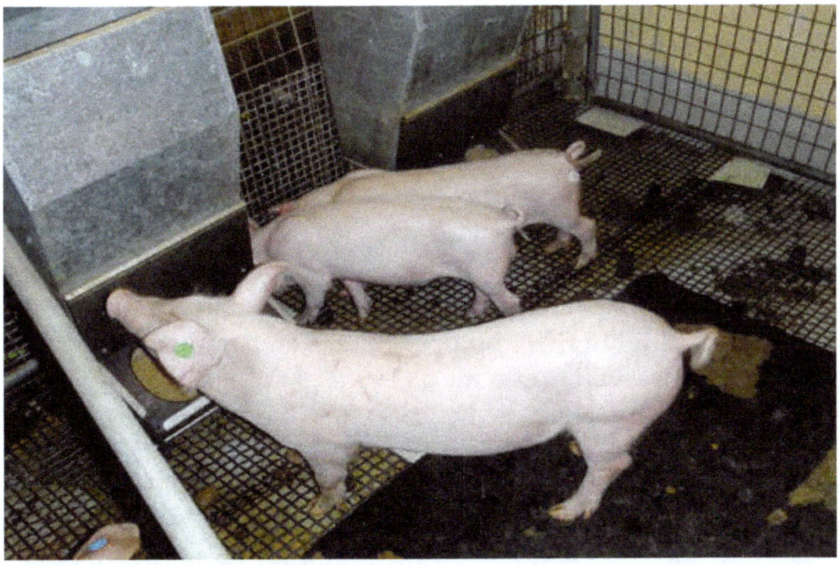

Figure 2. Littermates from litter 8 in D55 at 77 days old—note the stunting of two chronically infected littermates (8-01 and 8-05) compared with the larger non-persistently or chronically infected animal (8-03).

3.2.3. Group D75

Losses in the preweaning period were the result of savaging ($n = 18$), overlay ($n = 2$), splay leg ($n = 1$), runt ($n = 1$) and poor mothering/milk production ($n = 2$) and occurred in the first week of life (Table 1). Pigs surviving to weaning did not exhibit any signs of disease and 98% of the infected pigs were seropositive at birth [22].

After weaning, several pigs lost condition compared to others in the group and one developed a skin infection. Otherwise, no disease was observed. No postweaning mortalities occurred and 23 pigs in this group were reared up to 8 weeks of age.

3.2.4. Group D90

Preweaning losses (29%) in this group were higher compared to the D55 and D75 groups (Table 1) and were clinically different from the D35 group. Only 50% of the infected pigs were seropositive at birth, presumably because of the short interval between infection and birth [22]. While some losses due to savaging ($n = 4$) and overlay ($n = 1$) were recorded, some pigs also exhibited tachypnoea and dyspnoea prior to death or euthanasia. Sudden death was recorded for seven apparently healthy pigs between 2 and 5 days of age without any prior signs (19-03, 19-07, 20-04, 22-03, 22-05, 22-06 and 22-08).

Six pigs developed a notable increase in respiratory rate and effort (19-02, 20-06, 21-02, 21-03, 21-09 and 23-11). The earliest onset of respiratory signs was at 4 days and the latest at 7 days old. Three pigs were euthanased due to the severity of their clinical signs. Two pigs, one of which was thinner than its littermates, died 5 days after the detection of an increased respiratory rate. Finally, one pig continued to exhibit an increased respiratory rate when stressed and was thinner than its littermates through to weaning and subsequently to 5 weeks age.

Twenty pigs from this group were weaned and reared up to 5 weeks of age. No disease was evident in these animals.

3.2.5. Uninfected Litters

No disease was observed with the exception of diarrhoea in one pig. The only preweaning losses were due to overlay ($n = 2$), splay leg ($n = 3$), runt ($n = 1$) and accident ($n = 1$) (Table 1). While there was no statistical difference in birth weight between the infected and uninfected litters, the mean weight for the uninfected litters at approximately 7 and 14 days of age was 0.5–0.8 kg and 0.6–1.1 kg greater, respectively.

3.3. *Necropsy Findings*

Table 2 summarises the most common gross pathology findings observed following in utero infection with Bungowannah virus at different stages of gestation. The viral load in tissues at necropsy was dependent on the stage of gestation that infection occurred in, whether the pig was able to mount an immune response in utero and the age of the pig at necropsy [22].

3.3.1. Group D35

Subcutaneous oedema was observed in nine pigs and was most commonly observed ventrally and around the head and neck, giving rise to palpebral oedema and the impression of a Roman nose (Figure 1a,c). Petechiae were observed on the hearts of two stillborn pigs. Purpura (pigs 0 to 3 days old) were most easily identified on the ears, head, ventral abdomen and sometimes on the dorsal body (Figure 1a,b). Petechiae were observed on the pleural surface of the lungs of an overlain pig. White pin-point foci were observed throughout the brain of one stillborn pig (12-09) and a region of presumptive necrosis was observed in the left cerebral hemisphere of another (17-11). Other observations at necropsy in the preweaning period included haemorrhages on the tonsils ($n = 2$) and tongue ($n = 1$), mottled orange liver ($n = 3$) and the absence of facial whiskers ($n = 1$). Red mottled lungs were commonly observed and presumptively attributed to hypostasis. Thoracic and abdominal effusions in stillborn pigs were associated with autolysis. Fibrinous adhesions were observed in the thorax and or abdomen of two pigs that died at 12 and 15 days (both had previously been treated for diarrhoea).

A range of lesions was observed in the PI pigs that survived past weaning. These animals remained viraemic throughout their life, shed high levels of the virus and had high quantities of the virus in all tissues examined at their necropsies [22]. All became severely stunted, with weights ranging at time of euthanasia from 4.0 kg at 34 days to 13.2 kg at 77 days. Two animals (14-04, 14-09) showed evidence of a bleeding disorder, including the presence of clots in the abdominal cavity and serosanguinous fluid/effusion in the thoracic and/or abdominal cavities; blood streaks were observed in the stomach contents of one of these two pigs. Other changes that indicated a bleeding disorder or vasculitis in the PI pigs included red/haemorrhagic inguinal, mesenteric and/or lumbar lymph nodes in four animals; petechiae were occasionally observed on a number of organs, including the heart ($n = 3$), kidney ($n = 2$) (Figure 3a), liver ($n = 1$), serosal surface of the intestines/colon ($n = 2$), peritoneal surface ($n = 1$), cerebellum ($n = 1$) and oropharynx ($n = 1$). Other abnormalities observed included ulcerated tonsils (16-07) (Figure 3b), increased pericardial fluid ($n = 4$; up to 20 mL), cobblestone pattern to the liver ($n = 1$), mild pulmonary interlobular oedema ($n = 4$) and fibrin tags on intestinal serosa ($n = 1$). The facial mass observed in three pigs (Figure 1g) was firm with an intimate connection between the skin and the subcutis. There was no evidence of wounds in the skin or oral cavity connecting with the mass. Mild subcutaneous oedema was detected in the neck of one pig.

No abnormalities were detected in the two pigs that were not PI (17-02 and 17-06) [22]. At 75 days of age, their mean weight was 30.75 kg. Only low quantities of Bungowannah virus were detectable in these two animals at necropsy [22].

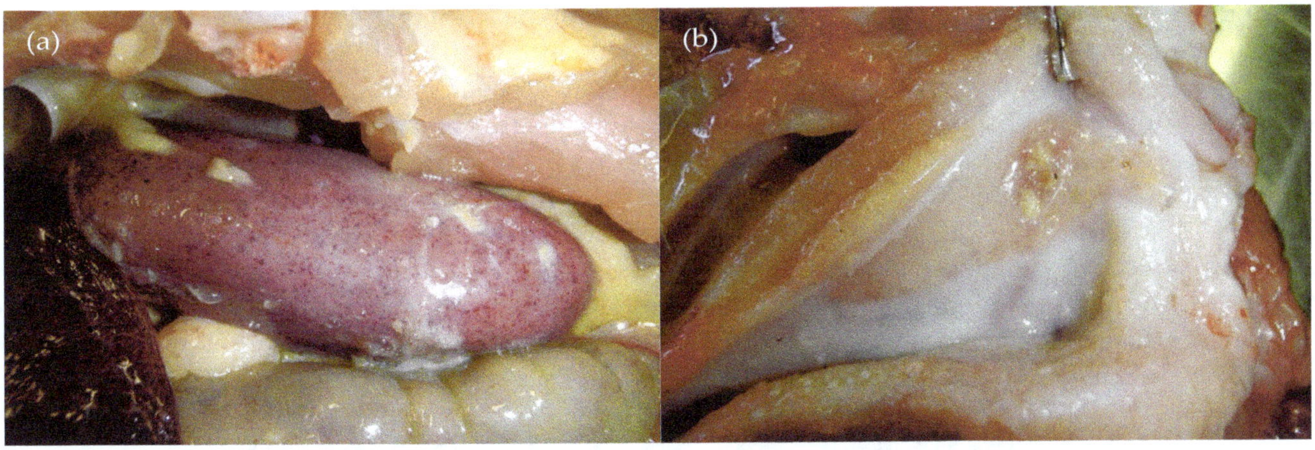

Figure 3. Necropsy findings from D35: (**a**) petechiation of a kidney (17-03—same pig as Figure 1e,f) and (**b**) ulcerated tonsil (16-07).

3.3.2. Group D55

Serosanginous pleural and abdominal fluid, as well as mild subcutaneous oedema, was noted in two stillborn pigs that exhibited autolytic changes. Pericardial petechiation was observed in one stillborn pig. Mild interlobular pulmonary oedema and congestion was observed in the lungs of six animals (ages 2–22 days) and was considered to be due to hypostasis. One animal had fibrinous pleural and abdominal adhesions, and another, fibrinous adhesions between the spleen and the liver; both suffered a preweaning death. Other lesions included a cobblestone pattern on the liver, kidney enlargement, oedematous spiral colon and dark blood clots in the colon.

The two chronically infected pigs (8-01 and 8-05) [22] were reared to 11 months of age. Few abnormalities were observed at necropsy. The testes of 8-01 were soft on palpation, fluid collected from the epididymis was of low opacity and sperm were not observed via a microscopic examination, suggesting infertility. The highest viral load detected throughout this study was in the epididymal semen of this animal (9.8 $\log_{10}$ copies/mL) [22]. Pig 8-05 was female and penned with 8-01 from 4 months old. From 8 months old, she was observed in oestrus approximately every 3 weeks and did not become pregnant. This was confirmed at necropsy, and an examination of her ovaries showed many follicles and multiple corpora lutea, indicating reproductive maturity.

3.3.3. Group D75

No significant gross pathology was observed for this group. Occasionally petechiae in the heart wall ($n = 2$; stillborn pigs) and consolidated lung lobules ($n = 6$; presumptively due to hypostasis) were observed. Serosanginous pleural and abdominal fluid was noted in two stillborn pigs that exhibited autolytic changes. Bungowannah virus was cleared relatively rapidly from this group, with only low viral loads generally detected after 21–28 days of age [22].

3.3.4. Group D90

Serosanguinous thoracic or abdominal effusions were observed in stillborn pigs with autolytic changes ($n = 3$). Occasional petechiation of the pericardium was also observed ($n = 1$). Two stillborn pigs had fibrin tags in the peritoneal cavity and equivocally enlarged hearts (18-07, 18-08), while another had red tonsils.

Of the preweaning mortalities, four of the five pigs observed to have increased respiratory rates exhibited cardiomegaly (20-06, 21-02, 21-03, 21-09) based on subjective observation of an increased base to apex height and increased sternal contact (Figure 4a), and two 5 mm white foci were observed in the superficial myocardium of 20-6. The fifth pig had a marked haemorrhagic pericardial effusion (>50 mL) and blood clots in the abdominal cavity (19-02) (Figure 4b). Thoracic and/or abdominal effusions ($n = 2$), fibrin tags in the thoracic and/or abdominal cavity ($n = 2$), liver enlargement ($n = 4$), reddened inguinal and mesenteric lymph nodes ($n = 3$) and oedema of the spiral colon ($n = 3$) were also observed amongst these five cases. The lungs of the most severely affected pigs did not deflate and a large amount of fluid/froth drained from the lungs after death. Viral RNA was detected in the hearts of all pigs sampled in the first 10 days of life [22]. The pigs that died suddenly (19-03, 19-07, 20-04, 22-03, 22-05, 22-06 and 22-08) appeared to be behaving normally and eating well prior to death. Bruising to suggest they had been overlain was not observed. A range of changes was observed, including subcutaneous oedema of the ventral neck ($n = 2$), pericardial effusion ($n = 1$), fibrin tags in thoracic and/or abdominal cavities ($n = 2$), blood clots in the abdominal cavity ($n = 2$), petechiae and haemorrhages on the kidney ($n = 1$), red/haemorrhagic mesenteric and/or inguinal lymph nodes ($n = 3$), haemorrhages on the spiral colon and caecum ($n = 2$) and oedema of the spiral colon ($n = 1$).

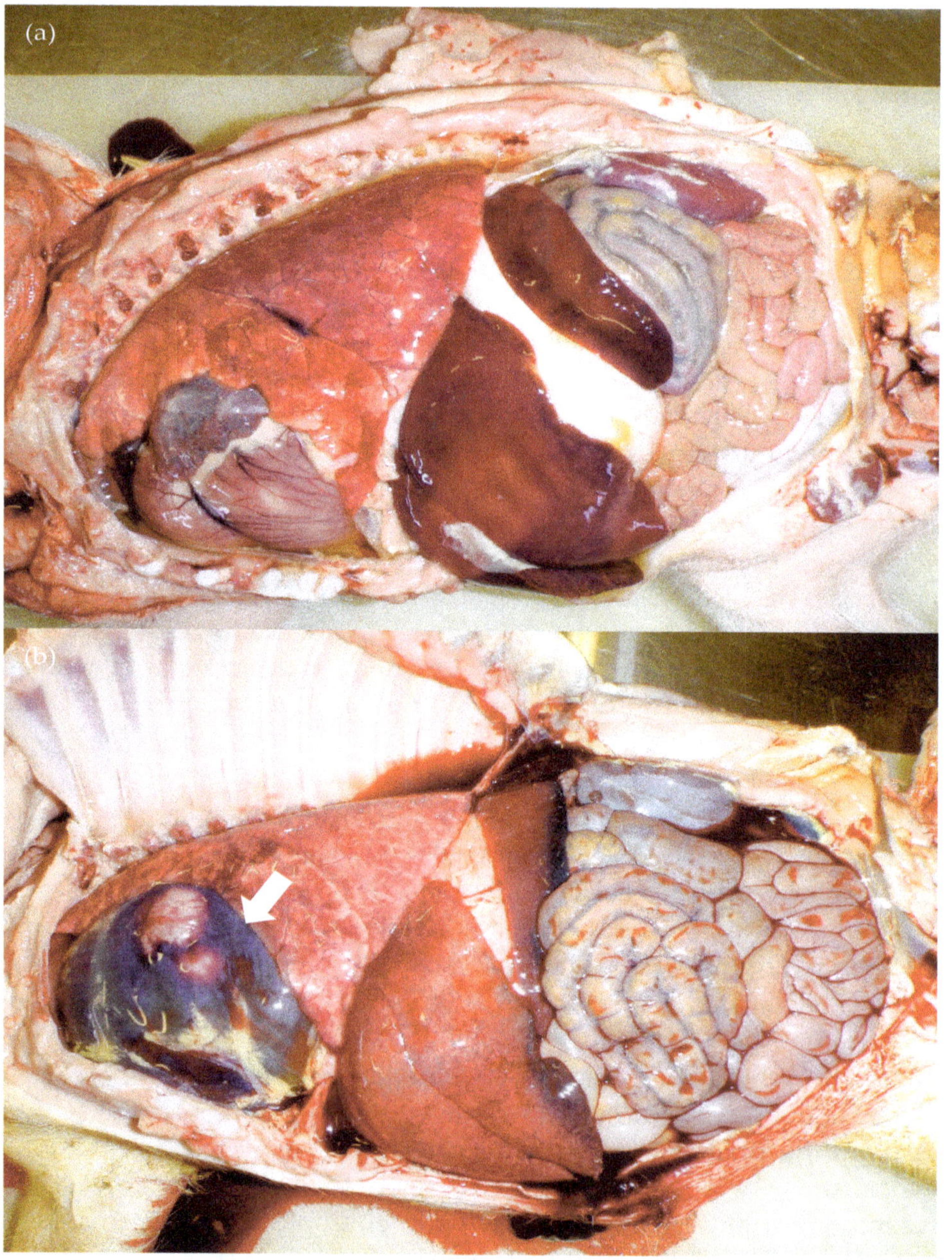

Figure 4. Necropsy findings from D90: (**a**) cardiac and hepatic enlargement (20-06; 7 days old) and (**b**) free blood in the unopened pericardial sac (arrow) and abdomen (19-02; 12 days old).

From weaning to termination of the monitoring at 5 weeks of age, few gross lesions were observed. Bungowannah virus was cleared most rapidly from this group with virus shedding and the viral loads in tissues were only at low levels from 11 days of age or often not detected at all [22]. Interlobular pulmonary oedema was observed in two animals and fine fibrin tags were observed in the peritoneal cavity of five animals. The pig that exhibited an increased respiratory rate after exercise and survived to 5 weeks old (23-11) also showed mild interlobular pulmonary oedema and a smaller than expected thymus, but did not have definite cardiac enlargement. However, the ventricular walls appeared thinner than normal, suggesting possible cardiac dilation.

3.3.5. Uninfected Litters

No significant abnormalities were observed at necropsy in pigs from this group. The ages of pigs examined ranged from stillborn to 21 days old. The most frequent changes observed were reddening of the lungs (presumptively due to hypostasis), with some interlobular oedema in four pigs. Other changes observed included petechial haemorrhages on the pericardium, tonsil and skull of an overlain pig, a moderate increase in the amount of thoracic fluid of stillborn pigs, circular skin deficits over the left carpus of two stillborn pigs in litter 9 and moderately enlarged inguinal lymph nodes in a splay-legged pig.

4. Discussion

In this study, the clinical signs and gross pathological lesions observed during the outbreak of the porcine myocarditis syndrome were reproduced in the progeny of pregnant pigs experimentally infected with Bungowannah virus. The disease and lesions associated with in utero Bungowannah virus infection at different gestational ages were further characterised. Infection of the foetus at 35 or 90 days gestation resulted in the most severe clinical and pathological effects.

Losses in the field due to PMC were characterised by increased stillbirths, preweaning losses and to a lesser extent, mummified foetuses. At the peak of the outbreak on the farm, on the most severely affected production unit (a gilt unit), preweaning losses approached 50%, stillbirths 40% and mummified foetuses 10–15%, although losses did vary across production units [1,27]. The results of the current study indicated that Bungowannah virus is capable of causing these effects and, depending on the presence of sows at critical stages of pregnancy, could cause significant reproductive losses if introduced into a naïve piggery. The two most critical time-points for exposure of the pregnant pig in relation to disease appears to be around 35 and 90 days of gestation. Our observations following infection at these stages of gestation are consistent with events observed during the early stages of the PMC outbreak, which suggests that the introduction of the virus occurred at a single time-point. The first losses observed were sudden death at 2–3 weeks of age, which is consistent with the outcomes of experimental infection at around 90 days gestation. These initial losses were followed approximately 4 weeks later by a marked increase in the number of stillborn pigs, which would indicate infection at around 40–50 days gestation if 90 days is considered the critical time-point for sudden death at 2–3 weeks of age [20,27].

The description of porcine myocarditis syndrome arose from the fact that early in the field outbreak, affected animals often had an enlarged/dilated heart with evidence of congestive heart failure and non-suppurative myocarditis [1]. Based on the results of this study, it appears that the cardiac enlargement previously reported occurs principally following infection in late gestation (approximately 90 days) and results in a moderate increase in preweaning losses. This was the only challenge group where the previously described [1] multifocal, non-suppurative myocarditis with myonecrosis was observed [28]. Based on these findings, it is clear that the outcome of infection with Bungowannah virus and the associated pathological changes are more extensive than the original field description "porcine myocarditis syndrome" would suggest. Clinically, similar to the field cases, sudden death or increased respiratory rate and effort were observed. Unlike the field situation, cyanosis of the snout and ears and excessive vocalisation before death were not observed during the course of this study.

The cardiorespiratory signs and sudden deaths observed have not been reported for CSFV, APPV or Linda viruses, the other pestiviruses primarily infecting pigs. Postnatal deaths are uncommon following infection after 90 days gestation with low virulence strains of CSFV [13,29].

The reproductive effects of in utero infection with Bungowannah virus were most severe following infection around 35 days gestation and are presumably a consequence of the foetus being unable to mount an immune response to the virus at this stage of gestation [22]. These effects included a marked increase in preweaning mortalities (particularly in the first few days of life) and mummified foetuses, as well as a moderate to marked increase in stillbirths, all of which suggests that these effects in the field were the result of infection around 35 days of gestation, reducing by day 55. These clinical findings are similar to those observed following in utero infections with low virulence strains of CSFV that, prior to 70 days gestation, are characterised by high prenatal mortality due to stillborn and mummified foetuses, and increased postnatal mortality with weak-born pigs, although congenital deformities were not observed for Bungowannah virus [13,29–31]. The increased levels of stillbirths following exposure of the dam at 55, 75 or 90 days gestation during this study, when compared with industry targets, suggests that Bungowannah virus may have also caused a mild to moderate increase in the stillbirth rate at these time-points, although a greater number of pregnant animals would need to be studied to confirm this finding.

Subcutaneous oedema that spread principally over the head and thorax was observed in a proportion of stillborn pigs during the PMC outbreak [1]. Experimentally, this clinical sign was only observed following Bungowannah virus infection in early gestation (approximately 35–55 days). While purpura was not reported in the field, it was observed in 31% of live and stillborn pigs born to dams infected at around 35 days gestation in the current study. Purpura/petechiae/haemorrhages and subcutaneous oedema have also been described following in utero infection with CSFV in foetuses infected before 70 days gestation [13,29–31].

Other clinical similarities between infection with Bungowannah virus at 35 days gestation and in utero CSFV infection prior to 70 days include weak-born pigs that may exhibit or develop poor sucking ability, alopecia, ascites/hydrothorax, petechiae/haemorrhages in organs other than the skin, pallor, diarrhoea, conjunctivitis, anorexia, lethargy or cyanosis of the snout and ears, with some of these changes being observed postweaning [13,29–31]. In contrast, the clinical signs following experimental Bungowannah virus infection at 55 days more closely parallel what is observed when in utero infection with CSFV occurs between 70 and 90 days gestation, which is associated with fewer prenatal deaths [29–31], although some melaena and diarrhoea was observed in the preweaning period. It is not clear whether the diarrhoea and melaena were increased compared to D75 and D90 pigs due to in utero Bungowannah virus infection or is unrelated.

Following the initial postnatal losses in the D35 group, the next major clinical effect noted following Bungowannah virus infection at either 35 or 55 days of gestation was variability in pig size within a litter postweaning. This disparity in size was noted in those pigs that were born seronegative to Bungowannah virus and, on the basis of PCR results, were considered to be persistently infected [22]. Persistent infections with CSFV are recognised following in utero infection before approximately 70 days gestation and with decreasing frequency up to 90 days gestation [13,29,30]. Clinically, CSFV PI pigs that survive past weaning may present similarly to chronic cases of classical swine fever (CSF), where after an initial, albeit slow recovery, they eventually relapse and die. Initially, they may be indistinguishable from uninfected pigs, but at a variable time (usually weeks to months) after weaning, they often develop severe runting and growth retardation, or "late-onset CSF", characterised by increasing anorexia and lethargy, pyrexia, conjunctivitis, dermatitis, locomotion disturbances and intermittent diarrhoea [13,15,30,31]. These clinical signs were generally consistent with those observed in pigs infected with Bungowannah virus at D35 that were considered PI. With the exception of a slightly slower growth rate, these pigs often appeared normal while still suckling, but at a variable time after weaning, developed severe growth retardation. Pallor (due to anaemia) and conjunctivitis were the most frequently observed clinical signs. Ataxia and locomotion disturbances were not observed. In contrast, those pigs that were infected at D55 and were born viraemic, seronegative and survived past weaning, while clearly stunted compared to their littermates, were generally disease-free. Whether this would be the case in the field, where there is greater exposure to pathogens, is not clear.

Two of the pigs (8-01 and 8-05) in the D55 group that were initially considered PI were raised until 11 months of age. Unexpectedly, these two animals seroconverted at approximately 6 months of age and cleared their viraemia, at which point, their growth rate increased [22]. After seroconversion, the gilt started cycling at around 8 months of age, which is older than expected and was presumably delayed due to her stunted growth. These animals are similar to the chronically infected pigs described when pigs were experimentally infected in utero with BDV or BDV-like viruses, or BVDV [14,16]. Similar to our study they also noted an improved growth rate after seroconversion. The reason for this improvement is not clear but it is suggested that the effect on growth is the result of a continuing process and not of an irreversible lesion acquired in early development [14].

Stunting is also observed in cattle PI with BVDV, although some animals may appear normal for several years before succumbing to a disease predominantly induced as a result of the persistent BVDV infection. While not observed during the course of this study, it is important to determine whether pigs persistently or "chronically" infected with Bungowannah virus can remain clinically normal for prolonged periods, as these animals are an ongoing source of infection in the herd and their selection as breeding animals could result in disastrous consequences if they were to be introduced into a naïve herd.

Congenital tremors were not observed in this study or in the field following Bungowannah virus infection. Aside from the absence of congenital tremors, the outcomes of infection of Bungowannah virus and CSFV after foetal infection in early gestation are remarkably similar and presumably have a similar pathogenesis. To date, Bungowannah virus has only been identified in Australia, but as its origin remains unknown, it should be considered in the differential diagnosis in reproductive investigations, especially if CFSV is suspected but has been excluded by laboratory testing.

It was not possible to weigh live animals once they reached 5 kg; therefore, all weights postweaning were obtained at the time of necropsy. In retrospect, weekly weights would have been useful to compare animal weights within litters and in relation to infection and serological status at birth. Any comments on stunting in this manuscript are unfortunately subjective rather than objective and relative to that challenge group cohort/littermates only. Additionally, while qRT-PCR results were typically available within a couple of days after sample collection, the serology (peroxidase-linked assay) was batch-tested at a convenient time [22]. The availability of these results may have been useful when selecting animals to follow postweaning, particularly for the D55 group, to better understand the impact of these "chronic" infections on growth rates. As each treatment group was reared individually and at separate times, direct comparisons regarding weight are difficult; in addition, direct comparisons against commercial growth targets are not appropriate.

5. Conclusions

This study demonstrates that in utero infection with Bungowannah virus was able to produce the clinical signs and gross pathology observed during the field outbreak and has the potential to be a significant reproductive pathogen of the pig, as well as impacting on postnatal mortality, principally in the first few weeks of life. The outcome of infection was dependent on the stage of gestation at which infection occurs. Maternal infection at around 35 days gestation resulted in high pre- and postnatal mortalities, which reduced when infected at about day 55. Reproductive effects and clinical signs were similar to those observed following in utero infection with low virulence strains of CSFV. Increased preweaning mortalities, cardiorespiratory clinical signs and gross lesions in the heart of the progeny of sows infected at around 90 days gestation suggests that infection in late gestation was required for the development of cardiac pathology. Persistent infections resulted in the development of clinical signs and lesions similar to "late-onset" CSFV.

Author Contributions: Conceptualization, D.S.F. and P.D.K.; methodology, D.S.F. and P.D.K.; investigation, D.S.F.; resources, D.S.F. and P.D.K.; data curation, D.S.F.; writing—original draft preparation, D.S.F.; writing—review and editing, D.S.F. and P.D.K.; visualization, D.S.F. and P.D.K.; supervision, P.D.K.; project administration, D.S.F. and P.D.K.; funding acquisition, P.D.K. All authors have read and agreed to the published version of the manuscript.

Acknowledgments: We gratefully acknowledge the staff of the Virology Laboratory at the Elizabeth Macarthur Agricultural Institute (EMAI) for technical assistance and assistance with sample collection, and both farm and laboratory staff, especially Glenda Macnamara, for their care of the animals used in this study. We thank Damien Collins for assistance with statistical analysis, and Sarah Gestier for constructive feedback on the gross pathology descriptions in the manuscript.

References

1. McOrist, S.; Thornton, E.; Peake, A.; Walker, R.; Robson, S.; Finlaison, D.; Kirkland, P.; Reece, R.; Ross, A.; Walker, K.; et al. An infectious myocarditis syndrome affecting late-term and neonatal piglets. *Aust. Vet. J.* **2004**, *82*, 509–511. [CrossRef]
2. Kirkland, P.D.; Frost, M.J.; Finlaison, D.S.; King, K.R.; Ridpath, J.F.; Gu, X. Identification of a novel virus in pigs-Bungowannah virus: A possible new species of pestivirus. *Virus Res.* **2007**, *129*, 26–34. [CrossRef] [PubMed]
3. Hause, B.M.; Collin, E.A.; Peddireddi, L.; Yuan, F.; Chen, Z.; Hesse, R.A.; Gauger, P.C.; Clement, T.; Fang, Y.; Anderson, G. Discovery of a novel putative atypical porcine pestivirus in pigs in the USA. *J. Gen. Virol.* **2015**, *96*, 2994–2998. [CrossRef] [PubMed]
4. Lamp, B.; Schwarz, L.; Hogler, S.; Riedel, C.; Sinn, L.; Rebel-Bauder, B.; Weissenbock, H.; Ladinig, A.; Rumenapf, T. Novel Pestivirus Species in Pigs, Austria, 2015. *Emerg. Infect. Dis.* **2017**, *23*, 1176–1179. [CrossRef] [PubMed]
5. Moennig, V.; Liess, B. Pathogenesis of intrauterine infections with bovine viral diarrhea virus. *Vet. Clin. N. Am. Food Anim. Pract.* **1995**, *11*, 477–487. [CrossRef]
6. Roeder, P.L.; Jeffrey, M.; Cranwell, M.P. Pestivirus fetopathogenicity in cattle: Changing sequelae with fetal maturation. *Vet. Rec.* **1986**, *118*, 44–48. [CrossRef]
7. Baker, J.C. The Clinical Manifestations of Bovine Viral Diarrhea Infection. *Vet. Clin. N. Am. Food A* **1995**, *11*, 425–445. [CrossRef]
8. McGowan, M.R.; Kirkland, P.D. Early reproductive loss due to bovine pestivirus infection. *Br. Vet. J.* **1995**, *151*, 263–270. [CrossRef]
9. Garcia-Perez, A.L.; Minguijon, E.; Estevez, L.; Barandika, J.F.; Aduriz, G.; Juste, R.A.; Hurtado, A. Clinical and laboratorial findings in pregnant ewes and their progeny infected with Border disease virus (BDV-4 genotype). *Res. Vet. Sci.* **2009**, *86*, 345–352. [CrossRef]
10. Arruda, B.L.; Arruda, P.H.; Magstadt, D.R.; Schwartz, K.J.; Dohlman, T.; Schleining, J.A.; Patterson, A.R.; Visek, C.A.; Victoria, J.G. Identification of a Divergent Lineage Porcine Pestivirus in Nursing Piglets with Congenital Tremors and Reproduction of Disease following Experimental Inoculation. *PLoS ONE* **2016**, *11*, e0150104. [CrossRef]
11. Trautwein, G.; Hewicker, M.; Liess, B.; Orban, S.; Grunert, E. Studies on Transplacental Transmissibility of a Bovine Virus Diarrhoea (BVD) Vaccine Virus in Cattle III. Occurrence of Central Nervous System Malformations in Calves Born from Vaccinated Cows. *J. Vet. Med. Ser. B* **1986**, *33*, 260–268. [CrossRef] [PubMed]
12. Nettleton, P.F. Border disease. In *Infectious Diseases of Livestock*, 2nd ed.; Coetzer, J.A.W., Tustin, R.C., Eds.; Oxford University Press Southern Africa: Cape Town, South Africa, 2004; Volume 2, pp. 970–974.
13. Van Oirschot, J.T. Experimental production of congenital persistent swine fever infections: I. Clinical, pathological and virological observations. *Vet. Microbiol.* **1979**, *4*, 117–132. [CrossRef]
14. Paton, D.J.; Done, S.H. Congenital infection of pigs with ruminant-type pestiviruses. *J. Comp. Pathol.* **1994**, *111*, 151–163. [CrossRef]
15. Van Oirschot, J.T.; Terpstra, C. A congenital persistent swine fever infection. I. Clinical and virological observations. *Vet. Microbiol.* **1977**, *2*, 121–132. [CrossRef]
16. Terpstra, C.; Wensvoort, G. A congenital persistent infection of bovine virus diarrhoea virus in pigs: Clinical, virological and immunological observations. *Vet. Q.* **1997**, *19*, 97–101. [CrossRef]
17. Young, G.A.; Kitchell, R.L.; Luedke, A.J.; Sautter, J.H. The effect of viral and other infections of the dam on fetal development in swine. I. Modified live hog cholera viruses; immunological, virological, and gross pathological studies. *J. Am. Vet. Med. Assoc.* **1955**, *126*, 165–171.

18. Leforban, Y.; Vannier, P.; Cariolet, R. Pathogenicity of border disease and bovine viral diarrhoea for pig: Experimental study on the vertical and horizontal transmission of the viruses. In Proceedings of the 11th International Pig Veterinary Society Congress, Lausanne, Switzerland, 1–5 July 1990; p. 204.
19. Postel, A.; Hansmann, F.; Baechlein, C.; Fischer, N.; Alawi, M.; Grundhoff, A.; Derking, S.; Tenhundfeld, J.; Pfankuche, V.M.; Herder, V.; et al. Presence of atypical porcine pestivirus (APPV) genomes in newborn piglets correlates with congenital tremor. *Sci. Rep.* **2016**, *6*, 27735. [CrossRef]
20. Finlaison, D.S.; King, K.R.; Frost, M.J.; Kirkland, P.D. Field and laboratory evidence that Bungowannah virus, a recently recognised pestivirus, is the causative agent of the porcine myocarditis syndrome (PMC). *Vet. Microbiol.* **2009**, *136*, 259–265. [CrossRef]
21. Finlaison, D.S.; Cook, R.W.; Srivastava, M.; Frost, M.J.; King, K.R.; Kirkland, P.D. Experimental infections of the porcine foetus with Bungowannah virus, a novel pestivirus. *Vet. Microbiol.* **2010**, *144*, 32–40. [CrossRef]
22. Finlaison, D.S.; Kirkland, P.D. The outcome of porcine foetal infection with Bungowannah virus is dependent on the stage of gestation at which infection occurs. Part 1: Serology and virology. *Viruses* **2020**, *12*, 691. [CrossRef]
23. Finlaison, D.S.; King, K.R.; Gabor, M.; Kirkland, P.D. An experimental study of Bungowannah virus infection in weaner aged pigs. *Vet. Microbiol.* **2012**, *160*, 245–250. [CrossRef] [PubMed]
24. R Core Team. *R: A Language and Environment for Statistical Computing*; R Foundation for Statisical Computing: Vienna, Austria, 2019; Available online: http://www.R-project.org (accessed on 1 April 2019).
25. Butler, D.G.; Cullis, B.R.; Gilmour, A.R.; Gogel, B.J. *ASReml-R Reference Manual, release 3 ed.*; Queensland Department of Primary Industries and Fisheries: Brisbane, Australia, 2009.
26. Friendship, R.M.; Lumsden, J.H.; McMillan, I.; Wilson, M.R. Hematology and biochemistry reference values for Ontario swine. *Can. J. Comp. Med.* **1984**, *48*, 390–393. [PubMed]
27. Finlaison, D.S. Studies of the Porcine Myocarditis Syndrome. Ph.D. Thesis, University of Sydney, Sydney, Australia, 2010.
28. Finlaison, D.S.; Gestier, S.; Kirkland, P.D. The outcome of porcine foetal infection with Bungowannah virus is dependent on the stage of gestation at which infection occurs—Histopathology. in preparation.
29. Frey, H.R.; Liess, B.; Richter-Reichhelm, H.B.; von Benten, K.; Trautwein, G. Experimental transplacental transmission of hog cholera virus in pigs. I. Virological and serological studies. *Zentralbl. Veterinarmed. B* **1980**, *27*, 154–164. [CrossRef] [PubMed]
30. Meyer, H.; Liess, B.; Frey, H.R.; Hermanns, W.; Trautwein, G. Experimental transplacental transmission of hog cholera virus in pigs. IV. Virological and serological studies in newborn piglets. *Zentralbl. Veterinarmed. B* **1981**, *28*, 659–668. [CrossRef]
31. Hermanns, W.; Trautwein, G.; Meyer, H.; Liess, B. Experimental transplacental transmission of hog cholera virus in pigs. V. Immunopathological findings in newborn pigs. *Zentralbl. Veterinarmed. B* **1981**, *28*, 669–683. [CrossRef]

7

Investigation of Macrolide Resistance Genotypes in *Mycoplasma bovis* Isolates from Canadian Feedlot Cattle

Andrea Kinnear [1], Tim A. McAllister [2], Rahat Zaheer [2], Matthew Waldner [1], Antonio C. Ruzzini [1,3], Sara Andrés-Lasheras [2], Sarah Parker [1], Janet E. Hill [1] and Murray D. Jelinski [1,*]

1 Western College of Veterinary Medicine, University of Saskatchewan, Saskatoon, SK S7N 5B4, Canada; andrea.kinnear@usask.ca (A.K.); matthew.waldner@usask.ca (M.W.); antonio.ruzzini@usask.ca (A.C.R.); sarah.parker@usask.ca (S.P.); janet.hill@usask.ca (J.E.H.)

2 Lethbridge Research and Development Centre, Agriculture and Agri-Food Canada, Lethbridge, AB T1J 4B1, Canada; tim.mcallister@canada.ca (T.A.M.); rahat.zaheer@canada.ca (R.Z.); sara.andreslasheras@canada.ca (S.A.-L.)

3 College of Medicine, Department of Biochemistry, Microbiology and Immunology, University of Saskatchewan, Saskatoon, SK S7N 5E5, Canada

* Correspondence: murray.jelinski@usask.ca;

Abstract: *Mycoplasma bovis* is associated with bovine respiratory disease (BRD) and chronic pneumonia and polyarthritis syndrome (CPPS) in feedlot cattle. No efficacious vaccines for *M. bovis* exist; hence, macrolides are commonly used to control mycoplasmosis. Whole genome sequences of 126 *M. bovis* isolates, derived from 96 feedlot cattle over 12 production years, were determined. Antimicrobial susceptibility testing (AST) of five macrolides (gamithromycin, tildipirosin, tilmicosin, tulathromycin, tylosin) was conducted using a microbroth dilution method. The AST phenotypes were compared to the genotypes generated for 23S rRNA and the L4 and L22 ribosomal proteins. Mutations in domains II (nucleotide 748; *E. coli* numbering) and V (nucleotide 2059 and 2060) of the 23S rRNA (*rrl*) gene alleles were associated with resistance. All isolates with a single mutation at Δ748 were susceptible to tulathromycin, but resistant to tilmicosin and tildipirosin. Isolates with mutations in both domain II and V (Δ748Δ2059 or Δ748Δ2060) were resistant to all five macrolides. However, >99% of isolates were resistant to tildipirosin and tilmicosin, regardless of the number and positions of the mutations. Isolates with a Δ748 mutation in the 23S rRNA gene and mutations in L4 and L22 were resistant to all macrolides except for tulathromycin.

Keywords: antimicrobial; susceptibility; resistance; genotype; rRNA; macrolides; feedlot; beef; cattle

---

1. Introduction

Mycoplasma bovis is associated with various diseases of cattle such as pneumonia, mastitis, arthritis, otitis media, conjunctivitis, and reproductive disorders [1,2]. In feedlot cattle, *M. bovis* infections commonly manifest as bovine respiratory disease (BRD) and chronic pneumonia and polyarthritis syndrome (CPPS) [3,4]. Furthermore, *M. bovis* infections often respond poorly to antimicrobial therapy, resulting in a chronic infection [5]. This lack of a response frequently results in prolonged antimicrobial therapy, which indiscriminately selects for antimicrobial resistance in the pathogens that comprise the BRD complex [6]. Mycoplasmosis in the feedlot results in economic losses due to reduced production performance, increased treatment costs, and death loss [2,6]. In addition, feedlot cattle with polyarthritis may become severely lame, which is a significant animal welfare issue.

As there are currently no effective vaccines for *M. bovis*, antimicrobials remain the primary means for the prevention and control of mycoplasmosis [2,7]. This has led to a number of *M. bovis* antimicrobial susceptibility studies in Canada [8–11], United States [12], Japan [13] and Europe [7,14–19]. These studies suggest that *M. bovis* will continue to become increasingly resistant to antimicrobials. This situation is exacerbated by the limited number of antimicrobials available for treating mycoplasma infections. *Mycoplasma* spp. lack a cell wall and the ability to synthesize folate, rendering them intrinsically resistant to all β-lactams and sulfonamides [2]. In addition, most aminoglycosides either lack label claims for BRD, or the formulations are not amenable for use in feedlot cattle. This narrows the selection of antimicrobials to those that target protein synthesis or DNA replication, and that have been formulated to maintain therapeutic blood levels for several days. The main class of antimicrobials that meet these criteria is the macrolides.

Macrolides have been formulated to be administered parenterally or in-feed; however, only one macrolide, tylosin tartrate (TYLT), is registered in Canada for in-feed use. Tylosin is typically administered throughout the feeding period, and is used to control liver abscesses [9]. The other four main macrolides used in the feedlot are: tilmicosin (TIL), tildipirosin (TIP), tulathromycin (TUL), and gamithromycin (GAM). All of which are formulated as long-acting injectable antimicrobials, and depending on the drug, may have label claims for the control (metaphylaxis) and treatment of BRD. A distinctive pharmacological characteristic of macrolides that makes them ideally suited for use in feedlot cattle is their predilection to concentrate in the pulmonary epithelial fluid [20]. This is notable because BRD is the most prevalent and costly disease of feedlot cattle [21]. Thus, the macrolides' pharmacokinetic and pharmacodynamic profiles are particularly well suited for metaphylaxis therapy for BRD in feedlots [22]. In western Canada, cattle deemed to be a high risk for developing BRD often receive TUL at the time of arrival to the feedlot; whereas, low risk cattle may receive either no antimicrobials or a long-acting oxytetracycline [23]. Lastly, unlike other BRD pathogens, antimicrobial resistance in *M. bovis* is not associated with antimicrobial resistance genes [24], but rather resistance arises from mutations in ribosomal RNAs [25].

Macrolides are a member of the macrolide–lincosamide–streptogramin B (MLS_B) superfamily, all of which exert a bacteriostatic effect by disrupting protein synthesis [26]. Specifically, they bind with domains II and V of 23S rRNA, which is a component of 50S ribosomal subunit [27,28]. Ribosomal proteins L4 and L22 are positioned in close proximity to these macrolide binding sites [28,29]. Mutations within 23S rRNA and the L4 and L22 ribosomal proteins are associated with macrolide resistance [25,30]. This mechanism of resistance is not unique to *M. bovis* [13,31,32], having been reported in a variety of bacterial species, including other *Mycoplasma* spp. [33,34], *Neisseria gonorrhoeae* [30], *Streptococcus* spp. [35,36], *Francisella tularensis* [37], *Escherichia coli* [38], *Chlamydia trachomatis* [39], and *Haemophilus influenzae* [40].

A limitation of antimicrobial susceptibility testing (AST) for *M. bovis* is the lack of established clinical breakpoints from the Clinical and Laboratory Standards Institute (CLSI) and the European Committee on Antimicrobial Susceptibility Testing (EUCAST). As a result, researchers have extrapolated *M. bovis* clinical breakpoints from human *Mycoplasma* spp. and other bovine respiratory pathogens for which clinical breakpoints have been established [9,11,12,15,41–43]. Another challenge with performing AST on *M. bovis* is its very fastidious culture requirements, which is related to its reduced genome and limited biosynthetic capacity [44]. These requirements, coupled with relatively slow nonprolific growth, have encouraged the development of rapid molecular testing techniques for predicting antimicrobial susceptibility for *M. bovis* [13,45]. Utilization of a genotypic approach to assess antimicrobial susceptibility of *M. bovis* could allow for more expeditious evaluation of antimicrobial efficacy and evidence-based selection of antimicrobials to enable judicious use of antimicrobials, which are all principles of antimicrobial stewardship. Additionally, a genotypic approach could be more amenable as a standardized approach to assess antimicrobial susceptibility in *M. bovis* than culture-based techniques, as it would not be susceptible to variable results due to growth conditions. To support these efforts, this study assessed the concordance between genotypes known to confer macrolide resistance to AST phenotypes. Specifically, the study compared the 23S rRNA, L4, and L22 genotypes of *M. bovis* isolates to the AST results of five macrolides commonly used in western Canadian feedlot cattle to control and treat BRD.

2. Results

2.1. Culture and Reference Antimicrobial Susceptibilities

A total of 126 *Mycoplasma bovis* isolates were derived from 96 head of feedlot cattle from 21 feedlots over 12 production years, 2006 to 2018 (Table 1). Thirty head of cattle provided paired lung/joint isolates ($n = 60$), 14 provided a lung sample, 5 provided a joint isolate, and 47 isolates came from the nasopharynx. Nasopharyngeal isolates were derived from healthy ($n = 30$), diseased ($n = 15$), and dead ($n = 2$) cattle. Phenotypically resistant isolates to the macrolides tested were derived from samples taken from healthy, diseased, and dead cattle (Table 2). Production years were used to define the sampling cohort, as animals often enter the feedlot in the fall and remain until the following calendar year. Thus, the 2018 production year included samples obtained between 1 November 2018 and 30 June 2019.

Table 1. *Mycoplasma bovis* isolates (n = 126) by anatomical location, health status, and production year.

	Production Year								
	2006	**2007**	**2008**	**2014**	**2015**	**2016**	**2017**	**2018**	**Total**
Anatomical Location									
Joint		1	1	1	1	14	11	6	35
Lung				3	3	17	15	6	44
Nasopharynx	5	28					9	5	47
Total	5	29	1	4	4	31	35	17	126
Health Status									
Healthy	2	14					9	5	30
Diseased	3	12							15
Dead		3	1	4	4	31	26	12	81
Total	5	29	1	4	4	31	35	17	126

Table 2. Number of *Mycoplasma bovis* isolates (n = 126) with a resistant (R) or susceptible (S) phenotype by health status.

Health Status		Phenotype (% Resistant)					
		GAM	**TIL**	**TIP**	**TUL**	**TYLT**	**Total**
Healthy	R/S (%R)	19/11 (63.3)	30/0 (100)	30/0 (100)	11/19 (36.7)	22/8 (73.3)	30
Diseased	R/S (%R)	9/6 (60.0)	15/0 (100)	15/0 (100)	9/6 (60.0)	11/4 (73.3)	15
Dead	R/S (%R)	78/3 (96.3)	80/1 (98.8)	81/0 (100)	72/9 (88.9)	78/3 (96.3)	81
Total	R/S (%R)	106/20 (84.1)	125/1 (99.2)	126/0 (100)	92/34 (73.0)	111/15 (88.1)	126

GAM—gamithromycin, TIL—tilmicosin, TIP—tildipirosin, TUL—tulathromycin, and TYLT—tylosin.

Mycoplasma bovis PG45 (*Mycoplasma bovis* ATCC® 25523) was resequenced and possessed the equivalent 23S rRNA genotype at positions 748, 2059, and 2060, as reported in the published reference genome [46]. Compared to the published reference genome, no nonsynonymous mutations in L4 and L22 ribosomal proteins were observed in this resequenced isolate. The following minimum inhibitory concentration (MIC) values, defined as the lowest concentration of antimicrobial to visibly inhibit growth, were determined from AST of five PG45 replicates: GAM, 8–16; TIP, 4–8; TIL, 1; TUL, 0.25; and TYLT, 1–2 μg/mL. Due to these genotypic and phenotypic findings, *M. bovis* PG45 was considered to be a susceptible wildtype isolate.

2.2. *Genome Sequencing and Assembly*

Draft genomes of the 126 isolates were assembled from an average 210,113 paired reads (range: 55,951 to 414,042); average read length of 217 bp (range: 166 to 233 bp). This produced assemblies with an average N50 of 18,690 bp (range: 1780 to 34,113 bp), an average coverage depth of 45.3 (range 12.2 to 89.1), and an average of 579 contigs (range: 171 to 1639).

2.3. *23 S rRNA Gene*

Among the 126 isolates analyzed, mutations (single nucleotide polymorphisms, SNPs) were located in hairpin 35 of domain II (nucleotide 748; *E. coli* numbering used throughout) and the peptidyl transferase loop of domain V (nucleotide 2059 and 2060) of the 23S rRNA (*rrl*) gene alleles. The 23S rRNA genotype was assigned based on alleles observed at position 748, 2059, and 2060 (Table 3). As there are up to two copies of the *rrl* gene reported for *M. bovis*, an isolate was categorized as having a change (Δ) if a mutation occurred in at least one copy of the gene. The *M. bovis* PG45 reference genome was considered as the reference (wildtype) and two isolates (1.6%) were identical to this 23S rRNA genotype. Most isolates (73.0%; 92/126) had mutations in domains II and V (Δ748Δ2059 or Δ748Δ2060); whereas, 25.4% (32/126) had a single mutation in domain II (Δ748). There were no isolates with lone mutations in domain V. All isolates with a single mutation at Δ748 were susceptible to TUL (MIC ≤ 16 μg/mL); resistant to TIP and TIL (MIC ≥ 8 μg/mL); and either susceptible (MIC ≤ 4 μg/mL) or resistant (MIC ≥ 8 μg/mL) to GAM and TYLT (Figure 1a). Isolates that had accumulated mutations in both domain II and V (Δ748Δ2059 or Δ748 Δ2060) were resistant to all five macrolides (Table 3 and Figure 1b).

No dose dependent effect was apparent within a given genotype (i.e., Δ748 only) for those with a single mutant allele (i.e., G748A) or a combined mutant/wildtype allele (i.e., G748, G748A). The MIC values for isolates with Δ748 only 23S rRNA genotype, with a single mutant allele, ranged from 1 to 128 μg/mL for GAM and TYLT, and 0.25 to 8 μg/mL for TUL. Isolates with combined alleles had consistently lower MIC values of 8, 8–16, and 0.25 μg/mL for GAM, TYLT, and TUL, respectively, which were within the MIC range for isolates with a single mutant allele. For isolates with the Δ748Δ2059 23S rRNA genotype, those with combined alleles had MIC values ranging from 8 to ≥128 μg/mL for TYLT compared to ≥128 μg/mL with a single mutant allele. Regardless of allelic composition, the MIC values for isolates with Δ748Δ2060 23S rRNA genotypes were ≥64 μg/mL.

The 23S rRNA genotypes were grouped based on the presence of mutations in domain II only versus domain II and V. The results were reported as % resistant with 95% confidence interval (95% CI) for a proportion (Table 4). The two isolates with wildtype 23S rRNA genotypes were susceptible to TUL and TYLT (0, 0–0.66), and 1 of 2 were resistant to GAM and TIL (0.5, 0.09–0.91). Isolates with mutations in domain II only (Δ748 only) had a similar proportion of isolates resistant to GAM (0.41, 0.26–0.58) and TYLT (0.59, 0.42–0.74) compared to TUL (0, 0–0.11). An additional mutation in domain V at positions 2059 (Δ748Δ2059) or 2060 (Δ748Δ2060) resulted in all isolates being resistant to all five macrolides. All isolates were resistant TIP, regardless of genotype.

Table 3. Comparison of 23S rRNA genotypes and the number (%) of *Mycoplasma bovis* isolates (n = 126) resistant to the five macrolides tested.

Genotype	23S rRNA Gene Alleles⁺ Domain II 748	Domain V 2059	Domain V 2060	Percent (n) of Isolates	Phenotype# (% Resistant) GAM	TIL	TIP	TUL	TYLT
Wildtype*	G748	A2059	A2060	1.6 (2)	1 (50)	1 (50)	2 (100)	0 (0)	0 (0)
	Total			1.6 (2)	1 (50)	1 (50)	2 (100)	0 (0)	0 (0)
Δ748 only	G748, G748A‡			4.0 (5)	5 (100)	5 (100)	5 (100)	0 (0)	5 (100)
	G748A			21.4 (27)	8 (29.6)	27 (100)	27 (100)	0 (0)	14 (51.9)
	Total			25.4 (32)	13 (40.6)	32 (100)	32 (100)	0 (0)	19 (59.4)
Δ748Δ2059	G748, G748A‡	A2059, A2059G‡		0.8 (1)	1 (100)	1 (100)	1 (100)	1 (100)	1 (100)
	G748A	A2059, A2059G‡		2.4 (3)	3 (100)	3 (100)	3 (100)	3 (100)	3 (100)
	G748A	A2059, A2059C‡		2.4 (3)	3 (100)	3 (100)	3 (100)	3 (100)	3 (100)
	G748A	A2059, A2059T‡		7.1 (9)	9 (100)	9 (100)	9 (100)	9 (100)	9 (100)
	G748A	A2059G		49.2 (62)	62 (100)	62 (100)	62 (100)	62 (100)	62 (100)
	Total			61.9 (78)	78 (100)	78 (100)	78 (100)	78 (100)	78 (100)
Δ748Δ2060	G748A		A2060, A2060C‡	0.8 (1)	1 (100)	1 (100)	1 (100)	1 (100)	1 (100)
	G748A		A2060C	7.9 (10)	10 (100)	10 (100)	10 (100)	10 (100)	10 (100)
	G748A		A2060G	2.4 (3)	3 (100)	3 (100)	3 (100)	3 (100)	3 (100)
	Total			11.1 (14)	14 (100)	14 (100)	14 (100)	14 (100)	14 (100)

* *Mycoplasma bovis* PG45 is designated as wildtype genotype. # GAM—gamithromycin, TIL—tilmicosin, TIP—tildipirosin, TUL—tulathromycin, and TYLT—tylosin. ‡ Representative of a combined wildtype and mutant allele. ⁺ Positioning of the alleles is based on *Escherichia coli* numbering.

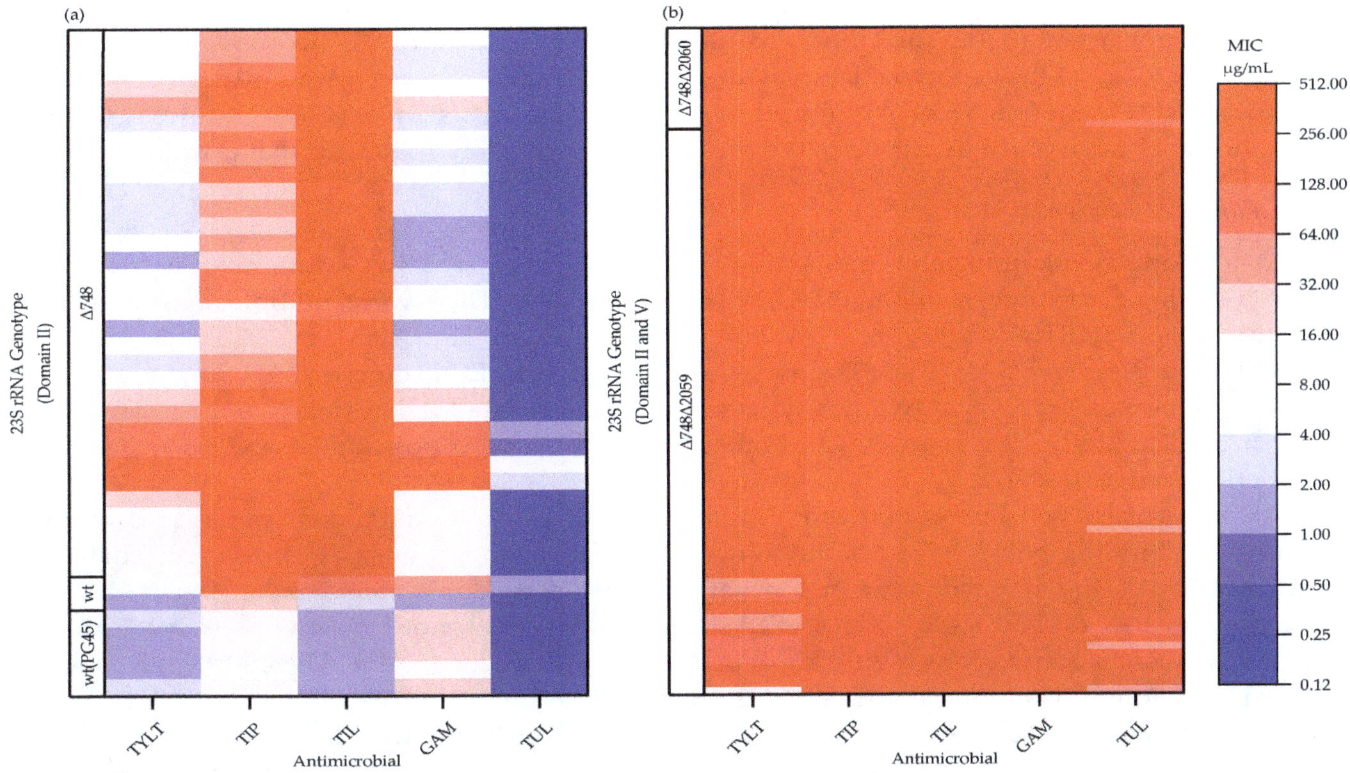

Figure 1. Minimum inhibitory concentrations (MIC) of *Mycoplasma bovis* isolates (n = 126) for tylosin (TYLT), tilmicosin (TIL), tildipirosin (TIP), gamithromycin (GAM), and tulathromycin (TUL), and the corresponding 23S rRNA genotype: (**a**) wildtype (wt) or mutations in domain II only (Δ748); (**b**) mutations in domain II and V (Δ748Δ2059, Δ748Δ2060). The MIC values for the five *M. bovis* PG45 replicates [wt(PG45)] are presented. TYLT, TIL, and TIP have a 16-membered core structure; whereas, GAM and TUL have a 15-membered core structure.

Table 4. Number and proportion of *Mycoplasma bovis* isolates (n = 126) resistant (R) or susceptible (S) by 23S rRNA genotype. The 95% binomial proportion confidence interval (Wilson score) is an interval estimate of the probability of the isolate being resistant if it has a particular 23S rRNA genotype.

		23S rRNA Genotype⁺			
		Wildtype	**Δ748 only**	**Δ748Δ2059**	**Δ748Δ2060**
TUL	R/S	0/2	0/32	78/0	14/0
Proportion (95% CI)		0 (0–0.66)	0 (0–0.11)	1 (0.95–1)	1 (0.78–1)
GAM	R/S	1/1	13/19	78/0	14/0
Proportion (95% CI)		0.50 (0.09–0.91)	0.41 (0.26–0.58)	1 (0.95–1)	1 (0.78–1)
TYLT	R/S	0/2	19/13	78/0	14/0
Proportion (95% CI)		0 (0–0.66)	0.59 (0.42–0.74)	1 (0.95–1)	1 (0.78–1)
TIL	R/S	1/1	32/0	78/0	14/0
Proportion (95% CI)		0.50 (0.09–0.91)	1 (0.89–1)	1 (0.95–1)	1 (0.78–1)
TIP	R/S	2/0	32/0	78/0	14/0
Proportion (95% CI)		1 (0.34–1)	1 (0.89–1)	1 (0.95–1)	1 (0.78–1)
Total		2	32	78	14

GAM—gamithromycin, TIL—tilmicosin, TIP—tildipirosin, TUL—tulathromycin, and TYLT—tylosin. ⁺ Positioning of the alleles is based on *Escherichia coli* numbering.

The level of agreement in the classification of resistance between the presence of a mutation in domain V in the 23S rRNA genotype and phenotype (MIC values) varied by macrolide. The kappa correlation coefficient was perfect (1.000) for TUL, moderate (0.676) for GAM, weak (0.536) for TYLT, essentially nonexistent (0.042) for TIL, and could not be determined for TIP because all isolates were resistant regardless of the genotype. Despite these differences, all isolates with a mutation in domain V of the 23S rRNA genotype (Δ748Δ2059 and Δ748Δ2060) were resistant to all macrolides. However, mutations in domain V also occurred in the presence of a mutation in domain II at position 748.

2.4. L4 and L22 Ribosomal Proteins

All isolates had a nonsynonymous mutation Gln93His (*M. bovis* PG45 number; equivalent to Gln90His using *E. coli* numbering) in the L22 ribosomal protein. There were multiple nonsynonymous L4 mutations: Ser18Thr, Thr43Ala, Ala44Thr, Glu50Thr, Ala51Thr, Ala51Ser, Ser55Ala, Thr57Ala, Val69Ala, Ala70Thr, Glu75Ala, Ala86Thr, and Ala101Thr (*M. bovis* PG45 numbering) with three different nonsynonymous mutations at two positions in proximity to the MLS_B binding pocket Gly185Arg, Gly185Ala, Thr186Pro (*M. bovis* PG45 numbering; equivalent to position 64 and 65 using *E. coli* numbering, respectively).

Twelve isolates had a nonsynonymous mutation in the L4 ribosomal protein in residues proximal to the MLS_B binding pocket. Four had two nonsynonymous mutations Gly185Ala and Thr186Pro, and eight had a single nonsynonymous mutation Gly185Arg (Table 5). All isolates had Gln93His mutations in L22 as well. All isolates with the two nonsynonymous mutations (Gly185Ala and Thr186Pro) also had mutations in domain II of the 23S rRNA gene (Δ748). The eight isolates with a single nonsynonymous mutation (Gly185Arg) had various 23S rRNA genotypes: wildtype ($n = 1$), Δ748 ($n = 1$), and Δ748Δ2059 ($n = 6$). Overall, isolates with a Δ748 mutation in the 23S rRNA gene and mutations in L4 and L22 near the MLS_B binding pocket were resistant (MICs ≥16 μg/mL) to GAM, TIL, TIP and TYLT; but susceptible (MICs ≤ 8 μg/mL) to TUL.

Table 5. Presence of ribosomal protein mutations in different 23S genotype groups and corresponding minimum inhibitory concentrations (MIC) values.

23S rRNA Genotype⁺	MIC (μg/mL)					Ribosomal Proteins‡	
	GAM	TIL	TIP	TUL	TYLT	L4	L22
wildtype (PG45)	8–16	1	4–8	0.25	1–2	Gly185, Thr186	Gln93
wildtype	32	64	>128	1	4	Gly185Arg	Gln93His
Δ748	128	>256	>128	2	128	Gly185Ala, Thr186Pro	Gln93His
	128	>256	>128	8	128	Gly185Ala, Thr186Pro	Gln93His
	64	>256	>128	0.5	64	Gly185Ala, Thr186Pro	Gln93His
	64	>256	>128	1	64	Gly185Ala, Thr186Pro	Gln93His
	16	256	128	0.25	32	Gly185Arg	Gln93His
Δ748Δ2059	>256	>256	>128	>256	>128	Gly185Arg	Gln93His
	>256	>256	>128	256	>128	Gly185Arg	Gln93His
	>256	>256	>128	>256	>128	Gly185Arg	Gln93His
	>256	>256	>128	128	64	Gly185Arg	Gln93His
	>256	>256	>128	128	64	Gly185Arg	Gln93His
	>256	>256	>128	32	64	Gly185Arg	Gln93His

⁺ Positioning of the alleles is based on *Escherichia coli* numbering. ‡ Positioning of amino acids is based on *Mycoplasma bovis* PG45 numbering.

3. Discussion

This study was unique in that it assessed the concordance between the genotypes and phenotypes of *M. bovis* for antimicrobial resistance (AMR) to five macrolides used to control and treat bovine respiratory disease in feedlot cattle. Of note was the inclusion of TUL, which is the most commonly used antimicrobial for BRD prophylaxis, but a pharmaceutical that has not been assessed in previous genotype–phenotype AMR studies [13,31,32,47]. This is salient because even though macrolides have a similar antibacterial mode of action, they differ in the size of the macrocyclic lactone ring and associated side-chains [48]. As a result, each macrolide has a slightly different binding affinity for domains II and V of 23S rRNA. Thus, one or more mutations within these domains may lead to very different antimicrobial susceptibility testing (AST) results. Exemplars are TUL, TIL, and TIP, where a single mutation in domain II (Δ748) conferred resistance to TIL and TIP, but not to TUL. This is consistent with the modeling of the *E. coli* ribosome, wherein TUL interacts primarily at A2058 of 23S rRNA, but is too small to span the ribosomal tunnel and interact with G748 in domain II [48]. This finding is of interest because previous genotype studies did not include TUL.

Within the 23S rRNA gene, mutations in domain V occurred at position 2059 or 2060, but not both. In contrast, Lerner et al. [31] identified two isolates with mutations in both *rrl* alleles in domain V, but at different positions (2058 and 2059). Furthermore, others have reported mutations at position 2058 in *M. bovis* [31,47,49], an outcome that was not found in the current study. Isolates with differing alleles at a given position in domain V were resistant to all five macrolides, which is consistent with a previous study in which *Mycoplasma* spp. having a heterozygous mutation in domain V conferred resistance [33]. Additionally, mutations at position 2060 have been reported in *M. bovis* isolates that are resistant to lincomycin [32], an antimicrobial with a mechanism of action similar to macrolides [7,26]. These differences in position, albeit in close proximity to one another, could reflect differences in the selective pressure of specific antimicrobials as a result of differences in use across production systems. Despite these differences, the increased resistance of *M. bovis* to macrolides as a result of mutations in domain II and domain V is consistent with previous reports [13,31,32,47].

Overall, concordance was observed between 23S rRNA genotype and AMR phenotype, which highlights the utility of molecular targets as a viable alternative to in vitro AST. Isolates with combined mutations in domain II and V binding sites of 23S rRNA gene (Δ748Δ2059 and Δ748Δ2060) all demonstrated resistance to TUL, GAM, and TYLT. Whereas regardless of genotype, >99% of all isolates were resistant to TIP and TIL. The accumulation of SNPs in domain II and V of the 23S rRNA gene and the relationship to increasing MIC values, and therefore inferred resistance, has been reported for TYLT and TIL in *M. bovis* by Hata et al. [13]. Lui and Douthwaite [50] also demonstrated that monomethylation at positions G748 and A2058 acted synergistically to increase TYLT resistance. In both the Lerner et al. [31] study and the current study, the existence of mutations in both the II and V domains correlated with MICs for TYLT and TIL that were indicative of clinical resistance. However, it has also been reported that some *M. bovis* isolates with elevated MICs to TYLT and TIL only have a mutation in domain V, without a concurrent mutation at position 748 [31,47], while others had a change at 748 without a mutation in domain V [32].

Given that TIP and TIL are both derivatives of TYLT, the similarities in the level of resistance to these macrolides is not surprising. These three macrolides vary in the groups that decorate C5, C6, and C14 of their shared 16-membered core structure. As high levels of resistance (>99%) to both TIL and TIP was present, it was difficult to correlate phenotype and genotype. However, as per previous reports [9,10,16,17] the very high MIC values for these two antimicrobials indicate that they are unsuitable for treating mycoplasmosis in cattle.

The associations of mutations in the L4 and L22 ribosomal proteins with susceptibility phenotypes were less clear than those of domains II and V of the 23S rRNA gene. Zhao et al. [51] reported that mutations in these ribosomal proteins lead to increased macrolide resistance in *M. pneumonia*. In the current study, mutations in L4 and L22 were associated with elevated MICs for GAM, TYLT, TIP, and TIL. Given that these ribosomal proteins form the narrowest constriction of the protein exit tunnel [52], with both having loops that extend adjacent to macrolide binding sites [53], the presence of mutations is consistent with the AST phenotypes. All isolates (n = 126) also had mutations in L22 relative to the type strain, a result more prevalent than reported by Lerner et al. [31], where the nonsynonymous mutation Gln90His (*E. coli* numbering) in L22 was observed in 75% of isolates. Again, these differences across studies are likely related to increased antimicrobial selection pressure placed on the western Canadian isolates.

There was a very low prevalence of the *M. bovis* type strain PG45 genotype (1.6%) in this study compared to Hata et al. [13], who observed this genotype in 12.3% of 203 bovine isolates from Japan. Lerner et al. [31] found that this genotype in about half of the 54 isolates from cattle originating in the Middle East, Europe, and Australia. Variation in the proportion of wildtype *M. bovis* isolates circulating within cattle populations is undoubtedly related to differences in cattle production systems and antimicrobial use. In western Canada, most beef calves are weaned in the fall of the year and sold at auctions where they are commingled with cohorts from other farms. These newly weaned calves are then transported to feedlots where they are processed on-arrival. In addition to these stressors, these events occur when the weather can be also be inclement. Therefore, calves deemed to be at high-risk of developing BRD are administered macrolides, often TUL, on-arrival. Our data indicate that over time this practice has selected against wildtype genotypes and for the emergence of macrolide resistant genotypes. Significantly, not only has macrolide resistance in western Canadian feedlot cattle been increasing, it is also not uncommon to recover macrolide resistant *M. bovis* isolates from the nasopharynx of healthy cattle at feedlot arrival [11]. While feedlots could rotate macrolides with tetracyclines or florfenicol, as a strategy to reduce resistance, this practice requires timely AST data or otherwise it may exacerbate antimicrobial resistance.

The study had a number of potential weaknesses. The wildtype 23S rRNA genotype essentially served as a control group; however, there were only two isolates in this group. This was unfortunate since one of two wildtype isolates were resistant to GAM and TIL, and both resistant to TIP. Additionally, control testing of healthy animals was not performed at the time of sampling diseased or dead animals. However, this study was not intended as a survey of macrolide susceptibility, but rather an investigation of the relationship between genotype and phenotype. Therefore, the healthy animals were sampled with the intent of culturing phenotypically susceptible isolates to serve as a basis of comparison to the abundance of resistant isolates derived from dead cattle. The other weaknesses were that the isolates were not uniformly spread over all 12 production years, and most isolates came from dead animals that had received extensive antimicrobial therapy prior to death. The study, however, also had some notable strengths. The relatively large number of isolates came from cattle that were sourced from a broad geographic area; samples were collected over 12 production years; from multiple anatomical locations; and from healthy, diseased and dead cattle.

Conventional antimicrobial susceptibility testing for *M. bovis* is time-consuming and technically demanding, making it unsuitable for monitoring antimicrobial resistance in real-time within a feedlot. This is an issue because prudent use guidelines for antimicrobial use are predicated on AST. This study, and others, have shown a clear linkage between genotypes and macrolide resistance, providing an avenue for developing a rapid, accurate, and cost-effective molecular based test for *M. bovis*, similar to what has been done for *Mycoplasma genitalium* [34,54,55]. This test could be used to assess *M. bovis* isolates obtained from nasapharyngeal swabs, or for conducting pen-level AST surveillance by testing isolates found in shared watering bowls.

4. Materials and Methods

4.1. Animals and Sample Collection

Mycoplasma bovis isolates were cultured from a cross-section of clinical samples derived from different anatomical regions (nasopharynx, lung, and joint) of western Canadian feedlot cattle over 12 production years (2006–2018). Deep nasopharyngeal swabs from live cattle were taken in accordance with Animal Use Protocols (#20070023; #20170021) approved by the University of Saskatchewan's Animal Research Ethics Board and Lethbridge Research Center's Animal Care Committee (#1641).

Sampling was performed as described in Jelinski et al. [11]. Briefly, doubled-guarded uterine swabs (Reproduction Resources, Walworth, WI, USA) were used to obtain deep nasopharyngeal (DNP) samples from healthy and diseased cattle. The diseased cattle were identified by feedlot personnel trained in recognizing the clinical signs of BRD (dyspnea, depression, nasal discharge, anorexia, and fever). Swabs were immediately placed in Ames media (Mai, Ames Media, Product 49203, Spring Valley, WI, USA).

All other swabs or tissues were collected from animals purposively sampled by feedlot veterinarians recruited to provide clinical case material for the study. Samples were obtained by the veterinarians from animals that on postmortem examination were found to have pathological lesions consistent with *M. bovis* pneumonia or chronic pneumonia and polyarthritis syndrome (CPPS). Specifically, the lungs had gross pathology consistent with caseonecrotic pneumonia and/or chronic bronchopneumonia. A minimum 3 × 3 cm lung sample was excised and if septic arthritis was concurrently observed, then the diseased joints were sampled by swabbing, aspirating synovial fluid, or excising synovial tissue.

Tissue and fluid specimens were stored at –20 °C, and batch shipped by courier. Upon receipt, samples were stored at –80 °C until culturing. For each sample, the following metadata were recorded: date of sampling, type of sample (swab, tissue, joint fluid), anatomical location (nasopharynx, lung, joint), and disease status (healthy, diseased, dead).

4.2. *Mycoplasma* Culture and Isolation

Selective culture was performed on the DNP swabs and on swabs of the cut tissue surfaces as previously described by Jelinski et al. [11]. Due to the extended time span of sample collection, there were slight differences in isolation methods and media over the course of the study. Samples collected between 2006 to 2008 were cultured using Hayflick's media (made in-house), whereas in subsequent years samples were cultured using pleuropneumonia-like organism (PPLO) broth and agar (BD Difco, Fisher Scientific, Waltham, MA, USA), supplemented with 10 g/L yeast extract (BD Diagnostic Systems, Fisher Scientific, Waltham, MA, USA), and 20% horse serum (Invitrogen, Fisher Scientific) [11,56]. Where specified, the media was supplemented with 0.05% thallium (I) acetate, 500 U/mL penicillin G, and/or 0.5% sodium pyruvate (Sigma-Aldrich, St. Louis, MO, USA).

Cultures derived from samples were filtered through 0.45 and 0.20 µm filters (Basix, VWR International, Radnor, PA, USA), and were used to inoculate PPLO broth with 0.05% thallium (I) acetate, 500 U/mL penicillin G, and 0.5% sodium pyruvate, and grown in a 5% CO_2 atmosphere with 75% humidity at 37 °C. Cultures with visible growth were streaked onto PPLO agar with 0.05% thallium (I) acetate and 500 U/mL penicillin G and incubated for 3–6 days. An isolated colony with characteristic "fried-egg" morphology was picked, replated on PPLO agar, and incubated for 72 h. Up to three individual colonies per sample were used to inoculate separate aliquots of PPLO broth with 0.05% thallium (I) acetate and 500 U/mL penicillin G. After 48 h of growth, each culture was separately stored in PPLO with glycerol (20%, *v*/*v*) at –80 °C. From the three possible cultures, a single culture was chosen to inoculate PPLO media for DNA extraction and antimicrobial susceptibility testing.

4.3. DNA Extraction and Identification

Mycoplasma bovis isolates were grown in PPLO media for 48 h and the genomic DNA was extracted using the GenElute Bacterial Genomic DNA Kit (Sigma-Aldrich, St. Louis, MO, USA). The DNA was extracted following manufacturer's instructions for Gram negative bacteria with the final elution buffer replaced with 10 mM Tris (pH 8.5). Extracted genomic DNA was assessed for quality using gel electrophoresis and quantified fluorometrically using Qubit (thermo Fisher Scientific, Waltham, MA, USA). Cultures were confirmed as *M. bovis*, based on confirmation of the presence of *uvrC* [57] and sequencing of the 16S rRNA gene [58]. The 16S rRNA amplicon was purified using a QIAquick PCR purification kit (Qiagen, Nevlo, Netherlands) and sent to Macrogen (Seoul, South Korea) for Sanger sequencing with the amplification primers. Forward and reverse sequences were assembled and edited using the Staden Package (version 1.6-r, http://staden.sourceforge.net/). The resulting sequences were compared to the National Center for Biotechnology Information (NCBI) nonredundant nucleotide database (nr) using BLASTn.

4.4. Whole Genome Sequencing and Assembly

Genomic DNA was prepared for sequencing using Illumina Nextera XT DNA Library Preparation (Illumina Inc., San Diego, CA, USA) and sequenced on a Illumina MiSeq platform using the MiSeq v2 Reagent Kit to generate 250 bp paired-end reads. Illumina reads were trimmed using Trimmomatic v0.38 [59] with settings slidingwindow:5:15 leading:5 trailing:5 and minlen:50. Genomes were assembled with *M. bovis* PG45 as the reference genome (CP002188) using BWA-MEM v0.7.10-r789 [60] with default settings, producing SAM formatted assemblies. SAMtools [61] was used to convert the assemblies to BAM files and then sort and index for further processing. The Picard v2.18.4-SNAPSHOT [62] marked and removed duplicate reads from the BAM file. The Genome Analysis ToolKit v3.4-46-gbc02625 was used to perform local indel realignment and base quality score recalibration to improve the alignment quality, according to GATK best practices pipeline [63]. Consensus sequences for each assembly were created from each BAM file using bcftools [61]. This was performed by piping results from bcftools mpileup to bcftools call to create a vcf file for each BAM file. Each vcf file was used as input for vcfutils vcf2fq to generate a consensus fastq file. The fastq files were converted to fasta files using a bash script.

Genes encoding for 23S rRNA (*rrl3* and *rrl4*), L4 (*rplD*), and L22 (*rplV*) ribosomal proteins were identified using BLASTn [64] to compare *M. bovis* strain PG45 genes to the assembled genomes. For *rrl3* and *rrl4*, the closest matching sequence to the start of the genome being analyzed was identified as *rrl3*, the furthest as *rrl4*. As two start sites have been proposed for ribosomal protein L4, for the purposes of this study the position of *rplD* and overall numbering was based on locus ID MBOVPG45_0263. Extraction of gene sequences was performed using the start and ends of the match as reported by BLASTn for input to SAMtools faidx [61]. Genes of interest extracted from each isolate were aligned with the equivalent region in the *M. bovis* PG45 reference genome (CP002188.1) in Geneious Prime 2020.0.5 (https://www.geneious.com) using MUSCLE to identify SNPs with a minimum variant frequency of 0.01. For L4 and L22 ribosomal protein gene alignments, they were translated using the *Mycoplasma* spp. genetic code. To verify the nucleotide composition in *rrl3* and *rrl4* at positions within hairpin 35 in domain II and the peptidyl transferase loop in domain V within the MLS_B binding pocket [65], the SAM files were queried for ambiguity to determine the representative nucleotide(s). In cases of ambiguity, the percent of reads for a given allele was >20%. The raw paired reads for the isolates used in this study are available at NCBI SRA (www.ncbi.nlm.nih.gov/sra) with BioProject ID PRJNA642970.

The *M. bovis* sequences were aligned to their respective 23S rRNA (*rrlA*), L4 (*rplD*), or L22 ribosomal protein (*rplV*) genes isolated from the *E. coli* K12 substrain MG1655 genome to determine equivalent positioning to generate numbering to allow for comparison between different studies and bacterial species.

4.5. Antimicrobial Susceptibility Testing

Antimicrobial susceptibility (AST) was determined using a microdilution assay, in a Sensititre™ (Trek Diagnostics, Oakwood, GA, USA) plate format and a customized panel designed to assess the antimicrobials most commonly used in North American feedlots for the treatment and control of BRD. The panel consisted of ten antimicrobials as described by Jelinski et al. [11], five of which were macrolides: tildipirosin (TIP; 0.12–128 μg/mL), gamithromycin (GAM; 0.25–256 μg/mL), tulathromycin (TUL; 0.25–256 μg/mL), tilmicosin (TIL; 1–256 μg/mL), and tylosin tartrate (TYLT; 1–128 μg/mL). AlamarBlue (thermoFisher Scientific, DAL1100), a color redox indicator, was used to assess growth in each well based on a blue to pink color transition.

The AST procedure began by inoculating an *M. bovis* isolate previously stored at –80 °C in 20% glycerol into PPLO broth with 0.5% pyruvate and incubating for 72 h at 5% CO_2 with 75% humidity at 37 °C. Broth cultures were then subcultured into neat PPLO (without antibiotics) and incubated for 24 h. Following incubation, the optical density (OD) at 450 nm was determined using a NanoDrop One Spectrophotometer (Fisher Scientific, Waltham, MA, USA) and the culture adjusted to an $OD_{450} = 0.1$. The adjusted culture was diluted up to 100×, and 120 μL of the diluted culture used to inoculate 6 mL of PPLO in 2× alamarBlue. Each well of a Sensititre™ plate was inoculated to a final concentration of 10^3 to 5×10^5 CFU/mL with 50 μL of culture in 2× alamarBlue in 50 μL of media with each of antimicrobials within a series of Sensititre wells (final working concentration of alamarBlue: 1×; final well volume:

100 μL). Plates were sealed with a CO_2 permeable film, and incubated for 48–72 h. Minimum inhibitory concentrations (MICs) were determined by visual assessment of plates at 48 and 72 h, based on a blue to pink colour change. The *M. bovis* reference strain (*Mycoplasma bovis* ATCC® 25523™) was tested five times for quality control.

4.6. Clinical Breakpoints

As there are no established macrolide breakpoints for *M. bovis,* they were extrapolated from other members of the bacterial BRD complex (i.e., *Mannheimia haemolytica, Pasteurella multocida, Histophilus somni*) and human *Mycoplasma* spp., as described previously in Jelinski et al. [11]. The resistance breakpoints were ≥8 μg/mL for TIP, GAM, TIL, and TYLT, and ≥32 μg/mL for TUL.

4.7. Statistical Analysis

As *rrl3* and *rrl4* genes in the reference sequence for *M. bovis* PG45 differ by only a single nucleotide, alleles in each isolate could not be assigned to a specific locus. Instead, allele(s) at a given position were reported and isolates were grouped into genotypes according to the presence of mutation(s) in domain II and V. This created four 23S rRNA genotype groups: wildtype, Δ748 only, Δ748Δ2059, and Δ748Δ2060.

As phenotypically resistant and susceptible isolates were derived from cattle in each health status cohort (healthy, diseased, and dead), all isolates were analyzed together regardless of their source. Confidence intervals were calculated using the Wilson score interval method for estimating intervals for proportions. The confidence intervals were used to represent the antimicrobial resistance for a given 23S rRNA genotype using Epitools [66]. To assess the agreement in classification of resistance between the presence of a mutation in domain V of the 23S rRNA genotype and phenotype (MIC value), the Cohen's kappa statistic interpretation criteria (value, level of agreement): 0–0.20, none; 0.21–0.39, minimal; 0.40–0.59, weak; 0.60–0.79, moderate; 0.80–0.90, strong; >0.90, almost perfect [67] were calculated using a commercial statistical program (SPSS 26, IBM SPSS Statistics version 26, IBM Corporation, Armonk, NY, USA). All descriptive statistics were calculated using a commercial spreadsheet software (Microsoft Excel version 15; Microsoft Corporation, Redmond, Washington, WA, USA).

5. Conclusions

Given that antimicrobials are the primary preventative and therapeutic tool to combat *M. bovis* infections in feedlot cattle, ongoing assessment of antimicrobial susceptibility remains crucial to maintaining the utility of these drugs and facilitating antimicrobial stewardship practices. However, the comparatively slow growth of *M. bovis* yields longer turn-around times when exclusively using culture-based methods of assessment, which can impede timely decision making on antimicrobial use. In our study, we were able to identify mutations in domains II and V of the 23S rRNA genes that are associated with increased resistance to macrolides which show a clear linkage between genotype and phenotypic macrolide resistance (AST). These findings add strong support for utilizing rapid, accurate, and cost-effective molecular based tests for assessing the susceptibility of *M. bovis* to macrolides.

Author Contributions: Conceptualization, M.D.J., T.A.M.; Methodology, M.D.J., T.A.M., A.K., M.W., R.Z, S.A.-L., J.E.H., A.C.R.; Formal Analysis, A.K., M.W., R.Z., S.P.; Investigation, M.D.J., A.K., R.Z.; Resources, M.D.J., T.A.M., J.E.H.; Data Curation, M.D.J., A.K., M.W.; Writing—Original Draft Preparation, A.K., M.DJ., T.A.M.; Writing—Review and Editing, A.K., M.J., T.A.M., M.W., R.Z., S.A.-L., S.P., J.E.H., A.C.R.; Supervision, M.D.J., T.A.M., J.E.H. Funding Acquisition, M.D.J., T.A.M. All authors have read and agreed to the published version of the manuscript.

Acknowledgments: the authors would like to express their appreciation to: Karen Register, Research Microbiologist, USDA, Ames, IA and Manual Chirino-Trejo, Professor Emeritus, Western College of Veterinary Medicine, for their assistance and guidance in the processing of the samples. They also thank Karen Gesy

(University of Saskatchewan), Champika Fernando (University of Saskatchewan), and Rodrigo Ortega-Polo (Lethbridge Research and Development Centre) for their assistance in culturing, sequencing, and bioinformatics, respectively. We also wish to acknowledge and thank the veterinary practices that collected samples and the feedlot producers for allowing their cattle to be sampled.

References

1. Nicholas, R.A.J.; Ayling, R.D. Mycoplasma bovis: Disease, diagnosis, and control. *Res. Vet. Sci.* **2003**, *74*, 105–112. [CrossRef]
2. Maunsell, F.P.; Woolums, A.R.; Francoz, D.; Rosenbusch, R.F.; Step, D.L.; Wilson, D.J.; Janzen, E.D. Mycoplasma bovis infections in cattle. *J. Vet. Intern. Med.* **2011**, *25*, 772–783. [CrossRef]
3. Gagea, M.I.; Bateman, K.G.; Shanahan, R.A.; van Dreumel, T.; McEwen, B.J.; Carman, S.; Archambault, M.; Caswell, J.L. Naturally Occurring Mycoplasma Bovis—Associated Pneumonia and Polyarthritis in Feedlot Beef Calves. *J. Vet. Diagn. Investig.* **2006**, *18*, 29–40. [CrossRef]
4. Caswell, J.L.; Bateman, K.G.; Cai, H.Y.; Castillo-Alcala, F. Mycoplasma bovis in Respiratory Disease of Feedlot Cattle. *Vet. Clin. N. Am. Food Anim.* **2010**, *26*, 365–379. [CrossRef]
5. Krysak, D.E. Chronic pneumonia and polyarthritis syndrome in a feedlot calf. *Can. Vet. J.* **2006**, *47*, 1019–1022.
6. Caswell, J.L.; Archambault, M. Mycoplasma bovis pneumonia in cattle. *Anim. Health Res. Rev.* **2007**, *8*, 161–186. [CrossRef]
7. Lysnyansky, I.; Ayling, R.D. Mycoplasma bovis: Mechanisms of Resistance and Trends in Antimicrobial Susceptibility. *Front. Microbiol.* **2016**, *7*, 595. [CrossRef] [PubMed]
8. Hendrick, S.H.; Bateman, K.G.; Rosengren, L.B. The effect of antimicrobial treatment and preventive strategies on bovine respiratory disease and genetic relatedness and antimicrobial resistance of Mycoplasma bovis isolates in a western Canadian feedlot. *Can. Vet. J.* **2013**, *54*, 1146–1156. [PubMed]
9. Anholt, R.M.; Klima, C.; Allan, N.; Matheson-Bird, H.; Schatz, C.; Ajitkumar, P.; Otto, S.J.; Peters, D.; Schmid, K.; Olson, M.; et al. Antimicrobial Susceptibility of Bacteria That Cause Bovine Respiratory Disease Complex in Alberta, Canada. *Front. Vet. Sci.* **2017**, *4*, 207. [CrossRef] [PubMed]
10. Cai, H.Y.; McDowall, R.; Parker, L.; Kaufman, E.I.; Caswell, J.L. Changes in antimicrobial susceptibility profiles of Mycoplasma bovis over time. *Can. J. Vet. Res.* **2019**, *83*, 34–41. [PubMed]
11. Jelinski, M.; Kinnear, A.; Gesy, K.; Andrés-Lasheras, S.; Zaheer, R.; Weese, S.; McAllister, T.A. Antimicrobial Sensitivity Testing of Mycoplasma bovis Isolates Derived from Western Canadian Feedlot Cattle. *Microorganisms* **2020**, *8*, 124. [CrossRef] [PubMed]
12. Rosenbusch, R.F.; Kinyon, J.M.; Apley, M.; Funk, N.D.; Smith, S.; Hoffman, L.J. In Vitro Antimicrobial Inhibition Profiles of Mycoplasma Bovis Isolates Recovered from Various Regions of the United States from 2002 to 2003. *J. Vet. Diagn. Investig.* **2005**, *17*, 436–441. [CrossRef]
13. Hata, E.; Harada, T.; Itoh, M. Relationship between Antimicrobial Susceptibility and Multilocus Sequence Type of Mycoplasma bovis Isolates and Development of a Method for Rapid Detection of Point Mutations Involved in Decreased Susceptibility to Macrolides, Lincosamides, Tetracyclines, and Spectinomycin. *Appl. Environ. Microbiol.* **2019**, *85*, e00575-19. [CrossRef] [PubMed]
14. Ayling, R.D.; Baker, S.E.; Nicholas, R.A.J.; Peek, M.L.; Simon, A.J. Comparison of in vitro activity of danofloxacin, florfenicol, oxytetracycline, spectinomycin and tilmicosin against recent field isolates of Mycoplasma bovis. *Vet. Rec.* **2000**, *146*, 745–747. [CrossRef] [PubMed]
15. Gerchman, I.; Levisohn, S.; Mikula, I.; Lysnyansky, I. In vitro antimicrobial susceptibility of Mycoplasma bovis isolated in Israel from local and imported cattle. *Vet. Microbiol.* **2009**, *137*, 268–275. [CrossRef] [PubMed]
16. Gautier-Bouchardon, A.V.; Ferré, S.; Le Grand, D.; Paoli, A.; Gay, E.; Poumarat, F. Overall decrease in the susceptibility of Mycoplasma bovis to antimicrobials over the past 30 years in France. *PLoS ONE* **2014**, *9*, e87672. [CrossRef]
17. Sulyok, K.M.; Kreizinger, Z.; Fekete, L.; Hrivnák, V.; Magyar, T.; Jánosi, S.; Schweitzer, N.; Turcsányi, I.; Makrai, L.; Erdélyi, K.; et al. Antibiotic susceptibility profiles of Mycoplasma bovis strains isolated from cattle in Hungary, Central Europe. *BMC Vet. Res.* **2014**, *10*, 256. [CrossRef]

18. Heuvelink, A.; Reugebrink, C.; Mars, J. Antimicrobial susceptibility of Mycoplasma bovis isolates from veal calves and dairy cattle in the Netherlands. *Vet. Microbiol.* **2016**, *189*, 1–7. [CrossRef]
19. Klein, U.; de Jong, A.; Moyaert, H.; El Garch, F.; Leon, R.; Richard-Mazet, A.; Rose, M.; Maes, D.; Pridmore, A.; Thomson, J.R.; et al. Antimicrobial susceptibility monitoring of Mycoplasma hyopneumoniae and Mycoplasma bovis isolated in Europe. *Vet. Microbiol.* **2017**, *204*, 188–193. [CrossRef]
20. Mzyk, D.A.; Bublitz, C.M.; Martinez, M.N.; Davis, J.L.; Baynes, R.E.; Smith, G.W. Impact of bovine respiratory disease on the pharmacokinetics of danofloxacin and tulathromycin in different ages of calves. *PLoS ONE* **2019**, *14*, e0218864. [CrossRef]
21. Griffin, D. Economic Impact Associated with Respiratory Disease in Beef Cattle. *Vet. Clin. N. Am. Large Anim. Pract.* **1997**, *13*, 367–377. [CrossRef]
22. Nickell, J.S.; White, B.J. Metaphylactic Antimicrobial therapy for Bovine Respiratory Disease in Stocker and Feedlot Cattle. *Vet. Clin. N. Am. Food Anim.* **2010**, *26*, 285–301. [CrossRef] [PubMed]
23. Brault, S.A.; Hannon, S.J.; Gow, S.P.; Warr, B.N.; Withell, J.; Song, J.; Williams, C.M.; Otto, S.J.G.; Booker, C.W.; Morley, P.S. Antimicrobial Use on 36 Beef Feedlots in Western Canada: 2008–2012. *Front. Vet. Sci.* **2019**, *6*, 329. [CrossRef] [PubMed]
24. Owen, J.R.; Noyes, N.; Young, A.E.; Prince, D.J.; Blanchard, P.C.; Lehenbauer, T.W.; Aly, S.S.; Davis, J.H.; O'Rourke, S.M.; Abdo, Z.; et al. Whole-Genome Sequencing and Concordance Between Antimicrobial Susceptibility Genotypes and Phenotypes of Bacterial Isolates Associated with Bovine Respiratory Disease. *G3 Genes Genomes Genet.* **2017**, *7*, 3059–3071. [CrossRef] [PubMed]
25. Calcutt, M.J.; Lysnyansky, I.; Sachse, K.; Fox, L.K.; Nicholas, R.A.J.; Ayling, R.D. Gap analysis of Mycoplasma bovis disease, diagnosis and control: An aid to identify future development requirements. *Transbound. Emerg. Dis.* **2018**, *65*, 91–109. [CrossRef]
26. Zaheer, R.; Cook, S.R.; Klima, C.L.; Stanford, K.; Alexander, T.; Topp, E.; Read, R.R.; McAllister, T.A. Effect of subtherapeutic vs. Therapeutic administration of macrolides on antimicrobial resistance in Mannheimia haemolytica and enterococci isolated from beef cattle. *Front. Microbiol.* **2013**, *4*, 133. [CrossRef]
27. Hansen, L.H.; Mauvais, P.; Douthwaite, S. The macrolide–ketolide antibiotic binding site is formed by structures in domains II and V of 23S ribosomal RNA. *Mol. Microbiol.* **1999**, *31*, 623–631. [CrossRef]
28. Moore, P.B.; Steitz, T.A. The Structural Basis of Large Ribosomal Subunit Function. *Annu. Rev. Biochem.* **2003**, *72*, 813–850. [CrossRef]
29. Dinos, G.P. The macrolide antibiotic renaissance. *Br. J. Pharmacol.* **2017**, *174*, 2967–2983. [CrossRef]
30. Demczuk, W.; Martin, I.; Peterson, S.; Bharat, A.; Van Domselaar, G.; Graham, M.; Lefebvre, B.; Allen, V.; Hoang, L.; Tyrrell, G.; et al. Genomic Epidemiology and Molecular Resistance Mechanisms of Azithromycin-Resistant Neisseria gonorrhoeae in Canada from 1997 to 2014. *J. Clin. Microbiol.* **2016**, *54*, 1304–1313. [CrossRef]
31. Lerner, U.; Amram, E.; Ayling, R.D.; Mikula, I.; Gerchman, I.; Harrus, S.; Teff, D.; Yogev, D.; Lysnyansky, I. Acquired resistance to the 16-membered macrolides tylosin and tilmicosin by Mycoplasma bovis. *Vet. Microbiol.* **2014**, *168*, 365–371. [CrossRef] [PubMed]
32. Sulyok, K.M.; Kreizinger, Z.; Wehmann, E.; Lysnyansky, I.; Bányai, K.; Marton, S.; Jerzsele, Á.; Rónai, Z.; Turcsányi, I.; Makrai, L.; et al. Mutations Associated with Decreased Susceptibility to Seven Antimicrobial Families in Field and Laboratory-Derived Mycoplasma bovis Strains. *Antimicrob. Agents Chemother.* **2017**, *61*, e01983-16. [CrossRef] [PubMed]
33. Pereyre, S.; Gonzalez, P.; de Barbeyrac, B.; Darnige, A.; Renaudin, H.; Charron, A.; Raherison, S.; Bébéar, C.; Bébéar, C.M. Mutations in 23S rRNA Account for Intrinsic Resistance to Macrolides in Mycoplasma hominis and Mycoplasma fermentans and for Acquired Resistance to Macrolides in M. hominis. *Antimicrob. Agents Chemother.* **2002**, *46*, 3142–3150. [CrossRef] [PubMed]
34. Chrisment, D.; Charron, A.; Cazanave, C.; Pereyre, S.; Bebear, C. Detection of macrolide resistance in Mycoplasma genitalium in France. *J. Antimicrob. Chemother.* **2012**, *67*, 2598–2601. [CrossRef] [PubMed]
35. Canu, A.; Malbruny, B.; Coquemont, M.; Davies, T.A.; Appelbaum, P.C.; Leclercq, R. Diversity of Ribosomal Mutations Conferring Resistance to Macrolides, Clindamycin, Streptogramin, and Telithromycin in Streptococcus pneumoniae. *Antimicrob. Agents Chemother.* **2002**, *46*, 125–131. [CrossRef]
36. Jalava, J.; Vaara, M.; Huovinen, P. Mutation at the position 2058 of the 23S rRNA as a cause of macrolide resistance in Streptococcus pyogenes. *Ann. Clin. Microbiol. Antimicrob.* **2004**, *3*, 5. [CrossRef]

37. Karlsson, E.; Golovliov, I.; Lärkeryd, A.; Granberg, M.; Larsson, E.; Öhrman, C.; Niemcewicz, M.; Birdsell, D.; Wagner, D.M.; Forsman, M.; et al. Clonality of erythromycin resistance in Francisella tularensis. *J. Antimicrob. Chemother.* **2016**, *71*, 2815–2823. [CrossRef]
38. Zaman, S.; Fitzpatrick, M.; Lindahl, L.; Zengel, J. Novel mutations in ribosomal proteins L4 and L22 that confer erythromycin resistance in Escherichia coli. *Mol. Microbiol.* **2007**, *66*, 1039–1050. [CrossRef]
39. Zhu, H.; Wang, H.-P.; Jiang, Y.; Hou, S.-P.; Liu, Y.-J.; Liu, Q.-Z. Mutations in 23S rRNA and ribosomal protein L4 account for resistance in Chlamydia trachomatis strains selected in vitro by macrolide passage. *Andrologia* **2010**, *42*, 274–280. [CrossRef]
40. Peric, M.; Bozdogan, B.; Jacobs, M.R.; Appelbaum, P.C. Effects of an Efflux Mechanism and Ribosomal Mutations on Macrolide Susceptibility of Haemophilus influenzae Clinical Isolates. *Antimicrob. Agents Chemother.* **2003**, *47*, 1017–1022. [CrossRef]
41. CLSI. *Methods for Antimicrobial Susceptibility Testing for Human Mycoplasmas*; Approved Guideline; CLSI Document M43-A; Clinical and Laboratory Standards Institute: Wayne, PA, USA, 2011.
42. CLSI. *Performance Standards for Antimicrobial Disk and Dilution Susceptibility Tests for Bacteria Isolated from Animals*, 4th ed.; CLSI Supplement VET08; Clinical and Laboratory Standards Institute: Wayne, PA, USA, 2018.
43. Gautier-Bouchardon, A.V. Antimicrobial resistance in mycoplasma spp. *Microbiol. Spectrum.* **2018**, *6*, 425–446. [CrossRef]
44. Rottem, S. Interaction of Mycoplasmas with Host Cells. *Physiol. Rev.* **2003**, *83*, 417–432. [CrossRef] [PubMed]
45. Sulyok, K.M.; Bekő, K.; Kreizinger, Z.; Wehmann, E.; Jerzsele, Á.; Rónai, Z.; Turcsányi, I.; Makrai, L.; Szeredi, L.; Jánosi, S.; et al. Development of molecular methods for the rapid detection of antibiotic susceptibility of Mycoplasma bovis. *Vet. Microbiol.* **2018**, *213*, 47–57. [CrossRef] [PubMed]
46. Wise, K.S.; Calcutt, M.J.; Foecking, M.F.; Röske, K.; Madupu, R.; Methé, B.A. Complete Genome Sequence of Mycoplasma bovis Type Strain PG45 (ATCC 25523). *Infect. Immun.* **2011**, *79*, 982–983. [CrossRef]
47. Khalil, D.; Becker, C.A.M.; Tardy, F. Monitoring the Decrease in Susceptibility to Ribosomal RNAs Targeting Antimicrobials and Its Molecular Basis in Clinical Mycoplasma bovis Isolates over Time. *Microb. Drug Resist.* **2017**, *23*, 799–811. [CrossRef]
48. Andersen, N.M.; Poehlsgaard, J.; Warrass, R.; Douthwaite, S. Inhibition of Protein Synthesis on the Ribosome by Tildipirosin Compared with Other Veterinary Macrolides. *Antimicrob. Agents Chemother.* **2012**, *56*, 6033–6036. [CrossRef]
49. Kong, L.C.; Gao, D.; Jia, B.Y.; Wang, Z.; Gao, Y.H.; Pei, Z.H.; Liu, S.M.; Xin, J.Q.; Ma, H.X. Antimicrobial susceptibility and molecular characterization of macrolide resistance of Mycoplasma bovis isolates from multiple provinces in China. *J. Vet. Med. Sci.* **2016**, *78*, 293–296. [CrossRef]
50. Liu, M.; Douthwaite, S. Resistance to the macrolide antibiotic tylosin is conferred by single methylations at 23S rRNA nucleotides G748 and A2058 acting in synergy. *Proc. Natl. Acad. Sci. USA* **2002**, *99*, 14658–14663. [CrossRef]
51. Zhao, F.; Liu, J.; Shi, W.; Huang, F.; Liu, L.; Zhao, S.; Zhang, J. Antimicrobial susceptibility and genotyping of Mycoplasma pneumoniae isolates in Beijing, China, from 2014 to 2016. *Antimicrob. Resist. Infect. Control* **2019**, *8*, 18. [CrossRef]
52. Auerbach-Nevo, T.; Baram, D.; Bashan, A.; Belousoff, M.; Breiner, E.; Davidovich, C.; Cimicata, G.; Eyal, Z.; Halfon, Y.; Krupkin, M.; et al. Ribosomal Antibiotics: Contemporary Challenges. *Antibiotics* **2016**, *5*, 24. [CrossRef]
53. Diner, E.J.; Hayes, C.S. Recombineering Reveals a Diverse Collection of Ribosomal Proteins L4 and L22 that Confer Resistance to Macrolide Antibiotics. *J. Mol. Biol.* **2009**, *386*, 300–315. [CrossRef] [PubMed]
54. Pitt, R.; Fifer, H.; Woodford, N.; Alexander, S. Detection of markers predictive of macrolide and fluoroquinolone resistance in Mycoplasma genitalium from patients attending sexual health services in England. *Sex. Transm. Infect.* **2018**, *94*, 9–13. [CrossRef] [PubMed]
55. Day, M.; Cole, M.; Patel, H.; Fifer, H.; Woodford, N.; Pitt, R. P616 Predictive macrolide and fluoroquinolone resistance markers in mycoplasma genitalium from the UK and ireland. *Sex. Transm. Infect.* **2019**, *95*, A272. [CrossRef]
56. Register, K.B.; Thole, L.; Rosenbush, R.F.; Minion, F.C. Multilocus sequence typing of Mycoplasma bovis reveals host-specific genotypes in cattle versus bison. *Vet. Microbiol.* **2015**, *175*, 92–98. [CrossRef] [PubMed]

57. Register, K.B.; Boatwright, W.D.; Gesy, K.M.; Thacker, T.C.; Jelinski, M.D. Mistaken identity of an open reading frame proposed for PCR-based identification of Mycoplasma bovis and the effect of polymorphisms and insertions on assay performance. *J. Vet. Diagn. Investig.* **2018**, *30*, 637–641. [CrossRef] [PubMed]
58. Miles, K.; McAuliffe, L.; Ayling, R.D.; Nicholas, R.A.J. Rapid detection of Mycoplasma dispar and M. bovirhinis using allele specific polymerase chain reaction protocols. *FEMS Microbiol. Lett.* **2004**, *241*, 103–107. [CrossRef]
59. Bolger, A.M.; Lohse, M.; Usadel, B. Trimmomatic: A flexible trimmer for Illumina sequence data. *Bioinformatics* **2014**, *30*, 2114–2120. [CrossRef]
60. Li, H.; Durbin, R. Fast and accurate short read alignment with Burrows–Wheeler transform. *Bioinformatics* **2009**, *25*, 1754–1760. [CrossRef]
61. Li, H.; Handsaker, B.; Wysoker, A.; Fennell, T.; Ruan, J.; Homer, N.; Marth, G.; Abecasis, G.; Durbin, R. The Sequence Alignment/Map format and SAMtools. *Bioinformatics* **2009**, *25*, 2078–2079. [CrossRef] [PubMed]
62. Broad Institute; GitHub Repository. Picard Toolkit. Available online: http://broadinstitute.github.io/picard/ (accessed on 15 June 2020).
63. Van de Auwera, G.A.; Carneiro, M.O.; Hartl, C.; Poplin, R.; del Angel, G.; Levy-Moonshine, A.; Jordan, T.; Shakir, K.; Roazen, D.; Thibault, J.; et al. From FastQ Data to High-Confidence Variant Calls: The Genome Analysis Toolkit Best Practices Pipeline. *Curr. Protoc. Bioinf.* **2013**, *43*, 11. [CrossRef]
64. Camacho, C.; Coulouris, G.; Avagyan, V.; Ma, N.; Papadopoulos, J.; Bealer, K.; Madden, T.L. BLAST+: Architecture and applications. *BMC Bioinf.* **2009**, *10*, 421. [CrossRef] [PubMed]
65. Vester, B.; Douthwaite, S. Macrolide Resistance Conferred by Base Substitutions in 23S rRNA. *Antimicrob. Agents Chemother.* **2001**, *45*, 1–12. [CrossRef] [PubMed]
66. Sergeant; ESG. Epitools Epidemiological Calculators. Ausvet. Available online: http://epitools.ausvet.com.au. (accessed on 15 June 2020).
67. McHugh, M.L. Interrater reliability: The kappa statistic. *Biochem. Med.* **2012**, *22*, 276–282. [CrossRef]

8

A CRISPR/Cas9 Generated Bovine CD46-Knockout Cell Line—A Tool to Elucidate the Adaptability of Bovine Viral Diarrhea Viruses (BVDV)

Kevin P. Szillat, Susanne Koethe, Kerstin Wernike, Dirk Höper and Martin Beer *

Institute of Diagnostic Virology, Friedrich-Loeffler-Institut, Federal Research Institute for Animal Health, 17493 Greifswald-Insel Riems, Germany; Kevin.Szillat@fli.de (K.P.S.); Susanne.Koethe@fli.de (S.K.); Kerstin.Wernike@fli.de (K.W.); Dirk.Hoeper@fli.de (D.H.)

* Correspondence: Martin.Beer@fli.de.

Abstract: Bovine viral diarrhea virus (BVDV) entry into a host cell is mediated by the interaction of the viral glycoprotein E2 with the cellular transmembrane CD46 receptor. In this study, we generated a stable Madin–Darby Bovine Kidney (MDBK) CD46-knockout cell line to study the ability of different *pestivirus A* and *B* species (BVDV-1 and -2) to escape CD46-dependent cell entry. Four different BVDV-1/2 isolates showed a clearly reduced infection rate after inoculation of the knockout cells. However, after further passaging starting from the remaining virus foci on the knockout cell line, all tested virus isolates were able to escape CD46-dependency and grew despite the lack of the entry receptor. Whole-genome sequencing of the escape-isolates suggests that the genetic basis for the observed shift in infectivity is an amino acid substitution of an uncharged (glycine/asparagine) for a charged amino acid (arginine/lysine) at position 479 in the E^{RNS} in three of the four isolates tested. In the fourth isolate, the exchange of a cysteine at position 441 in the E^{RNS} resulted in a loss of E^{RNS} dimerization that is likely to influence viral cell-to-cell spread. In general, the CD46-knockout cell line is a useful tool to analyze the role of CD46 for pestivirus replication and the virus–receptor interaction.

Keywords: bovine viral diarrhea virus (BVDV); pestivirus; escape mutant; CD46; E^{RNS}; adaptation; CRISPR; knockout; MDBK; cell entry

1. Introduction

The genus *Pestivirus* belongs to the family *Flaviviridae* and contains several veterinary-relevant virus species with major animal welfare and economic importance like *pestivirus A* and *B* (bovine viral diarrhea virus types 1 and 2, BVDV-1 and -2), *pestivirus D* (border disease virus, BDV) and *pestivirus C* (classical swine fever virus, CSFV) [1–4]. The host range of the classical pestivirus species includes cloven-hoofed animals. However, in recent years, a continuously growing diversity of pestiviruses has been seen worldwide with atypical pestiviruses being isolated from host species like rat, bat and whale [5–8].

Pestiviruses are positive-sense, enveloped, single-stranded RNA viruses with a genome size of 12.3–13 kb [9]. The genome encodes eight nonstructural and four structural proteins in a single open reading frame (ORF) [10], of which the glycoproteins E^{RNS}, E1 and E2 play an important role in the initiation of BVDV uptake by the host cell [11,12]. It has been shown that E^{RNS} interacts with the cell surface heparan sulfate and E1–E2 heterodimers bind the cellular receptor CD46 and mediate clathrin-dependent endocytosis [11,13,14]. CSFV E^{RNS} interacts with the heparan sulfate of porcine cells and both CD46 and heparan sulfate, are major factors for the attachment of CSFV in vitro [15,16]. Interestingly, a shift to a dominant role of the E^{RNS}-mediated binding in CSFV was connected with a drastic in vivo attenuation [15]. Furthermore, dimerization of E^{RNS} is an important virulence factor and abrogation leads to attenuation [17]. E^{RNS} also plays a role in the control of the activation of beta interferon induced upon viral infection by inhibiting the double stranded RNA-induced response of cells [18]. Heparan sulfate has been further described to be important for cellular binding of different viruses, e.g., Schmallenberg virus, hepatitis E virus and rabies virus [19–22].

The binding partner of the pestivirus envelope protein E2, cellular CD46, is a type 1 transmembrane glycoprotein expressed on all nucleated cells that protects host cells from damage by the complement system by the inactivation of C3b and C4b complement products (reviewed in [23]). CD46 is known to serve as a binding partner for several human pathogens like certain adenoviruses, as well as for animal viruses like BVDV and CSFV [16,24]. In particular the two peptide domains $E_{66}QIV_{69}$ and $G_{82}QVLAL_{87}$ of the complement control protein module 1 (CCP1) are crucial for the binding of BVDV—preincubation of MDBK cells with an anti-CD46 serum leads to a strong reduction in infection efficiency [25]. In vitro studies have shown that BVDV spreads by direct cell-to-cell transmission from infected to uninfected cells, even in the presence of neutralizing antibodies against the virus and also if CD46 receptors are blocked by antibodies [26].

Interestingly, there is to our knowledge no bovine CD46-knockout cell line available, allowing e.g., the analysis of the interaction of bovine pestiviruses with receptor molecules. Due to rapid developments in the field of CRISPR/Cas9-mediated gene editing, genetically modified in vitro models like knockout cell lines can be generated in a straightforward manner in a relatively short amount of time [27]. By using ribonucleoprotein (RNP) complexes, target-specific guide RNAs (gRNAs) are complexed with the Cas9 protein and transfected into the target cell. Unlike delivery of mRNA or DNA, RNP-mediated editing does not depend on the host cell for the synthesis of Cas9 and gRNAs. Furthermore, the RNP-based approach reduces the risk of off-target effects and cell death due to the shortened half-life of the proteins inside the target cell [28,29]. We used the CRISPR/Cas9 RNP approach in this study to knockout the cellular receptor CD46 in the Madin–Darby Bovine Kidney (MDBK) cell line to establish a stable in vitro model. We used the generated cell line to passage different BVDV type 1 and 2 strains to study adaptation mechanisms of these viruses in a CD46-negative cellular environment.

2. Materials and Methods

2.1. Cells and Viruses

All cell lines used in this study were obtained from the Collection of Cell Lines in Veterinary Medicine (CCLV) at the Federal Research Institute for Animal Health, Insel Riems, Germany (FLI). Cells were cultured in minimal essential medium (MEM), supplemented with 10% fetal calf serum (FCS), at 37 °C and 5% CO_2. A Madin–Darby Bovine Kidney cell line (MDBK, RIE0261) was used to generate the CD46-knockout cell line, further referred to as CD46-MDBK. Bovine esophagus cells (KOP-R, RIE0244) were used to propagate and titrate virus stocks of the BVDV-1 strains Paplitz (1b, cytopathic), NADL (1a), D02/11-2 (1d) and BVDV-2 strain CS8644 (2a). All pestiviruses were obtained from the German National Reference Laboratory for BVD/MD (FLI).

2.2. Generation of a CD46-knockout Cell Line

2.2.1. Transfection of MDBK Cells and Clone Selection

The CRISPR/Cas9 RNP-mediated editing approach was used in this study to knockout the BVDV binding domains $E_{66}QIV_{69}$ and $G_{82}QVLAL_{87}$ of the cellular receptor CD46 in MDBK cells. CRISPR RNAs (crRNAs) were designed to introduce double-strand breaks (DBS) inside the CCP1 domain, spanning these binding domains (overview in Figure S1). Suitability of the crRNAs was confirmed by CRISPOR [30] and CHOPCHOP [31]. The crRNAs (crRNA-1: GGCTTCATAGAGACAAATCT and crRNA-3: TCATACACAATCTGCTCCCC) and all transfection reagents were purchased from Thermo Fisher Scientific (Waltham, MA, USA). Annealing of the crRNAs with the trans-activating crRNA (tracrRNA) was done following the manufacturer's protocol. MDBK cells were seeded one day prior to transfection and subsequently transfected according to the manufacturer's instructions, using Lipofectamine CRISPRMAX Cas9 transfection reagents (Thermo Fisher Scientific) and TrueCut Cas9 Protein v2 (Thermo Fisher Scientific). The nontarget control cell line (NTC) was generated under identical conditions, using nontarget control gRNAs (Thermo Fisher Scientific). Single cell dilution and subsequent polymerase chain reaction (PCR) of the monoclonal cell colonies were used to screen for a cell clone with the intended deletion.

2.2.2. Isolation of DNA, PCR and Sequencing

DNA was isolated using the QIAamp DNA Mini Kit (Qiagen, Hilden, Germany) according to the manufacturer's instructions. The PCR to confirm the knockout was performed using the QuantiTect Multiplex-PCR Kit (Qiagen) in combination with CD46-specific primers (forward primer CD46_CCP1_F: 5′-GAT GCT GTC TCT TCC ATT TAC T-3′; reverse primer CD46_CCP1_R: 5′-GCC TGA ATG CAT GGC TAT CT-3′) and the following conditions: 15 min, 95 °C; 45× (60 s, 95 °C; 30 s 58 °C and 30 s 72 °C); 5 min, 72 °C; 12 °C storage. The PCR amplicon of the wild-type MDBK cell line is 545 nucleotides long and covers the entire CCP1 domain.

PCR products were analyzed by gel electrophoresis and bands were extracted from the gel using the QIAquick Gel Extraction Kit (Qiagen) according to the manufacturer's instructions. Single cell colonies with the intended knockout mutation display a truncated amplicon with a size of around 400 nucleotides. The PCR gel extract was further sequenced using the IonTorrent platform, as described later.

2.3. Immunofluorescence (IF) Staining, Plaque Assay and Fluorescence-Activated Cell Sorting (FACS)

Expression of the CD46 receptor by NTC and CD46⁻MDBK was visualized by IF staining, using antibodies BVD/CA 26/2/5 and BVD/CA 17/2/1(1:16 dilution in tris-buffered saline with tween (TBST)). The antibodies are directed against CD46 and were kindly provided by Prof. Becher, Institute of Virology, University of Veterinary Medicine, Hannover [32]. Antimouse Alexa Fluor™488 F(ab′)2 (1:1000 in TBST, Life Technologies, Carlsbad, CA, USA) was used as conjugate. FACS and IF was used to study the impact of the CD46-knockout on pestivirus entry into the host cell. In brief, CD46⁻MDBK and NTC cells were seeded one day prior to infection. On the day of infection, the cells were incubated with the different pestivirus isolates for 1 h at 37 °C and 5% CO_2, multiplicity of infection (MOI) of 1. Confluent cells were used at this point to study the initial infectivity of the virus isolates and at later time points the cell-to-cell spread. Uninfected cells were used as a negative control and incubated with maintenance medium only (supplemented with penicillin and streptomycin). After the incubation period, all cells were washed and cultured for 24 h at 37 °C and 5% CO_2 in maintenance medium.

For the IF-staining of pestiviruses, cell supernatant was discarded, and cells were fixed at 80 °C for 2 h. Subsequently, fixed cells were incubated with a 1:500 dilution of antibody WB103/105 (APHA Scientific, Addlestone, UK) in TBST for 1 h at room temperature (RT). Cells were washed thrice with TBST and incubated with a 1:1000 dilution of antimouse Alexa Fluor™488 F(ab′)2 (Life Technologies) in TBST for 1 h at RT. Cells were washed thrice and finally covered with 1,4-Diazabicyclo [2.2.2]octane (DABCO) fluorescence preservation buffer (Sigma-Aldrich, St. Louis, MO, USA) containing propidium iodide (Sigma-Aldrich).

For the IF plaque assay, CD46⁻MDBK cells were seeded one day prior to infection into a 24-well plate. Subsequently, cells were infected with the stock virus (passage 0) and passage 15 of virus isolate Paplitz (BVDV-1b) at MOI = 0.1 and incubated for 1 h at 37 °C, 5% CO_2. Thereafter, the cells were washed once with maintenance medium and overlayed with a 1:1 mix of 4% agarose (Lonza, Basel, Switzerland) in aqua dest. and MEM (2× concentrated) supplemented with penicillin/streptomycin and gentamicin. The medium layer was removed after 48 h, cells were washed once with TBST and fixed with 4% paraformaldehyde (Sigma-Aldrich) for 20 min. Cells were washed once and permeabilized with 0.5% Triton X-100 in phosphate-buffered saline (PBS) for 5 min. Cells were washed again and treated as previously described for the IF staining of pestiviruses. The size of 50 virus plaques was measured manually by using the Nikon Eclipse Ti-U inverted microscope (Nikon GmbH, Düsseldorf, Germany) and NIS-Elements software (v. 4.50). The assay was performed in triplicate. The difference between the groups was statistically evaluated with a Mann-Whitney rank sum test as implemented in SigmaPlot (Version 11.0; Systat Software Inc., San Jose, CA, USA).

For FACS analysis, cell supernatant and trypsinized cells were collected in a FACS tube (Sarstedt, Nümbrecht, Germany) and centrifuged for 5 min at 800× *g*. Supernatant was discarded and cells fixed with 4% paraformaldehyde (Sigma-Aldrich) for 15 min at 4 °C. Cells were further permeabilized with 0.01% Digitonin (Sigma-Aldrich) for 10 min at 4 °C and washed with PBS. Cells were incubated with antibody WB103/105 (1:500 dilution in PBS) for 15 min at 4 °C. The cells were washed with PBS prior application of the anti-mouse Alexa Fluor™488 F(ab')2 (1:1000 dilution in PBS) for 15 min at 4 °C. Cells were washed and resuspended in PBS. A total of 10,000 events were acquired from each sample, using the FACSCalibur (BD Biosciences, Franklin Lakes, NJ, USA). Uninfected cells were stained and used as a negative control. They were included in each run separately to allow subtraction of the background signal (<2.0%). Experiments were performed in three independent replicates.

2.4. *Pestivirus Passaging*

The different pestivirus isolates were passaged on CD46⁻MDBK and NTC cells to study the ability of the viruses to escape CD46-dependent cell entry and as a control, respectively. Cells were seeded one day prior to infection into a 24-well plate and infected with passage 0 (MOI = 1) for 1 h at 37 °C and 5% CO_2. Passage 0 represents the virus stock grown from the initial virus isolates on KOP-R cells. Cells were washed once and incubated in 1 mL maintenance medium for 72 h before they were frozen at −20 °C. For the next virus passage, crude cell extract (noncleared mix of cells and supernatant) were thawed and 100 µL per well were used for infection of the next passage of CD46⁻MDBK and NTC cells. Virus titers of passage 15 were determined by endpoint titration on KOP-R cells and further tested in FACS and IF regarding their infectivity on CD46⁻MDBK.

2.5. *Sequencing, Sequence Assembly and Sequence Comparison*

Virus passages 0 and 15 of the virus isolates passaged on CD46⁻MDBK were processed using a modification of the protocol published by Wylezich and colleagues [33] and sequenced using the Ion Torrent S5XL platform. Briefly, RNA was extracted from the freeze-thawed crude cell extract using the RNAdvance kit (Beckman Coulter, Fullerton, CA, USA) following the manufacturer's instructions and further concentrated using the Agencourt RNAClean XP magnetic beads (Beckman Coulter). Afterwards, cDNA was synthesized using a combination of the SuperScript™ IV First-Strand cDNA Synthesis System (Thermo Fisher Scientific) and the NEBNext®Ultra™ II Non-Directional RNA Second Strand Synthesis Module (New England Biolabs, Ipswich, MA, USA). The generated cDNA was fragmented to 500 bp using the Covaris M220 Focused-Ultrasonicator (Covaris, Brighton, UK) before Ion Torrent-compatible libraries were generated using the GeneRead L Core Kit (Qiagen) and IonXpress Barcode Adapter (Thermo Fisher Scientific). After size selection, library quality was checked using the Agilent 2100 Bioanalyzer system (Agilent Technologies, Santa Clara, CA, USA). The library concentration was measured with the KAPA Library Quantification kit (Roche, Mannheim, Germany). Using an Ion Torrent S5 XL, libraries were sequenced on an Ion 530 chip in 400-bp mode according to the manufacturer's instructions (Thermo Fisher Scientific).

For sequence assembly, a random subset of 50,000 to 500,000 reads was assembled (Newbler v.3.0; 454/Roche). The complete data set was mapped against the assembled genome (Newbler v.3.0; 454/Roche) to confirm the sequence. Consensus sequences were annotated based on the NADL (BVDV-1a) reference strain (NC_001461) and amino acid (aa) sequences were annotated accordingly (E^{RNS}: aa 271-497, E1: aa 498-692 and E2: aa 693-1066). Sequences were aligned using the MAFFT alignment of the bioinformatic software Geneious Prime (v.2020.1.2; Biomatters Ltd., Auckland, New Zealand). The variant analysis for the detection of viral quasispecies was performed in Geneious Prime (v.2020.1.2; Biomatters Ltd., Auckland, New Zealand), using the 454Contigs.bam from the mapping of passage 0 and passage 15 reads against the consensus sequence of passage 0 (Newbler v.3.0./Roche). Single-nucleotide-polymorphisms were detected with a minimum variant frequency of 0.1.

2.6. Immunoblotting

Cell lysates of passage 15 (on CD46⁻MDBK cells) and passage 0 (on NTC cells) were prepared 72 h after infection of the cells. For this purpose, cells were harvested and incubated for 30 min on ice in lysis buffer (Na_2HPO_4, 1% Triton), supplemented with protease inhibitor (Roche). Proteins were separated under nonreducing conditions on a 10% SDS-polyacrylamide gel for 75 min at 130 mA and subsequently blotted onto a GE Healthcare Amersham™ Protan™ nitrocellulose membrane (Thermo Fisher Scientific). The membrane was blocked with Roti®Block (Carl Roth, Karlsruhe, Germany) for 1 h. For the detection of pestivirus E^{RNS}, the membrane was incubated with monoclonal antibodies HC/TC169/2/3 and BVD/C46/2/1 for 1 h (1:100 in Roti®Block, kindly provided by Prof. Becher, Institute of Virology, University of Veterinary Medicine Hannover). The POD-antimouse antibody (Dianova, Hamburg, Germany) was used as a secondary antibody, diluted 1:20,000 in phosphate buffered saline with tween (PBST). Proteins were detected by chemiluminescence, using SuperSignal™ West Pico PLUS Chemiluminescent Substrate (Thermo Fisher Scientific).

3. Results

3.1. Characterization of CD46⁻MDBK

After single cell dilution of the transfected cells, colonies were screened via PCR and the knockout cell was identified to carry a homozygous deletion in the target region. Deep sequencing of the PCR product confirmed the successful biallelic knockout of 120 and 134 nucleotides in the target region, spanning the BVDV binding domains $E_{66}QIV_{69}$ and $G_{82}QVLAL_{87}$ (Figure 1b). CD46⁻MDBK were propagated and the deletion was confirmed by PCR up to the last passage used for passaging of the virus isolates (CD46⁻MDBK passage 54) (Figure 1a). IF staining with the anti-CD46 antibodies BVD/CA 26/2/5 and BVD/CA 17/2/1 (data not shown) showed no fluorescence signal on CD46⁻MDBK, compared to NTC cells (Figure 1c).

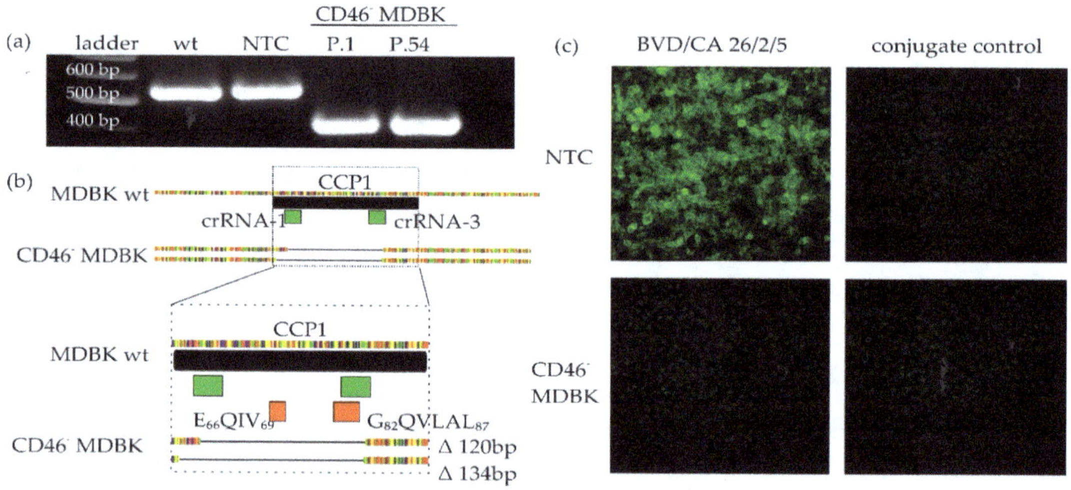

Figure 1. Characterization of CD46⁻MDBK cell line. (**a**) PCR amplification of knockout target region of MDBK wild-type (wt), nontarget control (NTC), CD46⁻MDBK passage 1 (P. 1) and passage 54 (P. 54) (**b**) Sequence comparison of wt and CD46⁻MDBK reveals a biallelic deletion of 120 and 134 nucleotides in the CCP1 region (black box), including the bovine viral diarrhea virus (BVDV) binding sides $E_{66}QIV_{69}$ and $G_{82}QVLAL_{87}$ (orange box). crRNAs are depicted in green (**c**) Staining of CD46 receptor using the anti-CD46 BVD/CA 26/2/5 antibody and conjugate only control on NTC (top) and CD46⁻MDBK (bottom). Magnification: 20×.

The functional knockout of the receptor was further confirmed via FACS and IF. The different BVDV isolates grew successfully on the NTC cells, whereas growth was strongly inhibited on the CD46⁻MDBK cells (Figure 2b,c). Based on the FACS data, the isolates used in this study (passage 0) infected 70–95% of the NTC cells, compared to less than 5% of the CD46⁻MDBK (Figure 2a).

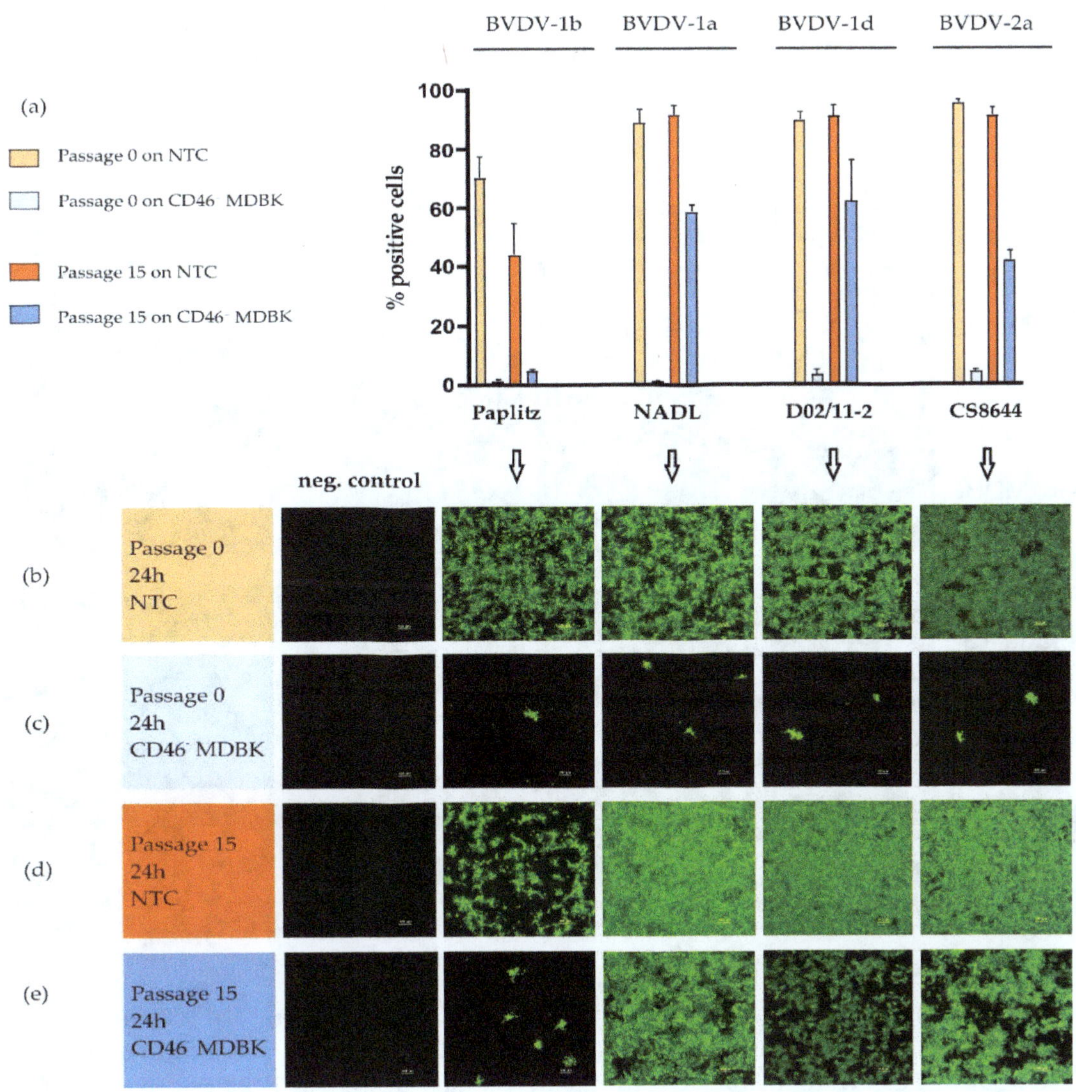

Figure 2. Detection of BVDV in the initial and the 15th passage on the indicated cell lines after incubation for 24 h. (**a**) Diagram depicting the percentages of positive cells in the fluorescence-activated cell sorting (FACS) analysis, conducted in triplicates. Immunofluorescence (IF) staining of (**b**) isolate passage 0 on non-target control (NTC), (**c**) passage 0 on CD46⁻MDBK (**d**) passage 15 on NTC and (**e**) passage 15 on CD46⁻MDBK. Scale bar 100 µm. Cells were incubated with the different pestivirus isolates (MOI = 1) for 1 h at 37 °C and subsequently washed and incubated for 24 h before analysis. Negative control: cells were incubated with maintenance medium only.

3.2. Adaption of Pestivirus Isolates by Passaging on CD46⁻MDBK Cells

The generated CD46⁻MDBK cell line was subsequently used to adapt different BVDV isolates to a host cell lacking the CD46 receptor. After 15 passages on the knockout cell line, the isolates NADL, D02/11-2 (BVDV-1d)and CS8644 (BVDV-2a) showed a strong increase in infectivity, from less than 5% positive cells (passage 0) to 40–60% (passage 15) on CD46⁻MDBKas measured by FACS analysis (Figure 2a). For all viruses, infectivity analyzed by IF staining was in line with the FACS data (Figure 2).

The cytopathic virus isolate Paplitz (cytopathic effect becomes apparent 3 to 5 days post infection) did not show a significant increase in CD46⁻MDBK cell infectivity after passaging based on the FACS results (from 1% positive cells with passage 0 virus to 4% with passage 15 virus, Figure 2a). Similarly, the IF staining did not show a strong increase in infectivity after incubation for 24 h on CD46⁻MDBK, when compared to the other isolates (Figure 2e). However, when the CD46⁻MDBK cells were incubated for 72 h, a complete infection of the cell layer was visible for all isolates (passage 15) (Figure 3d), that differed markedly from incubation for 72 h with the passage 0 virus (Figure 3b).

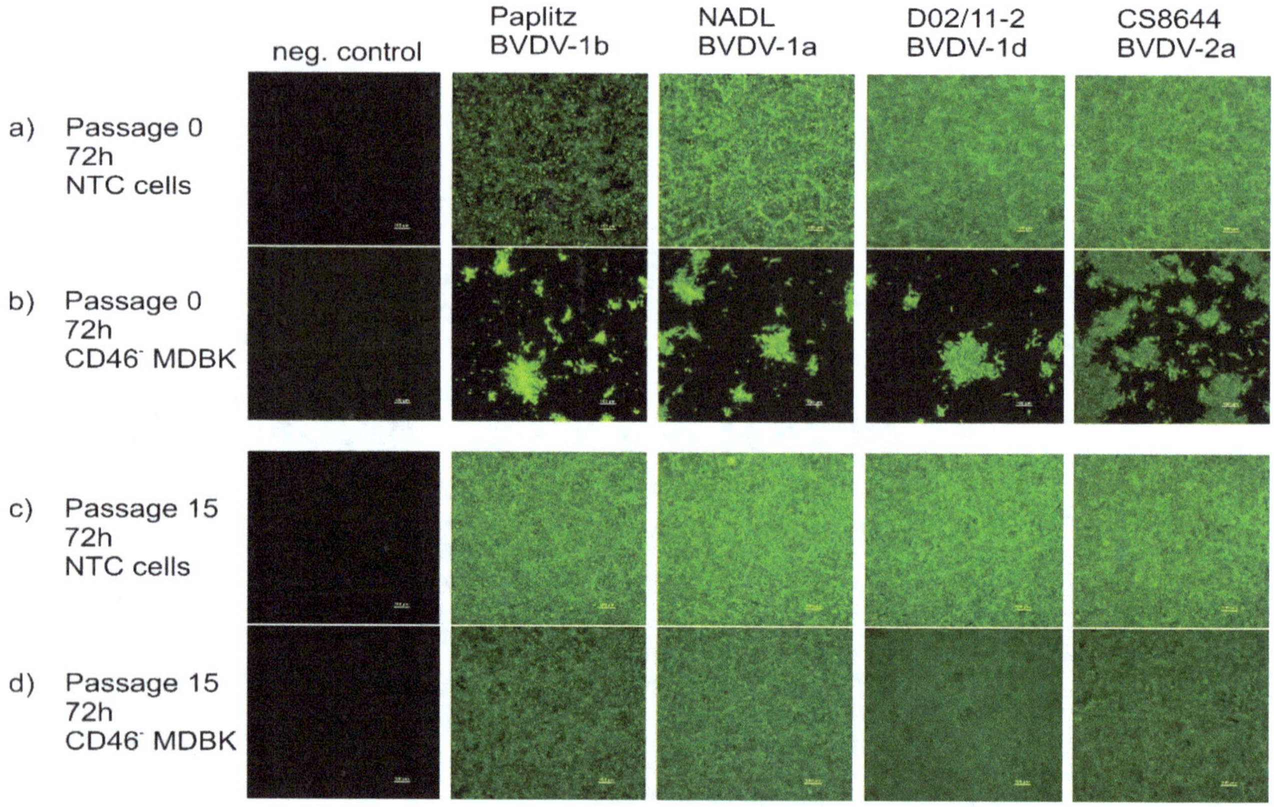

Figure 3. Comparison of the initial passage and passage 15 on non-target control (NTC) and CD46⁻MDBK after incubation for 72 h. Passage 0 on (**a**) NTC and (**b**) CD46⁻MDBK, passage 15 on (**c**) NTC and (**d**) CD46⁻MDBK. Cells were incubated with the designated pestivirus isolates (MOI = 1) for 1 h at 37 °C and subsequently washed and incubated for 72 h before analysis. Negative control: cells were incubated with maintenance medium only.

Therefore, passage 0 and 15 of virus isolate Paplitz (BVDV-1b) were further tested in a plaque assay, to investigate the underlying mechanism that led to a densely infected cell layer after 72 h. Virus plaques of passage 0 had an average area of 28,462 μm^2 (standard deviation (SD): 11,230 μm^2, median: 25,489 μm^2). Virus plaques of passage 15 were on average twice as big, with an average area of 55,985 μm^2 (SD: 21,349 μm^2, median: 53,725 μm^2) (Figure 4).

The difference between the plaque sizes of both groups was statistically significant ($p < 0.001$). In comparison, the plaque size of the other passage 0 virus isolates measures for NADL (BVDV-1a): 25,243 μm^2 (SD: 11,850 μm^2, median: 23,132 μm^2), D02/11-2 (BVDV-1d): 24,655 μm^2 (SD: 9181 μm^2, median: 24,011 μm^2) and for CS8644 (BVDV-2a): 52,072 μm^2 (SD: 21,839 μm^2, median: 50,417 μm^2). Based on these measurments, the Paplitz (BVDV-1b) passage 0 isolate is comparable to the plaque size of the other tested BVDV-1 strains.

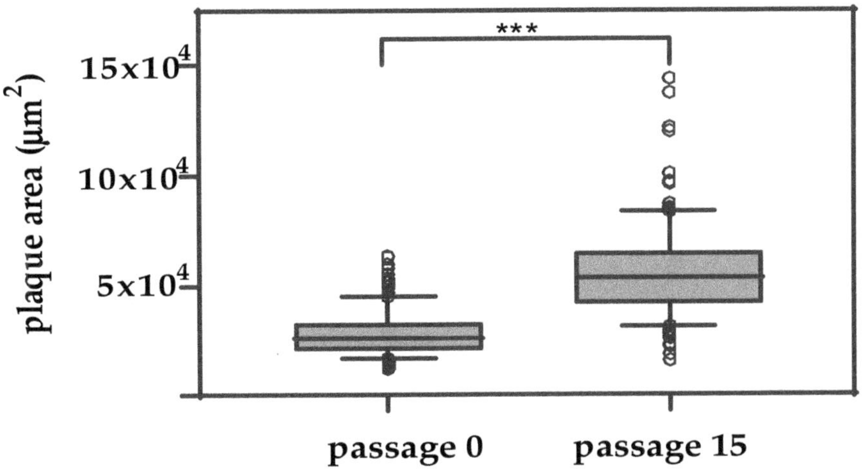

Figure 4. Comparison of plaque sizes of the initial passage and passage 15 of virus isolate Paplitz (BVDV-1b) on CD46⁻MDBK. Cells were incubated with a MOI = 0.1 for 1 h at 37 °C and subsequently washed and incubated for 48 h. The experiment was conducted in triplicate and 50 plaques were measured for each virus passage in each experiment (total n = 150 plaques/isolate). Whiskers indicate the 10% and 90% percentiles, respectively, and each outlier is depicted by a dot. The difference between the plaque sizes is statistically significant (*** $p < 0.001$).

3.3. Sequence Analysis after Virus Passaging on CD46⁻MDBK

In order to identify genetic adaptations that led to the observed shift in infectivity and virus-growth characteristics between the different virus passages, they were sequenced using next-generation sequencing. The genomic regions coding for the E^{RNS}, E1 and E2 proteins of the initial virus passage were compared to the 15th passage, since these regions are known to be involved in pestivirus entry into the host cell [11,14]. The graphical overview of the aligned sequences is depicted in Figure S2. After 15 passages, all virus isolates gained at least one aa substitution in the E^{RNS}-protein (Table 1).

Table 1. Overview of the amino acid substitution in E^{RNS}, E1 and E2 proteins based on the consensus sequences of the original BVDV isolates and their 15th passage on the CD46-deficient cell line. Amino acid positions with known effects are highlighted in bold.

Virus Strain	Amino Acid Position	Amino Acid Passage 0	Amino Acid Passage 15	Genome Region	Variant Frequency Passage 0	Variant Frequency Passage 15
Paplitz (BVDV-1b)	**441**	**Cystein**	**Arginine**	E^{RNS}	-	**98.7%**
	673	Alanine	Valine	E1	-	54.3%
	764	Glycine	Arginine	E2	-	99.7%
NADL (BVDV-1a)	450	Histidine	Leucine	E^{RNS}	-	100%
	479	**Glycine**	**Arginine**	E^{RNS}	-	**100%**
	677	Isoleucine	Methionine	E1	36.0%	100%
D02/11-2 (BVDV-1d)	**479**	**Asparagine**	**Lysine**	E^{RNS}	**42.1%**	**100%**
	631	Alanine	Valine	E1	-	91.6%
CS8644 (BVDV-2a)	423	Glycine	Arginine	E^{RNS}	-	75.3%
	477	Glutamine	Lysine	E^{RNS}	-	77.6%
	479	**Glycine**	**Arginine**	E^{RNS}	-	**99.4%**
	480	Isoleucine	Threonine	E^{RNS}	-	99.8%
	735	Histidine	Glutamine	E2	-	99.7%
	847	Isoleucine	Arginine	E2	-	99.4%
	880	Isoleucine	Valine	E2	-	95.8%

Virus isolates NADL (BVDV-1a), D02/11-2 (BVDV-1d) and CS8644 (BVDV-2a) displayed an aa exchange at the same position, namely 479 in the E^{RNS}. NADL (BVDV-1a) and CS8644 (BVDV-2a) exchanged the uncharged glycine with a charged arginine and D02/11-2 (BVDV-1d) exchanged the uncharged asparagine with a charged lysine. The cytopathic strain Paplitz (BVDV-1b) exchanged an uncharged cysteine for a charged arginine at position 441 in the E^{RNS} (Table 1). From the 15 mutations listed, two were already detected in the viral sequence reads from passage 0 as a minor population. Amino acid mutation in NADL (BVDV-1a) at position 677 and in D02/11-2 (BVDV-1d) at position 479 were identified with a sequence prevalence of 36% and 42%, respectively (Table 1). An important finding is that the minor population at aa position 479 of D02/11-2 (BVDV-1d) passage 0 is linked with another minor population in passage 0 that substitutes the original lysine at position 480 with an asparagine with a frequency of 39.9% (Table S1). During analysis of the actual reads of passage 0, it becomes apparent that reads are coding either for a lysine-asparagine or an asparagine-lysine (aa position 479 and 480) but not for a lysine-lysine or asparagine-asparagine (visualized in Figure S3).

3.4. E^{RNS} Dimerization of Virus Isolate Paplitz (BVDV-1b)

The formation of E^{RNS} dimers of virus isolate Paplitz (BVDV-1b) was analyzed, since the exchanged aa cysteine at position 441 was previously described to be important for dimerization of E^{RNS} [17]. Immunoblot analysis confirmed formation of E^{RNS} dimers (88-96 kDa) in virus passage 0, compared to monomer formation (48 kDa) of virus passage 15 (Figure 5).

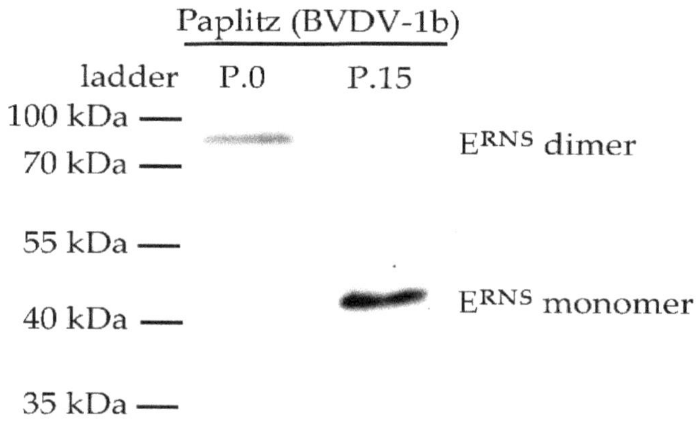

Figure 5. E^{RNS} formation of virus isolate Paplitz (BVDV-1b). Detection of E^{RNS} in the lysates of infected cells 72 h post infection using immunoblotting. Proteins were separated under nonreducing conditions. E^{RNS} of passage 0 (P.0) forms dimers (88–96 kDa), whereas passage 15 (P.15) forms monomers (44–48 kDa).

4. Discussion

The importance of bovine CD46 for pestivirus entry into a host cell has been already described in detail in the past and the two peptide domains $E_{66}QIV_{69}$ and $G_{82}QVLAL_{87}$ have been identified to be crucial [25,34,35]. However, for further analysis, bovine CD46-knock-out cells were needed. We therefore successfully knocked out the aforementioned domains and showed that this leads to a significant decrease in infectivity of the tested BVDV-1 and -2 isolates.

The strong reduction in infectivity on $CD46^{-}$MDBK is consistent with previous findings of Krey et al. [25], who showed reduced binding of pestivirus isolates in vitro by at least 70% (in 29 out of 30 isolates tested) after preincubation of MDBK cells with an anti-CD46 serum. Interestingly, we could show that the knockout of CD46 did not result in a complete loss of infectivity. A small percentage of less than 5% of the cells were still able to get infected by the tested BVDV isolates (passage 0). Therefore, a small fraction of the viruses most likely uses a CD46-independent route to enter the respective host cells.

After passaging the four different virus isolates 15 times on $CD46^{-}$MDBK, infectivity of the virus isolates NADL (BVDV-1a), D02/11-2 (BVDV-1d) and CS8644 (BVDV-2a) increased significantly when compared to passage 0 after incubation for 24 h. Sequencing of these passages showed that the isolates share the same aa exchange at position 479 after passaging. This aa exchange is of importance, since the same position (aa 476 in *pestivirus C* (CSFV) correlates to aa 479 in *pestivirus A/B*) has been shown to be crucial for CSFV interaction with membrane-associated heparan sulfate [36]. The exchange of an uncharged aa (glycine) to a positively charged aa (arginine) at this position has been described to increase virus replication in vitro of CSFV variants carrying this mutation [15,36]. It has been also suggested that this aa substitution (position 476 in CSFV; position 479 in BVDV-1 and -2) increases the positive charge of the E^{RNS} region and that this particular aa is exposed to the surface and involved into direct binding to the negatively charged heparan sulfate [36]. Reimann and colleagues [37] also associated the increased virus infectivity in vitro with the same aa substitution of glycine to arginine at position 479 in CP7_E2alf, a chimeric pestivirus constructed from a BVDV-1 backbone (strain CP7) and E2 from CSFV (strain Alfort). Overall, these findings indicate very clearly that the loss of the host cells CD46 favours the introduction of a positively charged aa at position 479 of the E^{RNS} in the pestivirus isolates studied. Even though the aa position 479 is in the amphipathic C-terminal end of the E^{RNS} that is important for membrane binding, it is likely that this aa substitution has no or only minor effects on lipid binding. Research has shown that the amphipathic helix has a robust lipid affinity that cannot be disturbed by mutating single amino acids [38].

The aa substitution at position 479 occurred most likely de novo in virus isolate NADL (BVDV-1a) and CS8644 (BVDV-2a), however, very low frequencies might be missed due to the sequencing depths. In case of virus isolate D02/11-2 (BVDV-1d), the minor variant of the aa substitution (asparagine for lysine) at position 479 can be detected already in passage 0 with a proportion of 42%. Therefore, we would expect the phenotype of this passage 0 virus isolate to show a higher infectivity than actually detected, since we postulate that this mutation is important for the change to a phenotype with higher infectivity. However, when we looked into the other minor variants of passage 0 virus isolate D02/11-2 (BVDV-1d), we found that a lysine at aa position 480 is substituted with an asparagine with a similar proportion of 39.9%. Furthermore, when looking into the actual reads of passage 0, we could see that the reads are coding either for a lysine-asparagine (in consensus) or an asparagine-lysine (in minor variant) at position 479–480 but not for a lysine-lysine or an asparagine-asparagine. We therefore assume that in case of D02/11-2 (BVDV-1d), both lysine at position 479 and 480 are necessary to increase the infectivity of the virus. This has probably been selected for since neither the lysine-asparagine nor the asparagine-lysine variant could be detected in passage 15.

We suggest that the aa exchange at position 479 may allow the virus isolates NADL (BVDV-1a), D02/11-2 (BVDV-1d) and CS8644 (BVDV-2a) to compensate for the loss of the potential binding side CD46 by an increased binding of heparan sulfate. This finding provides therefore additional evidence for previous assumptions concerning the role of the heparan sulfate binding and CD46 independent entry of pestiviruses [25]. Furthermore, it would be interesting to passage these mutated virus isolates (passage 15) in vivo, to study if the mutation at position 479 is selected against in vivo like it was shown for CSFV [15]. We would speculate that this is the case, considering the similarities of BVDV and CSFV cell entry in vitro regarding their dependency on CD46 and heparan sulfate [11,16,34].

Nevertheless, the cytopathic strain Paplitz (BVDV-1b) is of special interest, since the virus shows an altered and unexpected growth behaviour after passaging. It seems that the selection pressure from CD46-MDBK cell passaging does not result in an improved initial cell entry of the virus but rather changed the growth behaviour of the virus towards a markedly improved cell-to-cell spread after initial cell entry. The lower infectivity of Paplitz (passage 15) compared to Paplitz (passage 0) on the NTC cells might be explained by the special way of adaption of this strain to the CD46 deficient environment and the subsequent loss of E^{RNS} dimers. It can be hypothesized that this trade-off favours cell spread in CD46-deficient cells for the cost of reduced binding to CD46 and growth in NTC cells. Interestingly, one mutation identified in the E^{RNS} of Paplitz (BVDV-1b) results in the exchange of a cysteine at position 441, which is important for the formation of a intermolecular disulphide bond in the E^{RNS} of CSFV [17]. Mutation of this cysteine, that occurred most likely de novo, leads to a loss of dimerization of E^{RNS}

that results in case of CSFV in an attenuated virus that is still able to grow in cell culture [17] but also with larger plaque sizes due the reduced binding to heparan sulfate [39]. We could also demonstrate here the loss of E^{RNS} dimerization in the passage 15 variant. Paplitz (BVDV-1b) passages 0 and 15 are not able to enter the host cell faster after passaging, but once inside the cell, the virus grows differently than the initial passage 0 and shows an enhanced cell-to-cell spread. This change is likely influenced by substitution of the cystein at position 441, that leads to monomeric E^{RNS}. Further research should study if the adaption described for virus isolate Paplitz (BVDV-1b) is typical for cytopathic pestiviruses and if the other mutations identified in E1 and E2 might also play a role. It could be hypothesized that dimerizaton of E^{RNS} could have a function concering cell-to-cell spread of pestiviruses like BVDV-1.

In summary, we describe here the succesful generation of a stable CD46-knockout cell line and we demonstrated that the infectivity of different BVDV isolates strongly depends on CD46. At the same time, we showed that a fraction of the virus particles is still able to enter the host cell even in the absence of the CD46 receptor. The study also shows that forced adaption of the pestiviruses studied leads to compensatory mutations in the E^{RNS}, affecting the virus-host interplay. Forced adaption of virus isolates NADL (BVDV-1a), and CS8644 (BVDV-2a) and D02/11-2 (BVDV-1d) led to a mutation at aa position 479 probably increasing heparan sulfate binding. In contrast, isolate Paplitz (BVDV-1b) substituted a cystein at position 441 that led to a loss of E^{RNS}-dimer formation, that is further suggested to increase cell-to-cell spread of the virus. The newly generated cell line is now available for future research to elucidate the role of the CD46 receptor in the context of the pestivirus biology and growth cycle.

Supplementary Materials:
Supplementary Figure S1. Overview of the PCR amplicon, including the complement control protein 1 domain (CCP1, depicted in grey) with BVDV binding sides $E_{66}QIV_{69}$ and $G_{82}QVLA_{87}$ (both in orange), CRISPR RNAs (crRNA-1 and -3, depicted in yellow) and PCR primer (CD46_CCP1_F and _R, depicted in green). Supplementary Figure S2. Amino acid sequence alignment of passage 0 and 15 of the BVDV isolates. Differences between passages are depicted as a black gap in the alignment. The red box indicates the shared amino acid exchange at position 479 in virus passage 15 of NADL (BVDV-1a), D02/11-2 (BVDV-1b) and CS8644 (BVDV-2a). Supplementary Figure S3. Comparison of passage 0 and passage 15 sequence reads of D02/11-2 (BVDV-1b) at aa position 479 and 480 compared to consensus sequence passage 0. Two minor variants resulting in either a AAA-AAC or AAC-AAA codon (aa lysine-asparagine or asparagine-lysine). In comparison, passage 15 reads assemble only AAA-AAA (aa lysine-lysine) at position 479 and 480. The initial consensus sequence of passage 0 assembles AAC-AAA (aa lysine-asparagine). Supplementary Table S1. Overview of the variant analysis for passage 0 and 15 of virus isolate D02/11-2 (BVDV-1b). The variant of aa 479 and 480 is represented by nucleotide position 1437 and 1440 respectively and highlighted in bold.

Author Contributions: Conceptualization, M.B.; methodology, S.K., K.W., D.H. and M.B.; formal analysis, K.P.S., S.K., K.W., D.H. and M.B.; investigation, K.P.S., S.K., D.H. and K.W.; resources, D.H. and K.W.; writing—original draft preparation, K.P.S.; writing—review and editing, S.K., K.W., D.H. and M.B.; visualization, K.P.S. All authors have read and agreed to the published version of the manuscript.

Acknowledgments: The authors are grateful to Andrea Aebischer, Patrick Zitzow, Doreen Schulz and Bianka Hillmann for excellent technical assistance and support.

References

1. Edwards, S.; Fukusho, A.; Lefevre, P.C.; Lipowski, A.; Pejsak, Z.; Roehe, P.; Westergaard, J. Classical swine fever: The global situation. *Vet. Microbiol.* **2000**, *73*, 103–119. [CrossRef]
2. Richter, V.; Lebl, K.; Baumgartner, W.; Obritzhauser, W.; Käsbohrer, A.; Pinior, B. A systematic worldwide review of the direct monetary losses in cattle due to bovine viral diarrhoea virus infection. *Vet. J.* **2017**, *220*, 80–87. [CrossRef] [PubMed]
3. Braun, U.; Hilbe, M.; Peterhans, E.; Schweizer, M. Border disease in cattle. *Vet. J.* **2019**, *246*, 12–20. [CrossRef] [PubMed]

4. Smith, D.B.; Meyers, G.; Bukh, J.; Gould, E.A.; Monath, T.; Scott Muerhoff, A.; Pletnev, A.; Rico-Hesse, R.; Stapleton, J.T.; Simmonds, P.; et al. Proposed revision to the taxonomy of the genus Pestivirus, family Flaviviridae. *J. Gen. Virol.* **2017**, *98*, 2106–2112. [CrossRef] [PubMed]
5. Wu, Z.; Ren, X.; Yang, L.; Hu, Y.; Yang, J.; He, G.; Zhang, J.; Dong, J.; Sun, L.; Du, J.; et al. Virome analysis for identification of novel mammalian viruses in bat species from Chinese provinces. *J. Virol.* **2012**, *86*, 10999–11012. [CrossRef] [PubMed]
6. Firth, C.; Bhat, M.; Firth, M.A.; Williams, S.H.; Frye, M.J.; Simmonds, P.; Conte, J.M.; Ng, J.; Garcia, J.; Bhuva, N.P.; et al. Detection of zoonotic pathogens and characterization of novel viruses carried by commensal Rattus norvegicus in New York City. *mBio* **2014**, *5*, e01933–e02014. [CrossRef]
7. Blome, S.; Beer, M.; Wernike, K. New leaves in the growing tree of Pestiviruses. *Adv. Virus Res.* **2017**, *99*, 139–160.
8. Jo, W.K.; van Elk, C.; van de Bildt, M.; van Run, P.; Petry, M.; Jesse, S.T.; Jung, K.; Ludlow, M.; Kuiken, T.; Osterhaus, A. An evolutionary divergent pestivirus lacking the N^{pro} gene systemically infects a whale species. *Emerg. Microbes Infect.* **2019**, *8*, 1383–1392. [CrossRef]
9. Simmonds, P.; Becher, P.; Bukh, J.; Gould, E.A.; Meyers, G.; Monath, T.; Muerhoff, S.; Pletnev, A.; Rico-Hesse, R.; Smith, D.B.; et al. ICTV Virus Taxonomy Profile: Flaviviridae. *J. Gen. Virol.* **2017**, *98*, 2–3. [CrossRef]
10. Tautz, N.; Tews, B.A.; Meyers, G. The Molecular Biology of Pestiviruses. *Adv. Virus Res.* **2015**, *93*, 47–160.
11. Iqbal, M.; Flick-Smith, H.; McCauley, J.W. Interactions of bovine viral diarrhoea virus glycoprotein E^{rns} with cell surface glycosaminoglycans. *J. Gen. Virol.* **2000**, *81 Pt 2*, 451–459. [CrossRef]
12. Liang, D.; Sainz, I.F.; Ansari, I.H.; Gil, L.; Vassilev, V.; Donis, R.O. The envelope glycoprotein E2 is a determinant of cell culture tropism in ruminant pestiviruses. *J. Gen. Virol.* **2003**, *84 Pt 5*, 1269–1274. [CrossRef]
13. Grummer, B.; Grotha, S.; Greiser-Wilke, I. Bovine viral diarrhoea virus is internalized by clathrin-dependent receptor-mediated endocytosis. *J. Vet. Med. B Infect. Dis. Vet. Public Health* **2004**, *51*, 427–432. [CrossRef] [PubMed]
14. Ronecker, S.; Zimmer, G.; Herrler, G.; Greiser-Wilke, I.; Grummer, B. Formation of bovine viral diarrhea virus E1-E2 heterodimers is essential for virus entry and depends on charged residues in the transmembrane domains. *J. Gen. Virol.* **2008**, *89 Pt 9*, 2114–2121. [CrossRef]
15. Hulst, M.M.; van Gennip, H.G.; Vlot, A.C.; Schooten, E.; de Smit, A.J.; Moormann, R.J. Interaction of classical swine fever virus with membrane-associated heparan sulfate: Role for virus replication in vivo and virulence. *J. Virol.* **2001**, *75*, 9585–9595. [CrossRef] [PubMed]
16. Dräger, C.; Beer, M.; Blome, S. Porcine complement regulatory protein CD46 and heparan sulfates are the major factors for classical swine fever virus attachment in vitro. *Arch. Virol.* **2015**, *160*, 739–746. [CrossRef] [PubMed]
17. Tews, B.A.; Schürmann, E.M.; Meyers, G. Mutation of cysteine 171 of pestivirus E^{rns} RNase prevents homodimer formation and leads to attenuation of classical swine fever virus. *J. Virol.* **2009**, *83*, 4823–4834. [CrossRef] [PubMed]
18. Iqbal, M.; Poole, E.; Goodbourn, S.; McCauley, J.W. Role for bovine viral diarrhea virus E^{rns} glycoprotein in the control of activation of beta interferon by double-stranded RNA. *J. Virol.* **2004**, *78*, 136–145. [CrossRef] [PubMed]
19. Murakami, S.; Takenaka-Uema, A.; Kobayashi, T.; Kato, K.; Shimojima, M.; Palmarini, M.; Horimoto, T. Heparan sulfate proteoglycan is an important attachment factor for cell entry of Akabane and Schmallenberg viruses. *J. Virol.* **2017**, *91*, e00503–e00517. [CrossRef]
20. Kalia, M.; Chandra, V.; Rahman, S.A.; Sehgal, D.; Jameel, S. Heparan sulfate proteoglycans are required for cellular binding of the hepatitis E virus ORF2 capsid protein and for viral infection. *J. Virol.* **2009**, *83*, 12714–12724. [CrossRef]
21. Sasaki, M.; Anindita, P.D.; Ito, N.; Sugiyama, M.; Carr, M.; Fukuhara, H.; Ose, T.; Maenaka, K.; Takada, A.; Hall, W.W.; et al. The role of heparan sulfate proteoglycans as an attachment factor for rabies virus entry and infection. *J. Infect. Dis.* **2018**, *217*, 1740–1749. [CrossRef] [PubMed]
22. Thamamongood, T.; Aebischer, A.; Wagner, V.; Chang, M.W.; Elling, R.; Benner, C.; Garcia-Sastre, A.; Kochs, G.; Beer, M.; Schwemmle, M. A genome-wide CRISPR-Cas9 screen reveals the requirement of host cell sulfation for Schmallenberg virus infection. *J. Virol.* **2020**. [CrossRef] [PubMed]

23. Liszewski, M.K.; Atkinson, J.P. Complement regulator CD46: Genetic variants and disease associations. *Hum. Genom.* **2015**, *9*, 7. [CrossRef]
24. Cattaneo, R. Four viruses, two bacteria, and one receptor: Membrane cofactor protein (CD46) as pathogens' magnet. *J. Virol.* **2004**, *78*, 4385–4388. [CrossRef] [PubMed]
25. Krey, T.; Himmelreich, A.; Heimann, M.; Menge, C.; Thiel, H.J.; Maurer, K.; Rümenapf, T. Function of bovine CD46 as a cellular receptor for bovine viral diarrhea virus is determined by complement control protein 1. *J. Virol.* **2006**, *80*, 3912–3922. [CrossRef] [PubMed]
26. Merwaiss, F.; Czibener, C.; Alvarez, D.E. Cell-to-cell transmission is the main mechanism supporting bovine viral diarrhea virus spread in cell culture. *J. Virol.* **2019**, *93*, e01776–e01818. [CrossRef]
27. Doudna, J.A.; Charpentier, E. Genome editing. The new frontier of genome engineering with CRISPR-Cas9. *Science* **2014**, *346*, 1258096. [CrossRef]
28. Lin, S.; Staahl, B.T.; Alla, R.K.; Doudna, J.A. Enhanced homology-directed human genome engineering by controlled timing of CRISPR/Cas9 delivery. *Elife* **2014**, *3*, e04766. [CrossRef]
29. DeWitt, M.A.; Corn, J.E.; Carroll, D. Genome editing via delivery of Cas9 ribonucleoprotein. *Methods* **2017**, *121*, 9–15. [CrossRef] [PubMed]
30. Haeussler, M.; Schönig, K.; Eckert, H.; Eschstruth, A.; Mianne, J.; Renaud, J.B.; Schneider-Maunoury, S.; Shkumatava, A.; Teboul, L.; Kent, J.; et al. Evaluation of off-target and on-target scoring algorithms and integration into the guide RNA selection tool CRISPOR. *Genome Biol.* **2016**, *17*, 148. [CrossRef]
31. Labun, K.; Montague, T.G.; Krause, M.; Torres Cleuren, Y.N.; Tjeldnes, H.; Valen, E. CHOPCHOP v3: Expanding the CRISPR web toolbox beyond genome editing. *Nucleic Acids Res.* **2019**, *47*, W171–W174. [CrossRef] [PubMed]
32. Schelp, C.; Greiser-Wilke, I.; Wolf, G.; Beer, M.; Moennig, V.; Liess, B. Identification of cell membrane proteins linked to susceptibility to bovine viral diarrhoea virus infection. *Arch. Virol.* **1995**, *140*, 1997–2009. [CrossRef] [PubMed]
33. Wylezich, C.; Papa, A.; Beer, M.; Höper, D. A versatile sample processing workflow for metagenomic pathogen detection. *Sci. Rep.* **2018**, *8*, 13108. [CrossRef] [PubMed]
34. Maurer, K.; Krey, T.; Moennig, V.; Thiel, H.J.; Rümenapf, T. CD46 is a cellular receptor for bovine viral diarrhea virus. *J. Virol.* **2004**, *78*, 1792–1799. [CrossRef] [PubMed]
35. Alzamel, N.; Bayrou, C.; Decreux, A.; Desmecht, D. Soluble forms of CD46 are detected in Bos taurus plasma and neutralize BVDV, the bovine pestivirus. *Comp. Immunol. Microbiol. Infect. Dis.* **2016**, *49*, 39–46. [CrossRef] [PubMed]
36. Hulst, M.M.; van Gennip, H.G.; Moormann, R.J. Passage of classical swine fever virus in cultured swine kidney cells selects virus variants that bind to heparan sulfate due to a single amino acid change in envelope protein E^{rns}. *J. Virol.* **2000**, *74*, 9553–9561. [CrossRef] [PubMed]
37. Reimann, I.; Depner, K.; Trapp, S.; Beer, M. An avirulent chimeric Pestivirus with altered cell tropism protects pigs against lethal infection with classical swine fever virus. *Virology* **2004**, *322*, 143–157. [CrossRef]
38. Aberle, D.; Oetter, K.M.; Meyers, G. Lipid binding of the amphipathic helix serving as membrane anchor of Pestivirus glycoprotein E^{rns}. *PLoS ONE* **2015**, *10*, e0135680. [CrossRef]
39. van Gennip, H.G.; Hesselink, A.T.; Moormann, R.J.; Hulst, M.M. Dimerization of glycoprotein E^{rns} of classical swine fever virus is not essential for viral replication and infection. *Arch. Virol.* **2005**, *150*, 2271–2286. [CrossRef]

9

Molecular Survey and Phylogenetic Analysis of Atypical Porcine Pestivirus (APPV) Identified in Swine and Wild Boar from Northern Italy

Enrica Sozzi *, Cristian Salogni, Davide Lelli, Ilaria Barbieri, Ana Moreno, Giovanni Loris Alborali and Antonio Lavazza

Istituto Zooprofilattico Sperimentale della Lombardia e dell'Emilia Romagna "Bruno Ubertini" (IZSLER), Via Antonio Bianchi 7/9, 25124 Brescia, Italy; cristian.salogni@izsler.it (C.S.); davide.lelli@izsler.it (D.L.); ilaria.barbieri@izsler.it (I.B.); anamaria.morenomartin@izsler.it (A.M.); giovanni.alborali@izsler.it (G.L.A.); antonio.lavazza@izsler.it (A.L.)

* Correspondence: enrica.sozzi@izsler.it.

Abstract: Atypical porcine pestivirus (APPV) is a newly recognized member of the *Flaviviridae* family. This novel porcine pestivirus was first described in 2015 in the USA, where it has been associated with congenital tremor type A-II in new-born piglets. APPV is widely distributed in domestic pigs in Europe and Asia. In this study, a virological survey was performed in Northern Italy to investigate the presence of APPV using molecular methods. Testing of 360 abortion samples from pig herds revealed two APPV strains from distinct provinces in the Lombardy region and testing of 430 wild boar blood samples revealed three strains, one from Lombardy and two from Emilia Romagna. The nucleotide sequencing of a fragment of the nonstructural protein 3-coding region revealed a high similarity to the previously detected European strains (Spanish, German, and Italian) of APPV.

Keywords: pestivirus; pig; APPV; phylogenetic analysis; Italy

---

1. Introduction

Pestiviruses are highly variable single-stranded RNA genome viruses, belonging to the *Flaviviridae* family. Actually, based on molecular and epidemiological evidence, the genus Pestivirus includes eleven species, indicated with progressive letters from A to K. Thus, the "classical" species are A (Bovine viral diarrhea virus 1), B (Bovine viral diarrhea virus 2), C (Classical swine fever virus), and D (Border disease virus), whereas the new species are E to K [1]. In addition, other pestiviruses were described, likely as three additional species, respectively, in bats (bat-derived pestivirus) [2,3], sheep and goats (Tunisian sheep pestiviruses) [4], and pigs (Linda pestivirus) [5]. In the swine species only, in addition to Pestivirus C, three pestiviruses have been identified to date: (1) Pestivirus F (Bungowannah virus) reported only in Australia, as a cause of reproductive disorders, fetal death, and sudden death in piglets, [6]; (2) The Linda virus described in association with congenital tremors (CTs) in piglets in Austria and thereafter only occasionally reported, leaving its geographical spread and clinical relevance in pigs undefined [5]; and (3) Pestivirus K, commonly known as atypical porcine pestivirus (APPV), which is the most relevant due to the frequency of identification, clinical findings, and economic importance. In fact, it has been identified several times in North America [7,8], South America [9,10], Europe [11–13], and Asia [14,15], and it should be considered as stably present for a long time in domestic and wild pig populations [8,10,15,16]. This is true also for Italy, since in a previous survey, at least four APPV isolates were found between 2015–2017 and a quite high seroprevalence was detected in pig sera [15].

Although APPV has been repeatedly identified in asymptomatic animals, there is clear evidence that it is associated with CT syndrome type A-II (CT A-II) in newborns [7]. Clinically healthy pigs and wild boars may have an epidemiological role as vehicles of APPV, but, considering the different frequency of detection in wild boars, which was quite high in Germany and Serbia [17] and very low in Spain [18], the epidemiology of APPV may vary considerably from country to country with increases in livestock and wild populations, animal breeding, and world trade [18]. While one study described the economic losses caused by a 10% drop in the number of weaned piglets per sow [19], the full economic consequences of APPV outbreaks remain to be determined.

In this study, the presence of the APPV genome in pig fetuses and wild boars from both the Lombardy and Emilia Romagna regions of Northern Italy was determined, and the genetic characterizations of the identified strains are described.

2. Materials and Methods

2.1. Pigs

From 2016 to 2018, 360 fetuses of pigs from pig farms in the Lombardy region were examined at the IZSLER Diagnostic Laboratory in Brescia. All of the samples examined originated from field cases of spontaneous abortions in pig farms and sent to the general diagnostic laboratory of IZSLER to determine the presence of any infectious agent. In none of these cases was the presence of clinical signs referable to CT syndrome specifically reported. During necropsy, samples of organs (brain, lung, spleen, liver, and kidney) were taken from each aborted fetus, then collected into a single farm-specific pool and homogenized (10% w/v) in minimum essential medium (MEM; Gibco, Life Technologies, Paisley, UK) supplemented with an antibiotic (1000 U/mL penicillin, 1 mg/mL streptomycin; Gibco, Life Technologies, Paisley, UK) and anti-mycotic (2.5 μg/mL amphotericin B; Gibco, Life Technologies, Paisley, UK). After centrifugation, the supernatant was analyzed to identify any agents that cause abortions in swine. For bacteriological agents such as Brucella spp., Listeria spp., and Mycoplasma spp., the screening and pathogen identification were conducted according to Office International des Epizooties (OIE) standardized protocols [20]. The presence of Chlamydophila spp. was investigated by real-time Polymerase Chain Reaction (PCR) directly in biological samples [21] and typing by the PCR-restriction fragment length polymorphism (RFLP) assay, targeting the 16S ribosomal gene [22]. For Mycoplasma spp., the PCR method described by van Kuppeveld et al. [23] was used. Virological analyses for detecting the more common pig pathogens were conducted using a panel of PCR methods including porcine reproductive and respiratory syndrome virus (PRRSV) (AgPath-ID™ NA and EU PRRSV Multiplex© Applied Biosystems), porcine circovirus type 2 (PCV-2) [24], porcine parvovirus (PPV) [25], and porcine circovirus type 3 (PCV-3) [26]. The presence of pestiviruses was determined by using a pan-pestivirus real-time RT-PCR [27], and, considering its limited capacity in detecting APPV, by a APPV-specific real-time RT-PCR [19]. In addition, all the tested samples were inoculated on cell cultures (primary embryonic swine kidney cells, swine alveolar macrophages, and monkey kidney cell line MARC-145), which allow the isolation of a broad range of swine viruses. The inoculated cell monolayers were observed daily for 5–7 d for the appearance of a cytopathic effect and then sub-cultured to the second passage, at which time they were independently tested using an "in-house" sandwich enzyme-linked immunosorbent assay (ELISAs) for the presence of pestivirus [28] and PRRSV antigens [29]. Only those samples that were positive for APPV at the initial screening test using the APPV-specific real-time RT-PCR were further subcultured to improve the chance to isolate the APPV until the fifth passage, at which time, even in the absence of a cytopathic effect, they were assessed again with the APPV-specific real-time RT-PCR.

2.2. Wild Boars

In total, 430 blood samples of wild boars, killed during the 2017–2018 hunting season, were collected in the framework of the Lombardy and Emilia Romagna wildlife monitoring plans for classical swine fever (CSF) and Aujeszky disease and transferred to IZSLER for examination. Serum samples were tested for antibodies against swine vesicular disease virus [30,31], encephalomyocarditis virus [32], glycoprotein E of Aujeszky's disease virus [33], pestivirus (A–D) [34], swine influenza virus type A, subtypes H1N1, H1N2, and H3N2 [35,36], and finally for Brucella spp. (Svanovir Brucella–Ab C-ELISA©). Serological analyses were conducted with the methods currently in use at the IZSLER.

2.3. *Identification and Genomic Characterization of Atypical Porcine Pestivirus (APPV)*

For the investigation of the APPV genome, all samples, both the homogenates from fetal organs and the wild boar sera, were screened using the NS5B gene-specific real-time RT-PCR method [19]. Samples that tested positive were characterized by Sanger sequencing using RT-PCR that amplified a fragment of the NS3 region. The nucleotide sequences were aligned using the ClustalW method and compared with sequences present in GenBank [37] using MEGA6 software [38]. The maximum likelihood phylogenetic tree was constructed using IQ-tree software [39] by applying the TIM2+F+G4 model identified using ModelFinder selection [40].

3. Results

3.1. *Pigs*

The examination of the NS5B gene by real-time RT-PCR in the homogenized samples of pig fetuses identified two (0.6%) positive samples in two distinct farrow-to-finish farms, one from the province of Brescia in a pool containing the organs of three fetuses and the other from the province of Mantua in a pool containing the organs of two fetuses (Figure 1).

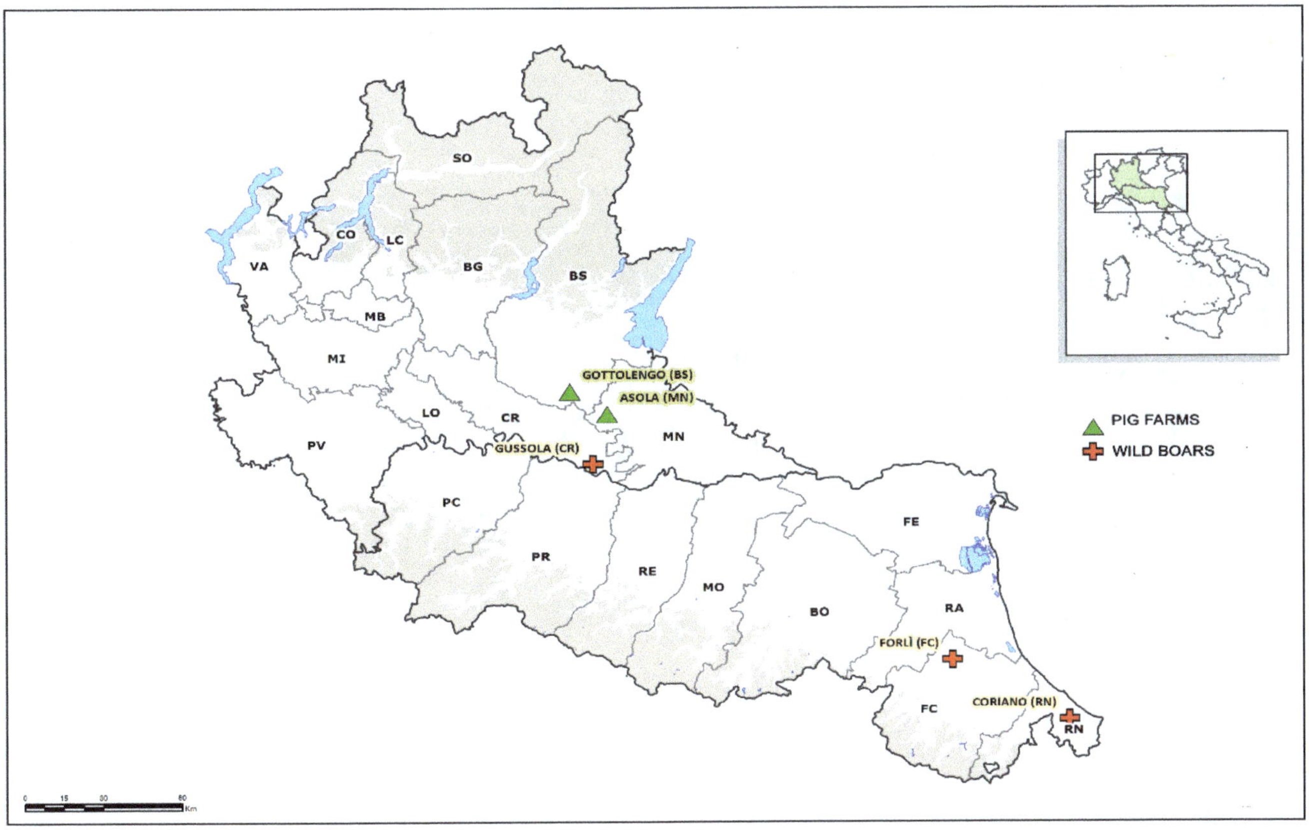

Figure 1. Geographical distribution of the pig farms and wild boar hunting sites where atypical porcine pestivirus (APPV) was identified.

At necropsy, none of these fetuses showed internal macroscopic lesions, and bacteriological investigations consistently produced negative results. Moreover, the molecular examinations for PRRSV, PCV-2, PPV, and pan-pestivirus were all negative, and only the real-time PCR for PCV-3 produced a positive result from a pool of fetuses that originated from the province of Brescia.

The two sequences obtained, APPV_Italy_SW_BS341729_2017 and APPV_Italy_SW_MN212160_2016, had a nucleotide similarity of 92.5% between them and clustered with APPVs previously identified in Europe. In particular, the phylogenetic tree constructed using the NS3 region (Figure 2) revealed that the two identified strains belong to distinct groups: (1) the APPV_Italy_SW_MN212160_2016 strain is related to both the 98/Sp06 strain identified in Spain in 2006 [16] (99.2% identity) and the German strain Bavaria S5/9 identified in 2015 [11] (96.8% identity); and (2) APPV_Italy_SW_BS341729_2017 forms a separate and closely related clade with two sequences identified in 2015 in pigs from Italy, Italy-164 and Italy-181 [15], with a nucleotide similarity of 95.5% and 99.2%, respectively.

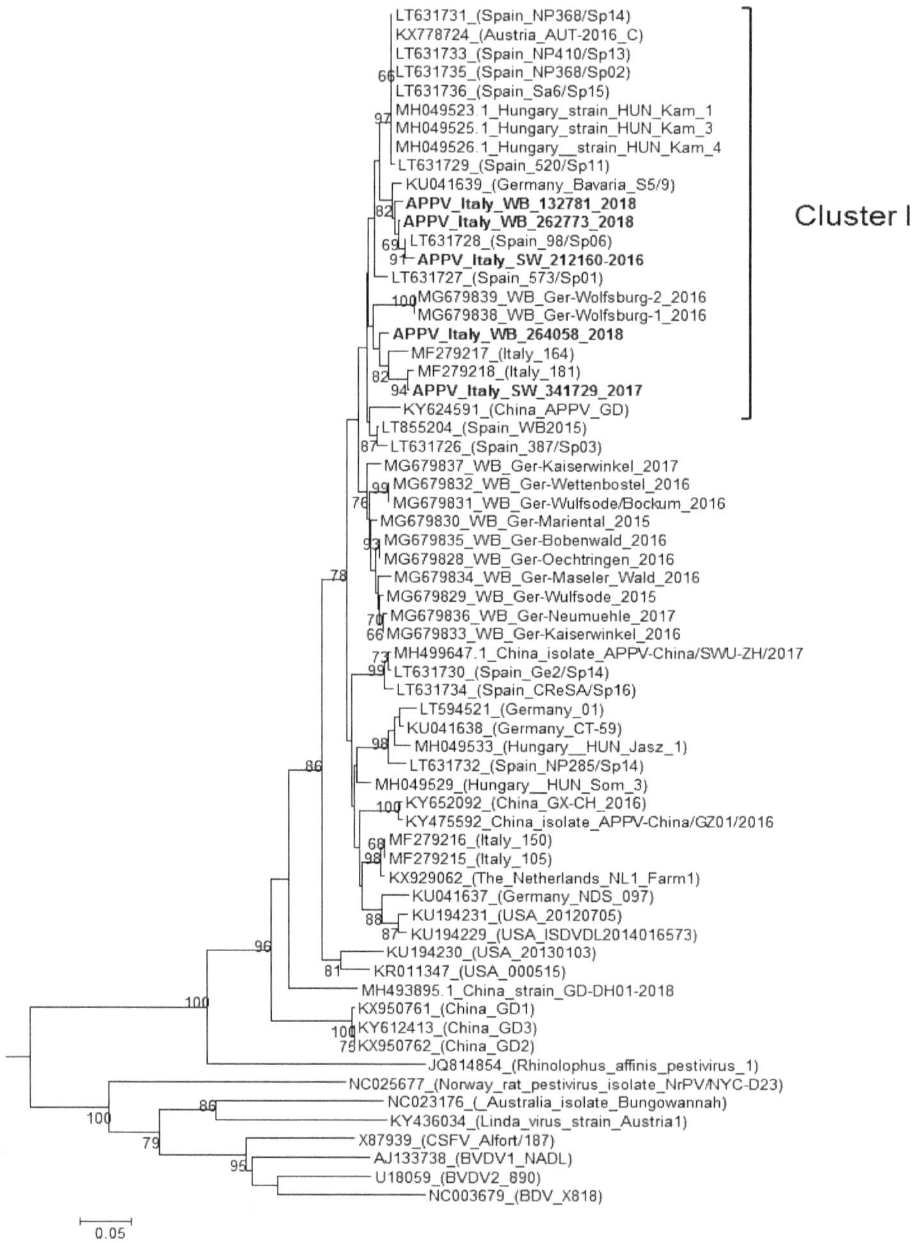

Figure 2. Phylogenetic tree based on a 645-nt fragment of the nonstructural protein 3-encoding region of the atypical porcine pestivirus (APPV) genome present in GenBank. A phylogenetic analysis using the maximum likelihood method including 1.000 bootstrap iterations was performed. Only bootstrap values ≥60 are indicated. Sequences in bold were generated in this study.

Despite the positive results of the real-time RT-PCR test, virological examinations of the organs of swine fetuses by inoculating cell cultures up to the fifth passage produced consistent negative results. Consequently, we did not succeed in isolating any APPV strains.

3.2. Wild Boars

All of the wild boar samples examined in this study including those that tested APPV-positive, originated from hunting activity, and thus, they were considered healthy based on their behavior before shooting and the absence of lesions on carcasses examined at slaughter. Out of the 430 blood samples examined, three (0.69%), originating from the Cremona Province in Lombardy (APPV_Italy_WB_CR264058_2018) and from two neighboring provinces, Rimini and Forlì in Emilia Romagna (APPV_Italy_WB_RN262773_2018 and APPV_Italy_WB_FC132781_2018, respectively) (Figure 1), screened positive for APPV. In agreement with the genomic characterization of the strains identified in pigs, the sequences of those identified in wild boars could be divided into two distinct clusters. The first included the two strains detected in Emilia Romagna (APPV_Italy_WB _RN262773_2018 and APPV_Italy_WB _FC132781_2018) and the sequence identified in the pig farm from Mantua Province in Lombardy (APPV_Italy_SW_MN212160_2016), which had identities of 95.6% and 96%, respectively; plus the previously characterized strains BavariaS5/9 and Spain 98/Sp06, with which the WB strains had a higher nucleotide identity of 98–99.2%.

The second cluster included the APPV_Italy_WB_CR264058_2018, the APPV Italy_SW_ BS341729_2017 (96.4% identity), the Italian pig strains, Italy-164 and Italy-181, which had nucleotide of 96.4% and 96%, respectively, and the strains identified in 2016 in Lower Saxony, Germany (94.3% identity).

For the collateral serological examinations, all APPV positive samples were negative for all serological tests employed except for: (a) one serum (APPV_Italy_WB_CR264058_2018) that tested positive for anti-Brucella spp. antibodies and (b) one (APPV_Italy_WB_FC132781_2018) that tested positive for glycoprotein E antibodies to the Aujeszky's disease virus.

The nucleotide sequences of the five APPV isolates were deposited in GenBank (NCBI) with the accession numbers MN736974–MN736978.

4. Discussion

The examination of 360 swine fetuses and 430 hunted wild boar blood samples identified APPVs in the area, two strains from the former and three strains from the latter. Based on the phylogenetic analysis performed, all five of these strains clustered with APPV strains previously identified in Spain and Germany. Although all of the sequences obtained can be grouped into the putative Cluster I described by Muñoz-González et al. [16], which should include viruses that have a common origin, the strains identified here could be further divided in two distinct sub-clusters.

Based on the absence of lesions on both fetuses and wild boars, we were keen to exclude a definite pathogenic role for APPV in these specific cases. However, it remains to be clarified whether the PCV-3 plus APPV (APPV_Italy_SW_BS341729_2017) co-infection, which was detected in the pool of fetuses originating from Brescia Province, may have had a synergistic effect in infected piglets, resulting in a clinical form characterized by abortion and natimortality. The very low prevalence of APPV found in the examined pig samples (0.6%) is largely different from the sole previous study on APPV in Italy [15], which reported a higher prevalence of viral detection (17.5%). This could be likely due to the sample types and selection, since we included in the survey only aborted pig fetuses with the aim of trying to establish if any correlation existed between the clinical case and the detection of APPV. A more specific monitoring program focused on the two APPV positive farms, and in general, to have systematically reported and analyzed cases of CT are anticipated in order to better define the prevalence of APPV in pig farms in Italy and clarify its effects.

Wild boars are susceptible to APPV infection, but their role in the epidemiology of the virus remains unknown. The low prevalence of APPV in the examined wild boar population is well correlated with the numbers reported by Colom-Cadena et al. [18] in Spain, but is in contrast to the high prevalence found in wild boars from northern Germany [17], where APPV seems to be endemic among wild boars in many areas. Considering the small number of strains isolated from the large geographical territory represented by the two regions (Lombardy and Emilia Romagna) and the lack of any particular geographic distribution of the clustered strains, it is impossible to draw epidemiological interpretations on APPV diffusion or on transmission between domestic pigs and wild boars.

5. Conclusions

APPV appears to be well established in the domestic swine populations of different countries in Europe, America, and Asia. Indeed, although identifying APPV has only become possible during the last few years due to the progressive refinement of diagnostic techniques, retrospective studies have indicated its circulation for many years. Based on the available genomic characterization data in the literature and the prevalence in domestic pigs, APPV exhibits a high genetic diversity among viral strains detected in different countries and tends to form independent clusters according to geographic locations. This study confirms the presence and distribution of APPV in populations of domestic and wild pigs present in the Lombardy and Emilia Romagna regions of Italy, which are under the jurisdiction of IZSLER. The high homology levels with strains identified in Germany and Spain reinforce the hypothesis that Italian strains have a European origin, and they confirm the likely determining role in the spread of infection being the commercial trade in pigs among different countries. The detection of new pestiviruses indicates the need to monitor for their presence and distribution using a systematic surveillance and diagnostic approach. In fact, the accurate and constant characterization of circulating strains is necessary to update the serological and virological tests, which in turn may be used to collect more detailed epidemiological information regarding APPV such as routes of entry and dissemination, and genetic evolution.

Author Contributions: C.S. and G.L.A. performed necropsy and routine laboratory examinations; E.S., I.B., D.L., and A.M. performed the laboratory work and analyzed the data; E.S., A.M., D.L., and A.L. interpreted the results and designed the figures; E.S. and A.L. wrote the manuscript. All the authors critically analyzed, revised, and approved the manuscript.

Acknowledgments: The authors would like to thank Loredana Zingarello and Debora Campagna for their excellent technical assistance.

References

1. Smith, D.B.; Meyers, G.; Bukh, J.; Gould, E.A.; Monath, T.; Scott Muerhoff, A.; Pletnev, A.; Rico-Hesse, R.; Stapleton, J.T.; Simmonds, P.; et al. Proposed revision to the taxonomy of the genus Pestivirus, family Flaviviridae. *J. Gen. Virol.* **2017**, *98*, 2106–2112. [CrossRef] [PubMed]
2. Wu, Z.Q.; Ren, X.W.; Yang, L.; Hu, Y.F.; Yang, J.; He, G.M.; Zhang, J.P.; Dong, J.; Sun, L.L.; Du, J.; et al. Virome analysis for identification of novel mammalian viruses in bat species from Chinese provinces. *J. Virol.* **2012**, *86*, 10999–11012. [CrossRef] [PubMed]
3. Wu, Z.Q.; Liu, B.; Du, J.; Zhang, J.P.; Lu, L.; Zhu, G.J.; Han, Y.L.; Su, H.X.; Yang, L.; Zhang, S.Y.; et al. Discovery of diverse rodent and bat pestiviruses with distinct genomic and phylogenetic characteristics in several Chinese provinces. *Front. Microbiol.* **2018**, *9*, 2562. [CrossRef] [PubMed]
4. Liu, L.L.; Xia, H.; Wahlberg, N.; Belák, S.; Baule, C. Phylogeny, classification and evolutionary insights into pestiviruses. *Virol.* **2009**, *385*, 351–357. [CrossRef] [PubMed]
5. Lamp, B.; Schwarz, L.; Högler, S.; Riedel, C.; Sinn, L.; Rebel-Bauder, B.; Weissenböck, H.; Ladinig, A.; Rümenapf, T. Novel pestivirus species in pigs, Austria, 2015. *Emerg. Infect. Dis.* **2017**, *23*, 1176–1179. [CrossRef]
6. Kirkland, P.D.; Frost, M.J.; Finlaison, D.S.; King, K.R.; Ridpath, J.F.; Gu, X. Identification of a novel virus in pigs—Bungowannah virus: A possible new species of pestivirus. *Virus Res.* **2007**, *129*, 26–34. [CrossRef]

7. Arruda, B.L.; Arruda, P.H.; Magstadt, D.R.; Schwartz, K.J.; Dohlman, T.; Schleining, J.A.; Patterson, A.R.; Visek, C.A.; Victoria, J.G. Identification of a Divergent Lineage Porcine Pestivirus in Nursing Piglets with Congenital Tremors and Reproduction of Disease following Experimental Inoculation. *PLoS ONE* **2016**, *11*, e0150104. [CrossRef]
8. Hause, B.M.; Collin, E.A.; Peddireddi, L.; Yuan, F.; Chen, Z.; Hesse, R.A.; Gauger, P.C.; Clement, T.; Fang, Y.; Anderson, G. Discovery of a novel putative atypical porcine pestivirus in pigs in the USA. *J. Gen. Virol.* **2015**, *96*, 2994–2998. [CrossRef]
9. Gatto, I.R.H.; Harmon, K.; Bradner, L.; Silva, P.; Linhares, D.C.L.; Arruda, P.H.; de Oliveira, L.G.; Arruda, B.L. Detection of atypical porcine pestivirus in Brazil in the central nervous system of suckling piglets with congenital tremor. *Transbound Emerg. Dis.* **2018**, *65*, 375–380. [CrossRef]
10. Mósena, A.C.S.; Weber, M.N.; da Cruz, R.A.S.; Cibulski, S.P.; da Silva, M.S.; Puhl, D.E.; Hammerschmitt, M.E.; Takeuti, K.L.; Driemeier, D.; de Barcellos, D.E.S.N.; et al. Presence of atypical porcine pestivirus (APPV) in Brazilian pigs. *Transbound Emerg. Dis.* **2018**, *65*, 22–26. [CrossRef]
11. Postel, A.; Hansmann, F.; Baechlein, C.; Fischer, N.; Alawi, M.; Grundhoff, A.; Derking, S.; Tenhündfeld, J.; Pfankuche, V.M.; Herder, V.; et al. Presence of atypical porcine pestivirus (APPV) genomes in newborn piglets correlates with congenital tremor. *Sci. Rep.* **2016**, *6*, 27735. [CrossRef] [PubMed]
12. Beer, M.; Wernike, K.; Dräger, C.; Höper, D.; Pohlmann, A.; Bergermann, C.; Schröder, C.; Klinkhammer, S.; Blome, S.; Hoffmann, B. High Prevalence of Highly Variable Atypical Porcine Pestiviruses Found in Germany. *Transbound Emerg. Dis.* **2017**, *64*, e22–e26. [CrossRef] [PubMed]
13. de Groof, A.; Deijs, M.; Guelen, L.; van Grinsven, L.; van Os-Galdos, L.; Vogels, W.; Derks, C.; Cruijsen, T.; Geurts, V.; Vrijenhoek, M.; et al. Atypical Porcine Pestivirus: A Possible Cause of Congenital Tremor Type A-II in Newborn Piglets. *Viruses* **2016**, *8*, 271. [CrossRef] [PubMed]
14. Yuan, J.; Han, Z.; Li, J.; Huang, Y.; Yang, J.; Ding, H.; Zhang, J.; Zhu, M.; Zhang, Y.; Liao, J.; et al. Atypical Porcine Pestivirus as a Novel Type of Pestivirus in Pigs in China. *Front. Microbiol.* **2017**, *8*, 862. [CrossRef] [PubMed]
15. Postel, A.; Meyer, D.; Cagatay, G.N.; Feliziani, F.; De Mia, G.M.; Fischer, N.; Grundhoff, A.; Milićević, V.; Deng, M.C.; Chang, C.Y.; et al. High Abundance and Genetic Variability of Atypical Porcine Pestivirus in Pigs from Europe and Asia. *Emerg. Infect. Dis.* **2017**, *23*, 2104–2107. [CrossRef] [PubMed]
16. Muñoz-González, S.; Canturri, A.; Pérez-Simó, M.; Bohórquez, J.A.; Rosell, R.; Cabezón, O.; Segalés, J.; Domingo, M.; Ganges, L. First report of the novel atypical porcine pestivirus in Spain and a retrospective study. *Transbound Emerg. Dis.* **2017**, *64*, 1645–1649. [CrossRef] [PubMed]
17. Cagatay, G.N.; Antos, A.; Meyer, D.; Maistrelli, C.; Keuling, O.; Becher, P.; Postel, A. Frequent infection of wild boar with atypical porcine pestivirus (APPV). *Transbound Emerg. Dis.* **2018**, *65*, 1087–1093. [CrossRef]
18. Colom-Cadena, A.; Ganges, L.A.; Muñoz-González, S.; Castillo-Contreras, R.; Alejandro Bohórquez, J.; Rosell, R.; Segalés, J.; Marco, I.; Cabezon, O. Atypical porcine pestivirus in wild boar (Sus scrofa), Spain. *Vet. Rec.* **2018**, *183*, 569.
19. Schwarz, L.; Riedel, C.; Högler, S.; Sinn, L.J.; Voglmayr, T.; Wöchtl, B.; Dinhopl, N.; Rebel-Bauder, B.; Weissenböck, H.; Ladinig, A.; et al. Congenital infection with atypical porcine pestivirus (APPV) is associated with disease and viral persistence. *Vet. Res.* **2017**, *48*, 1. [CrossRef]
20. OIE Manual for Terrestrial Animals 2016 cap 2.1.4 par B1, B1.1, B1.2, B1.3: Brucellosis [Brucella abortus, B. melitensis, B. suis (Infection with B. abortus, B. melitensis, B. suis)]—Diagnostic Techniques—Identification of the Agent—Staining Methods—Collection of Samples and Culture—Identification and Typing. Available online: https://www.oie.int/fileadmin/Home/eng/Health_standards/tahm/3.01.04_BRUCELLOSIS.pdf (accessed on 15 October 2019).
21. Ehricht, R.; Slickers, P.; Goellner, S.; Hotzel, H.; Sachse, K. Optimized DNA microarray assay allows detection and genotyping of single PCR-amplifiable target copies. *Mol. Cell Probes.* **2006**, *20*, 60–66. [CrossRef]
22. Vicari, N.; Santoni, R.; Vigo, P.G.; Magnino, S. A PCR-RFLP assay targeting the 16S ribosomal gene for the diagnosis of animal chlamydioses. In Proceedings of the 5th Meeting of the European Society for Chlamydia Research, Budapest, Hungary, 1–4 September 2004.
23. Van Kuppeveld, F.J.; van der Logt, J.T.; Angulo, A.F.; van Zoest, M.J.; Quint, W.G.; Niesters, H.G.; Galama, J.M.; Melchers, W.J. Genus- and species-specific identification of mycoplasmas by 16S rRNA amplification. *Appl. Environ. Microbiol.* **1992**, *58*, 2606–2615, Erratum in: *Appl. Environ. Microbiol.* **1993**, *59*, 655.

24. Olvera, A.; Sibila, M.; Calsamiglia, M.; Segalés, J.; Domingo, M. Comparison of porcine circovirus type 2 load in serum quantified by a real time PCR in postweaning multisystemic wasting syndrome and porcine dermatitis and nephropathy syndrome naturally affected pigs. *J. Virol. Methods* **2004**, *117*, 75–80. [CrossRef] [PubMed]
25. Kim, J.; Choi, C.; Han, D.U.; Chae, C. Simultaneous detection of porcine circovirus type 2 and porcine parvovirus in pigs with PMWS by multiplex PCR. *Vet. Rec.* **2001**, *149*, 304–305. [CrossRef] [PubMed]
26. Palinski, R.; Pineyro, P.; Shang, P.; Yuan, F.; Guo, R.; Fang, Y.; Byers, E.; Hause, B.M. A novel porcine circovirus distantly related to known circoviruses is associated with porcine dermatitis and nephropathy syndrome and reproductive failure. *J. Virol.* **2016**, *91*, 16. [CrossRef] [PubMed]
27. OIE Manual for Terrestrial Animals 2018 cap 3.4.7 par B1.2: Bovine Viral Diarrhea—Diagnostic Techniques—Detection of the Agent—Nucleic Acid Detection. Available online: https://www.oie.int/fileadmin/Home/eng/Health_standards/tahm/3.04.07_BVD.pdf (accessed on 15 October 2019).
28. Brocchi, E.; Cordioli, P.; Berlinzani, A.; Gamba, D.; De Simone, F. Development of a panel of anti-pestivirus monoclonal antibodies useful for virus identification and antibody assessment. In Proceedings of the second Symposium on Ruminant Pestiviruses, Annecy, France, 1–3 October 1992; Edwards, S., Ed.; Fondation Marcel Mérieux: Lyon, France, 1993; pp. 215–218.
29. Grazioli, S.; Pezzoni, G.; Cordioli, P.; Brocchi, E. Validation of a competitive ELISA for serodiagnosis of PRRS based on recombinant n-protein and monoclonal antibody. In Proceedings of the 8th International Congress of Veterinary Virology, Budapest, Hungary, 24–27 August 2009; Benkõ, M., Harrach, B., Eds.; Hungarian Academy of Sciences: Budapest, Hungary, 2009; p. 199.
30. Heckert, R.A.; Brocchi, E.; Berlinzani, A.; Mackay, D.K. An international comparative analysis of a competitive ELISA for the detection of antibodies to swine vesicular disease virus. *J. Vet. Diagn. Invest.* **1998**, *10*, 295–297. [CrossRef]
31. OIE Manual for Terrestrial Animals 2018 cap 3.8.8 par B2.2: Swine Vesicular Disease—Diagnostic Techniques—Serological Tests—Enzyme-Linked Immunosorbent Assay. Available online: https://www.oie.int/fileadmin/Home/eng/Health_standards/tahm/3.08.08_SVD.pdf (accessed on 15 October 2019).
32. Brocchi, E.; Carra, E.; Koenen, F.; De Simone, F. *Sviluppo di metodi ELISA basati sull'impiego di anticorpi monoclonali per la dimostrazione del virus della encefalomiocardite (EMCV) e dei relativi anticorpi*; La Selezione Veterinaria—Supplemento; IZSLER: Brescia, Italy, 2000; pp. 207–215.
33. OIE Manual for Terrestrial Animals 2018 cap 3.1.2 par B2.2: Aujeszky's Disease (Infection with Aujeszky's Disease Virus)—Diagnostic Techniques—Serological Tests—Enzyme-Linked Immunosorbent Assay (a Prescribed Test for International Trade). Available online: https://www.oie.int/fileadmin/Home/eng/Health_standards/tahm/3.01.02_AUJESZKYS.pdf (accessed on 15 October 2019).
34. OIE Manual for Terrestrial Animals 2019 cap 3.8.3 par B2.3: Classical Swine Fever (Infection with Classical Swine Fever Virus)—Diagnostic Techniques—Serological Tests—Enzyme-Linked Immunosorbent Assay (a Prescribed Test for International Trade). Available online: https://www.oie.int/fileadmin/Home/eng/Health_standards/tahm/3.08.03_CSF.pdf (accessed on 15 October 2019).
35. Kendall, A.P.; Pereira, M.S.; Skehel, J.J. *Concepts and Procedures for Laboratory-Based Influ-Enza Surveillance*; World Health Organization: Geneva, Switzerland, 1982; (Copies available from the WHO Collaborating Centre for Surveillance, Epidemiology and Control of Influenza, CDC, Atlanta, GA).
36. OIE Manual for Terrestrial Animals 2018 cap 3.8.7 par B2.1: Influenza A Virus of Swine–Diagnostic Techniques—Serological Tests—Haemagglutination Inhibition Test. Available online: https://www.oie.int/fileadmin/Home/eng/Health_standards/tahm/3.08.07_INF_A_SWINE.pdf (accessed on 15 October 2019).
37. GenBank® (NCBI). Available online: www.ncbi.nlm.nih.gov (accessed on 22 November 2019).
38. Tamura, K.; Stecher, G.; Peterson, D.; Filipski, A.; Kumar, S. MEGA6: Molecular evolutionary genetics analysis version 6.0. *Mol. Biol. Evol.* **2013**, *30*, 2725–2729. [CrossRef]
39. Nguyen, L.T.; Schmidt, H.A.; von Haeseler, A.; Minh, B.Q. IQ-TREE: A fast and effective stochastic algorithm for estimating maximum-likelihood phylogenies. *Mol. Biol. Evol.* **2015**, *32*, 268–274. [CrossRef]
40. Kalyaanamoorthy, S.; Minh, B.Q.; Wong, T.K.F.; von Haeseler, A.; Jermiin, L.S. ModelFinder: Fast model selection for accurate phylogenetic estimates. *Nat. Methods* **2017**, *14*, 587–589. [CrossRef]

10

Single-Round Infectious Particle Production by DNA-Launched Infectious Clones of Bungowannah Pestivirus

Anja Dalmann [1], Kerstin Wernike [1], Eric J. Snijder [2], Nadia Oreshkova [2], Ilona Reimann [1] and Martin Beer [1,*]

1 Institute of Diagnostic Virology, Friedrich-Loeffler-Institut, 17493 Greifswald-Insel Riems, Germany; anja.dalmann@fli.de (A.D.); kerstin.wernike@fli.de (K.W.)

2 Molecular Virology Laboratory, Department of Medical Microbiology, Leiden University Medical Center, 2333 ZA Leiden, The Netherlands; E.J.Snijder@lumc.nl (E.J.S.); nadia.oreshkova@wur.nl (N.O.)

* Correspondence: martin.beer@fli.de

Abstract: Reverse genetics systems are powerful tools for functional studies of viral genes or for vaccine development. Here, we established DNA-launched reverse genetics for the pestivirus Bungowannah virus (BuPV), where cDNA flanked by a hammerhead ribozyme sequence at the 5′ end and the hepatitis delta ribozyme at the 3′ end was placed under the control of the CMV RNA polymerase II promoter. Infectious recombinant BuPV could be rescued from pBuPV-DNA-transfected SK-6 cells and it had very similar growth characteristics to BuPV generated by conventional RNA-based reverse genetics and wild type BuPV. Subsequently, DNA-based E^{RNS} deleted BuPV split genomes (pBuPV$\Delta E^{RNS}/E^{RNS}$)—co-expressing the E^{RNS} protein from a separate synthetic CAG promoter—were constructed and characterized in vitro. Overall, DNA-launched BuPV genomes enable a rapid and cost-effective generation of recombinant BuPV and virus mutants, however, the protein expression efficiency of the DNA-launched systems after transfection is very low and needs further optimization in the future to allow the use e.g., as vaccine platform.

Keywords: Bungowannah virus; flavivirus; reverse genetics; single round infectious particle

---

1. Introduction

Bungowannah virus (BuPV) is an atypical pestivirus (species *Pestivirus F*) within the genus *Pestivirus* of the *Flavivirdae* family [1]. The virus was isolated for the first time in 2003 from a large Australian integrated pig farm during an outbreak of sudden death in young pigs, followed by an increase in stillbirth [2,3]. Although BuPV represents a potential threat to commercial pig farming, it has not yet been reported from any other region or country [4,5].

BuPV has a positive sense RNA genome that is approximately 12.6 kb in length. A single open reading frame, flanked by 5′ and 3′ non-translated regions, encodes a polyprotein, which is co- and post-translationally processed into structural proteins (C, E^{RNS}, E1, E2) and non-structural proteins (N^{PRO}, p7, NS2/NS3 (NS2, NS3), NS4A, NS4B, NS5A, NS5B) [2]. The envelope protein E^{RNS} as well as the non-structural protein N^{PRO} are unique to pestiviruses.

Genomic and antigenic properties of BuPV, as well as its broad in vitro host cell tropism, indicate remarkable distance to previously described pestiviruses [6–9]. In general, pestiviruses infect host-specific cells of ruminant, porcine, or sheep origin. Classical swine fever virus (CSFV) can only infect porcine cells efficiently, while bovine viral diarrhea virus (BVDV) and border disease virus (BDV) have the potential to infect broader host spectra [10–14]. However, only BuPV could infect cell lines of African green monkey, bat, human, and mouse origin [9].

To study the special characteristics of BuPV in detail, a robust reverse genetics system (RGS) is essential. For other pestiviruses, such as CSFV or BVDV, many RGSs based on cDNA copies of the viral genome cloned into plasmid or bacterial artificial chromosome (BAC) vectors have already been reported [15–20]. Furthermore, recombinant pestiviruses were generated by full-length genome RT-PCR-based amplification and direct RNA generation from the amplicons without cloning steps [21]. All these techniques have in common the use of a bacteriophage T7 or SP6 RNA polymerase promoter for in vitro transcription to synthesize infectious positive strand RNA, which is subsequently transfected into cells to produce infectious virus progeny.

Here, we report a first dual promoter DNA-launched BuPV RGS, which is based on a cDNA plasmid (pBuPV), with a cytomegalovirus (CMV) immediate-early promoter as well as the bacteriophage RNA polymerase T7 (T7) promoter upstream of the BuPV genome in a mammalian expression vector. For the generation of correct 5′ and 3′ ends, self-cleaving ribozyme sequences were inserted. This construct enables the transcription of the BuPV DNA by the CMV promoter in the nucleus and by the T7 promoter in the cytoplasm of polymerase expressing BSR cells (BSR-T7/5), where the latter serves as proof of principle to demonstrate that the modifications of the genome do not affect the transcription. This plasmid allows the rescue of infectious virus without in vitro RNA synthesis, and the virus can be passaged efficiently. We also established a split genome construct (pBuPVΔE^{RNS}/E^{RNS}) with a large deletion in the E^{RNS} gene, preventing the efficient generation of virus progeny, and a synthetic CAG promoter followed by the genomic region encoding the BuPV-E^{RNS} protein downstream the T7 termination signal (T7$_{term}$) for the expression of BuPV-E^{RNS} and the production of single-round infectious particles (SRIPs) via *trans*-complementation. The particles generated in this way should be able to pass through an additional replication cycle to infect surrounding cells, but are not expected to be capable of further propagation.

2. Materials and Methods

2.1. Cells and Viruses

SK-6 cells (RIE262, Collection of Cell Lines in Veterinary Medicine (CCLV), Friedrich-Loeffler-Institut, Insel Riems, Germany) and BSR-T7/5 cells, constitutively expressing the T7 polymerase (RIE583, CCLV) [22], were grown in Dulbecco's Modified Eagle Medium (DMEM) supplemented with 10% fetal calf serum (FCS) at 37 °C and 5% CO_2. rBuPV^{RNA} was generated after RNA transfection of SK-6 cells with in vitro transcribed RNA from the previously described synthetic cDNA clone pA/BV [9]. The virus was propagated in SK-6 cells and virus stocks were generated after three cell culture passages.

2.2. Plasmid Construction

All plasmids were prepared by standard molecular biological methods and plasmid DNA was purified by the Qiagen Plasmid Midi kit (Qiagen, Hilden, Germany). The identity of the constructs was confirmed by Sanger sequencing using the Big Dye® Terminator v1.1 Cycle sequencing kit (Applied Biosystems, Foster City, CA, USA) and appropriate primers. Nucleotide sequences were read with an automatic sequencer (3130 Genetic Analyzer; Applied Biosystems, Foster City, CA, USA) and analyzed using Geneious software (version 10.2.3.). Primers used for cloning procedures are shown in Table 1.

Table 1. Primer sequences for plasmid construction.

Construct	Primer	Sequence 5′-3′
pBV_opt	Ph_Donor_C-Erns_F	GCCTGCCTATTGGTCGTGCCCGTGGGCTCCACCAACGTGACACAATG
	Ph_Donor_Erns_R	TCACCCCTAAGTCTGCATCGTATCTGCATGTGACTGCGCACTC
	Ph_Donor_Erns_F	GTTGACGGTTACACCGAGGTGGTGGAGAAGGCCAGGTCAAGTGG
	Bungo_2534R	CGCTAATGCGTACATGAATTC
	Bungo_Npro_Mut_Donor_F	CTTTGTACAAACCAAGAGAGATGTGAGGGATCCAAGTGTGTA
	Bungo_1079R	GTGGCATCTGGTGGTCTAG
	Bungo_Donor_IV_F	GGCACTTGTATTGACAAAGAGGGTAGCGTGCAATGCTACATAGGGGA
	Bungo_Donor_IV_R_new	TCTTTAGTTCCCTCTTCGGCGCGTACTAAACCGACGAAGTAGACCAC
	Bungo_Donor_V_F	GCCTACACACACCCTGGAGGTGTAAGCAGTGTGATGCATGTCACCGC
	Bungo_6186_R	CACCGAACCTATGTATTTTTGACATCACTGCCAACTGTTC
	Bungo_Donor_VI_F	ATCACCAAATCCAACAAATTCTCGAGGGTGGGAAAGAATATGTCGGCCAAGCCTA
	Bungo_Donor_VI_R_new	GGACCCCCCATAGACCGTATTTCTTGATGTCACCGGCATGCTCTTGCAAGTATTC
	Bungo_Donor_VII_F	GGCCAGAAAAATTGCCAGTAGTAAGGGCCCAGACCAGTACCAAAG
	Bungo_Donor_VII_R	CTGGTTGACCACTTCCCCTTTGTCCTTCTCTTATGTAGACGTTTC
	Bungo_Donor_VIII_F	GTAGATGATTGGATGGAAGGAGATTATGTAGAAGAAAAAAGACC
	Bungo_Donor_VIII_R	GGCCCCTTGATCGCAAAGGCTTCGCCAAAACTTTTCTCAGTTATC
	Bungo_Donor_IX_F	GGTCAACCAGACACTAGCGCTGGAAATAGTATGTTGAATGTACT
	Bungo_Donor_IX_R	GACAAGCAGGCATATTCTTCGTACGAGGGGGTTCCAAGAATAC
pBuPV	Bungo_LLHR_F	CGTCGTTATACCTGATGAGTCCGTGAGGACGAAACCCGGAGTCCCGGGTCGTATAACGACAGTAGTTCAA
	Bungo_LLHR_R	TTCGGATGCCCAGGTCGGACCGCGAGGAGGTGGAGATGCCATGCCGACCCAGGGCTTTTTGGAACTGTGC
	pHaHd_F	TGGGTCGGCATGGCATCTCC
	pHaHd_R	GACCCGGGACTCCGGGTTTCGTCCTCACGGACTCATCAGGTATAACGACGACTAGCCAGCTTG
pBuPVΔE^{RNS}	Bungo_dERNS_F	CATCTAGCAGCAGACTATGAAAGTAAGATTGAAAACACCAAGA
	Bungo_2164R	CATCACGAAGTCCCTGTTGTC

The infectious clone pBuPV, the basis for DNA-launched BuPV, was constructed by multiple cloning steps. In a first step, donor splice sites, that were detected in the BuPV genome with a confidence >0.65 using the NetGene2 Server (http://www.cbs.dtu.dk/services/NetGene2 [23,24]; Table S1), were mutated in the full-length clone "pA/BV." For this, fusion PCR was applied, which is a restriction-free cloning method [7], using the Phusion® High-Fidelity PCR kit (New England Biolabs, Ipswich, MA, USA) and the primers Ph_Donor_C-Erns_F, Ph_Donor_Erns_R, Ph_Donor_Erns_F, Bungo_2534R, Bungo_Npro_Mut_Donor_F, Bungo_1079R, Bungo_Donor_IV_F, Bungo_Donor_IV_R_new, Bungo_Donor_V_F, Bungo_6186_R, Bungo_Donor_VI_F, Bungo_Donor_VI_R_new, Bungo_Donor_VII_F, Bungo_Donor_VII_R, Bungo_Donor_VIII_F, Bungo_Donor_VIII_R, Bungo_Donor_IX_F, and Bungo_Donor_IX_R (biomers.net GmbH, Ulm Germany), resulting in plasmid "pBV_opt."

For pBuPV generation, the well characterized plasmid pHaHd was used, which contains in addition to the CMV and T7 promoters, ribozyme sequences for the generation of correct genome sequences. In order to insert the optimized BuPV-specific cDNA into plasmid pHaHd [25] by linear-to-linear homologous recombination (LLHR) [26], plasmid pHaHd was linearized with *BglII* and used as template for PCR amplification of a linear vector fragment with the Phusion® High-Fidelity PCR kit and primers pHaHd_F and pHaHd_R. A full-length BuPV-specific PCR fragment was amplified by using plasmid DNA pBV_opt as template and primers Bungo_LLHR_F and Bungo_LLHR_R. To allow homologous recombination of the virus- and vector-specific fragments, 50 nucleotide-long vector specific homology arms were included in the primer sequences. Furthermore, for correct cleavage by the synthetic hammerhead ribozyme (HHr), five nucleotides complementary to the 5′ end of the BuPV-genome had to be inserted into primer Bungo_LLHR_F (Table 1). Thereafter, the PCR fragments were digested with *DpnI* to remove residual template DNA and gel purified (QIAquick Gel Extraction kit; Qiagen, Hilden, Germany). Subsequently, both PCR fragments were subjected to LLHR [26]. Recombination was performed by electroporation of both DNA fragments in the *E. coli* strain GB05-dir (Gene Bridges, Heidelberg, Germany). In brief, fresh overnight cultures in lysogeny broth (LB) medium were incubated at 37 °C for 1.5 h and RecE/RecT recombination was induced by L-Arabinose. After an additional incubation period at 37 °C for 30 min, the cells were washed two times with ice-cold water. A total of 100 ng of the amplified DNA fragments were added to the pelleted bacteria and electroporation was done at 1350 V, 50 μF, and 600 Ω by using the Gene pulser Xcell Electroporation System (Bio-Rad, Hercules, CA, USA).

Plasmid pBuPVΔE^{RNS} with a deletion of 448 bases within the E^{RNS} protein (aa 328–483) was generated by fusion PCR using pBuPV as DNA template and primer pair Bungo_dERNS_F and Bungo_2164R. For construction of the split genome plasmid pBuPV$\Delta E^{RNS}/E^{RNS}$, plasmid pCAGGS_BuPV-E^{RNS} [27] was digested with *SmaI* and *NotI* and the E^{RNS} comprising fragment was ligated into plasmid pBuPVΔE^{RNS}, digested with *PmeI* and *NotI*. Further details of the plasmid constructions are available on request.

2.3. cDNA Stability

The plasmid pBuPV was propagated for 10 passages in *E. coli*. Subsequently, the DNA was purified using the Qiagen Plasmid Mini kit (Qiagen, Hilden, Germany) and analyzed by *HindIII* digestion. DNA preparations of passages 5 and 10 were also used to transfect SK-6 or BSR-T7/5 cells and investigate for virus rescue.

2.4. Transfection and Virus Rescue

DNA transfections of plasmids pBuPV, pBuPVΔE^{RNS} and pBuPV$\Delta E^{RNS}/E^{RNS}$ (2 μg DNA each) into SK-6 (plasmid pBuPV) or BSR-T7/5 (all plasmids) cells were performed by using Lipofectamine™ 2000 Transfection Reagent (Invitrogen, Carlsbad, CA, USA) according to the manufacturer's protocol.

The transfected cells were seeded and incubated for three days at 37 °C and 5% CO_2. For recovery of infectious viruses, supernatants of the transfected cells were harvested three days post transfection (p.t.) and passaged on SK-6 cells. At the day of collection, replication of BuPV was monitored by immunofluorescence (IF) staining using monoclonal antibodies. Virus stocks of pBuPV were prepared after four cell culture passages. The identity of the recombinant viruses was confirmed by RT-PCR and sequence analysis using appropriate primers. For RT-PCR, total RNA of virus-infected cells was extracted using the QIAamp Viral RNA Mini kit (Qiagen, Hilden, Germany) according to manufacturer's instructions, and the cDNA was amplified using the OneStep RT-PCR kit (Qiagen, Hilden, Germany).

2.5. *Immunofluorescence Assay*

Transfected or infected cells were fixed and permeabilized with 80% acetone on ice for 15 min. After 30 to 45 min incubation with monoclonal antibodies specific for BuPV-E^{RNS} (682/43C3, diluted 1:20; M. Dauber, Friedrich-Loeffler-Institut, Insel Riems, Germany), for BuPV-E2 (682/45F12, diluted 1:20; M. Dauber, Friedrich-Loeffler-Institut, Insel Riems, Germany) or the pan-*Pestivirus* NS3 antibody WB112 (diluted 1:500; CVL, Weybridge, UK), the cells were washed twice with phosphate buffered saline (PBS). Thereafter, cell cultures were incubated with a goat anti-mouse Ig Alexa-488 conjugate (1:1000; Thermo Fischer scientific Inc., Waltham, MA, USA) for 30 min and analyzed by using a fluorescence microscope (Nikon Eclipse; Nikon GmbH, Düsseldorf, Germany).

2.6. *Virus Titration and Growth Kinetics*

SK-6 cells were infected with recombinant BuPV recovered from pBuPV ($rBuPV^{DNA}$) and recombinant BuPV recovered from pA/BV ($rBuPV^{RNA}$) at a multiplicity of infection (M.O.I.) of 1. Supernatants were collected at 0, 8, 24, 48, and 72 h post infection (p.i.), and virus titers were calculated as a 50% tissue culture infective dose per ml ($TCID_{50/mL}$) after IF staining.

3. Results and Discussion

Reverse genetics systems are important tools that enable the investigation of viral genes, viral replication cycles, or pathogenesis, and allow for the development of safe and efficacious vaccines. Infectious virus production from DNA plasmid transfections into mammalian cells using RNA polymerase I (pol I) or RNA pol II systems had been described for several RNA viruses [28–32]. These systems allow a simple and stable virus rescue, faster and less costly than conventional RNA-based reverse genetics. RGS using a pol I-promoter [33] or a pol II-promoter [34] were also described previously for the pestivirus CSFV. Both systems allowed the rescue of infectious CSFV with high virus titers. In our study, we established a dual promoter BuPV infectious clone "pBuPV" with both the CMV pol II promoter and the bacteriophage T7 promoter, which allows virus generation via DNA through the nucleus (CMV pol II promoter) or cytoplasmatic T7-based generation. The T7-based generation served as a proof of principle to demonstrate that the modifications of the genome do not affect the transcription.

In order to prevent the viral RNA from being spliced in the nucleus, donor splice sites with confidence >0.65 detected in N^{PRO}, C, E^{RNS}, E2, p7, and the other non-structural proteins were mutated in pA/BV (Table S1). Subsequently, the optimized BuPV-specific cDNA was used for construction resulting in plasmid pBuPV. In this construct, downstream of the CMV and bacteriophage T7 promoters, the BuPV genome termini were flanked by sequences coding for a synthetic HHr and hepatitis delta virus ribozyme (HDVr) to generate precise 5′- and 3′-terminal sequences. Downstream of the HDVr sequence, a T7 termination ($T7_{term}$) signal allows transcription termination (Figure 1A).

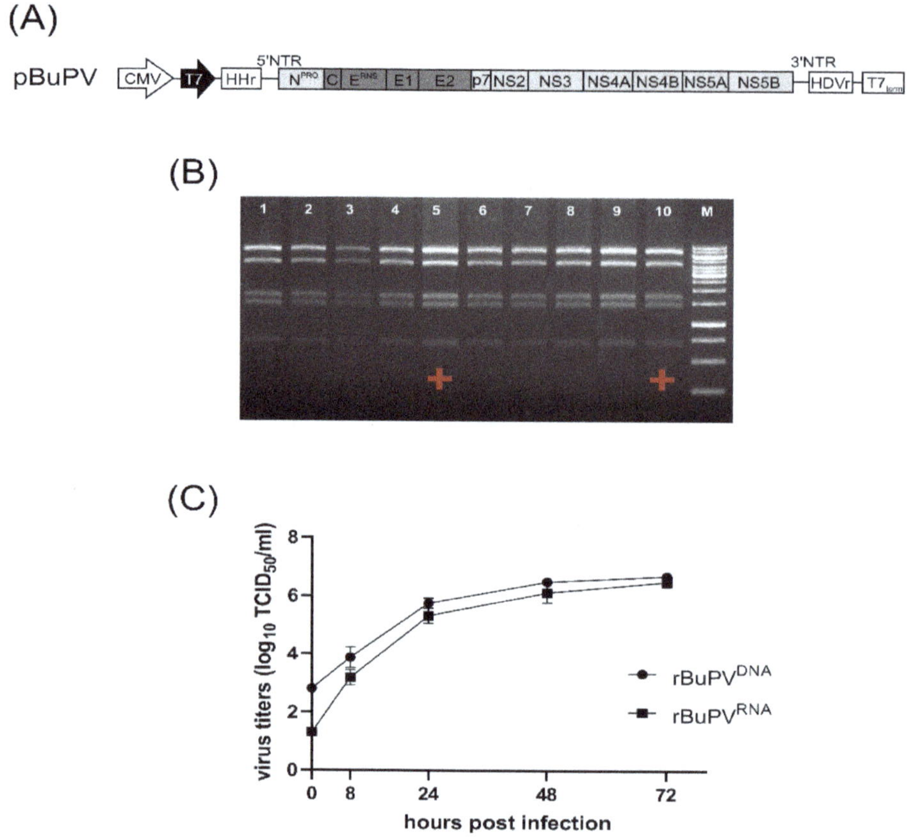

Figure 1. Plasmid pBuPV, genetic stability and rescue of recombinant rBuPV^{DNA}. (**A**) Schematic representation of the RNA Polymerase II-based plasmid pBuPV encoding full-length BuPV cDNA. Indicated are cytomegalovirus immediate-early (CMV) RNA Polymerase II promoter (open arrow), bacteriophage RNA polymerase T7 (T7) promoter (shaded arrow), hammerhead ribozyme (HHr), 3′ hepatitis delta virus ribozyme (HDVr), and T7 terminator sequence (T7$_{term}$). (**B**) Stability of the full-length cDNA clone pBuPV. The primary plasmid (P0) was passaged 10 times in *E. coli* DH10B (P1–P10) and investigated by restriction analysis using *Hind*III. + indicates generation of infectious rBuPV^{DNA} in rescue experiments. (**C**) Multi-step growth curves determined after infection of SK-6 cells with rBuPV^{DNA} (rescued by DNA transfection of pBuPV) or rBuPV^{RNA} (rescued by transfection of in vitro transcribed RNA of the infectious cDNA clone pA/BV) at an M.O.I. of 1 showed similar growth characteristics for both viruses.

The stability of plasmid pBuPV in bacteria was investigated by 10 serial cloning and passaging cycles in *E. coli* DH10B cells. Restriction enzyme analysis using *Hind*III provided some indication about the genetic stability of the construct, and the same restriction pattern for P0 (primary construct) and passages P1 to P10 were observed (Figure 1B). In transfection experiments, the DNA-launched recombinant rBuPV^{DNA} was analyzed for RNA replication, expression of BuPV proteins, and virus growth in both SK-6 and BSR-T7/5 cells. At 72 h p.t., CMV-driven expression of the BuPV proteins NS3 (anti-NS3), E2 (anti-E2), and E^{RNS} (anti-E^{RNS}) was detected by IF staining of the pBuPV-transfected SK-6 cells.

Bacteriophage T7 RNA polymerase (T7-RNA-Polymerase)-driven cytoplasmatic expression of all proteins could be observed as well after transfection in BSR-T7/5 cells; DNA-transfection of SK-6 cells and transfection in BSR-T7/5 cells resulted in single NS3, E2, and E^{RNS} expressing cells (Figure 2). Cell culture supernatants collected from both transfected cell lines were inoculated into fresh SK-6 cells and the presence of recombinant BuPV (rBuPV^{DNA}) particles in supernatants of both cell lines could be confirmed by IF analysis. The rescued rBuPV^{DNA} could be efficiently passaged in SK-6 cells (Figure 2). Virus rescue was possible, regardless of the bacterial passage number of pBuPV in *E. coli*, indicating once more the general stability of the plasmid (data not shown). Virus stocks produced from pBuPV-transfected SK-6 cells after four passages in SK-6 cells with a titer of $10^{6.25}$ $TCID_{50}/mL$ were used for growth kinetics analyses in comparison to rBuPV generated by the previously established T7-RNA-Polymerase based RGS [9]. Analysis of the multi-step growth curves in SK-6 cells revealed similar growth characteristics for both viruses, and final virus titers of $10^{6.6}$ $TCID_{50}/mL$ ($rBuPV^{DNA}$) and $10^{6.5}$ $TCID_{50}/mL$ ($rBuPV^{RNA}$) could be determined at 72 h p.i. (Figure 1C).

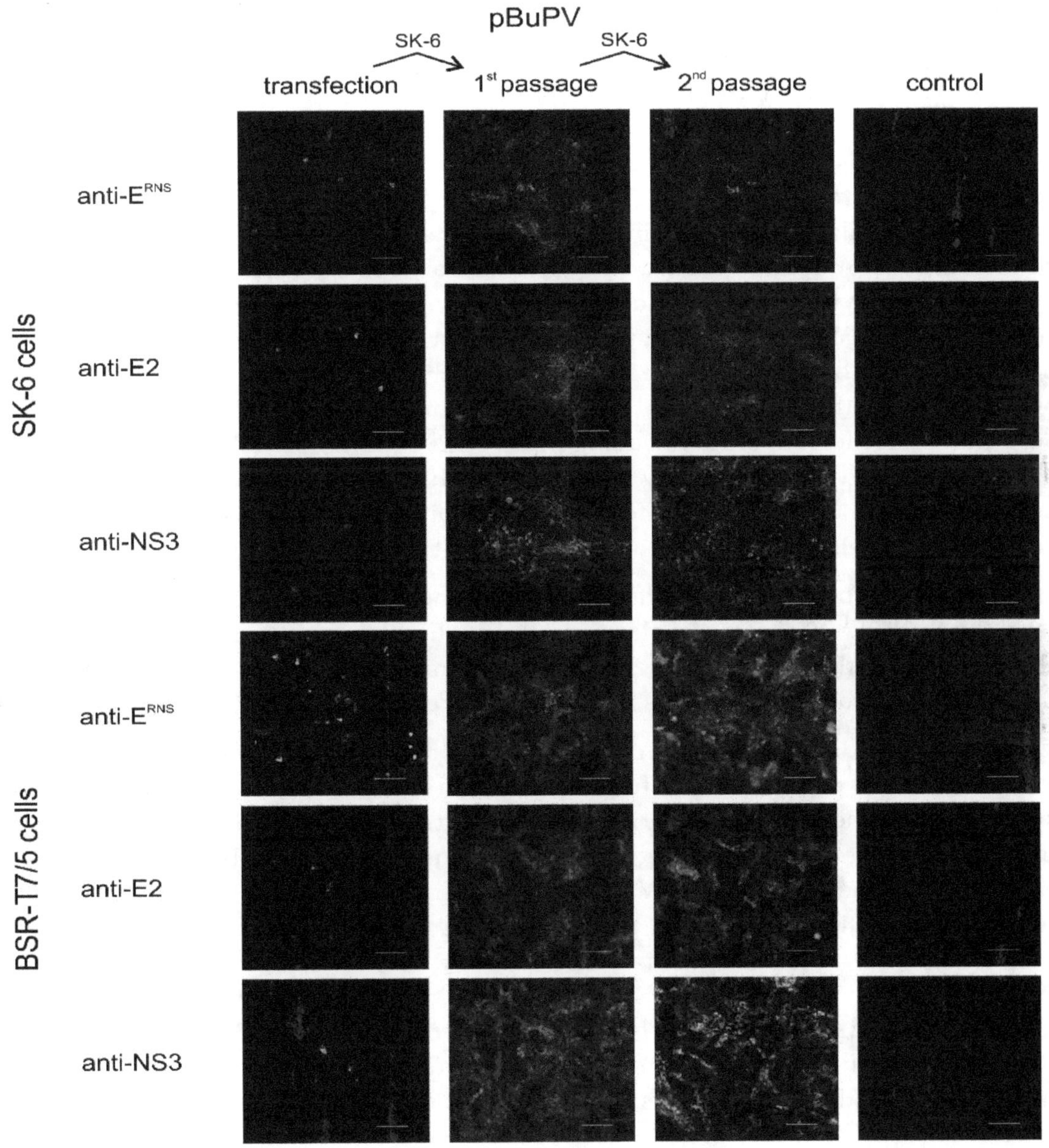

Figure 2. Rescue of $rBuPV^{DNA}$ in BSR-T7/5 and SK-6 cells. Cells were transfected with plasmid pBuPV. At 72 h p.t, IF staining with pan-pesti NS3-specific mab WB112 (anti-NS3), and E2-specific and E^{RNS}-specific mabs verified expression of NS3, E2 and E^{RNS} in transfected cells. At this time, recombinant virus in the supernatants was transferred to SK-6 cells (1st passage), and later on transferred for a 2nd passage. E2, E^{RNS} and NS3-positive cells indicated the generation of infectious progeny virus at 72 h p.i. in both transfected SK-6 and BSR-T7/5 cells. Scale bars indicate 100 μm.

In a next step, we were interested in the production of BuPV single-round infectious particles (SRIPs), since RNA-based SRIPs generating systems have already been described for several other flaviviruses [35–38]. SRIP production relies on the transfection of in vitro transcribed replicon

RNA with deletions within the genomic region encoding for one of the structural proteins C, E^{RNS}, E1, or E2 in cells stably expressing either the protein missing in the replicon or all structural proteins [39–43]. The packaged replicon particles are infectious, but progeny virus cannot spread from the infected cells, because the packaged replicon genome lacks the respective structural protein genes. In experimental animal studies, packaged replicon particles were proven to be appropriate for the development of non-transmissible, life attenuated pestivirus marker vaccine candidates [44–46]. However, the production of the replicon particles is time-consuming and needs the establishment of *trans*-complementing cell lines, which in many cases do not allow further passaging of the packaged pestivirus replicon particles.

Here, DNA-based SRIPs were produced as packaged BuPV replicon particles. Other DNA-based flavivirus SRIPs generating systems are mostly based on co-transfection of two expressing plasmids directly in eukaryotic cells, a subgenomic replicon plasmid, which lacks the structural protein-coding region, and a structural protein-expressing plasmid [35–38]. In addition, split genomes with two CMV promoters in back-to-back orientation, directing either the transcription of a capsid-deleted replicon RNA or the transcription of capsid-encoding mRNA had been described [47]. Since this strategy was described for the flavivirus West Nile virus, but had not been applied to pestiviruses up to now, we first constructed pBuPVΔE^{RNS}, which is a DNA-based replicon plasmid with a deletion of a large portion (codons 328–483) of the genome region encoding E^{RNS} (Figure 3A, upper panel). Subsequently, this plasmid was used for the establishment of the split genome construct pBuPV$\Delta E^{RNS}/E^{RNS}$ (Figure 3A, lower panel). In transfection experiments using pBuPVΔE^{RNS} and BSR-T7/5 cells, transient expression of NS3 could be detected at 24 h p.t. by IF staining, while expression of BuPV-E^{RNS} could not be observed (Figure 3C, panels c–d). No infectious recombinant BuPV could be recovered, even after serial passages in SK-6 cells (Figure 3C, panels k–l and s–t).

By insertion of a synthetic CAG promoter and the genomic region encoding the N-terminal signal sequence and the BuPV-E^{RNS} protein in plasmid pBuPVΔE^{RNS} downstream the $T7_{term}$ signal, the split genome plasmid pBuPV$\Delta E^{RNS}/E^{RNS}$ was generated (Figure 3A, lower panel). This construct is capable of transcribing two separate RNA species from two different promoters.

The CMV promoter directs the transcription of BuPV replicon RNA BuPVΔE^{RNS}, which expresses all non-structural protein genes and the structural protein genes *C*, *E1*, *E2*, and a truncated E^{RNS} gene (ΔE^{RNS}), whereas a synthetic CAG promoter [48] downstream of the BuPV replicon genome directs transcription of mRNA encoding full-length E^{RNS} for complementation. Together, the two promoters allow the expression of the complete BuPV genome including all structural proteins. The E^{RNS}-deleted replicon genome is amplified by the BuPV non-structural proteins NS3, NS4A, NS4B, NS5A, and NS5B and can be packaged by the structural proteins C, E^{RNS}, E1, and E2, essential for virus assembly, to generate SRIPs (Figure 3B). Secreted SRIPs are able to infect surrounding cells, where the replicon RNA can be replicated. As the structural proteins C, E1, and E2, but not BuPV-E^{RNS} can be expressed from this RNA by the non-structural proteins, the RNA cannot be packaged again into new particles and no further spread of the SRIPs is possible (Figure 3B) resulting in a self-restricted system.

To examine the ability of the split genome plasmid pBuPV$\Delta E^{RNS}/E^{RNS}$ to produce SRIPs, BSR-T7/5 cells were transfected with pBuPV$\Delta E^{RNS}/E^{RNS}$ and compared with cells transfected with the replicon plasmid pBuPVΔE^{RNS} and the full-length plasmid pBuPV. Autonomous replication of the newly synthesized BuPV RNA was shown by the expression of BuPV-NS3 in cells transfected with plasmids pBuPVΔE^{RNS} and full-length pBuPV. However, unexpectedly no NS3 expression was observed for the SRIPs, which might be due to the low transfection efficiency, especially since also only single positive cells could be shown for the other constructs. Expression of E^{RNS} could only be detected in cells transfected with pBuPV$\Delta E^{RNS}/E^{RNS}$ and the full-length pBuPV, but not in pBuPVΔE^{RNS} DNA transfected SK-6 cells (Figure 3C, panels a, c, and e). The observation that the SRIPs showed an increased E^{RNS} expression (Figure 3C, panel a) could be related to the fact that the inserted sequence was optimized for the expression system applied in this study.

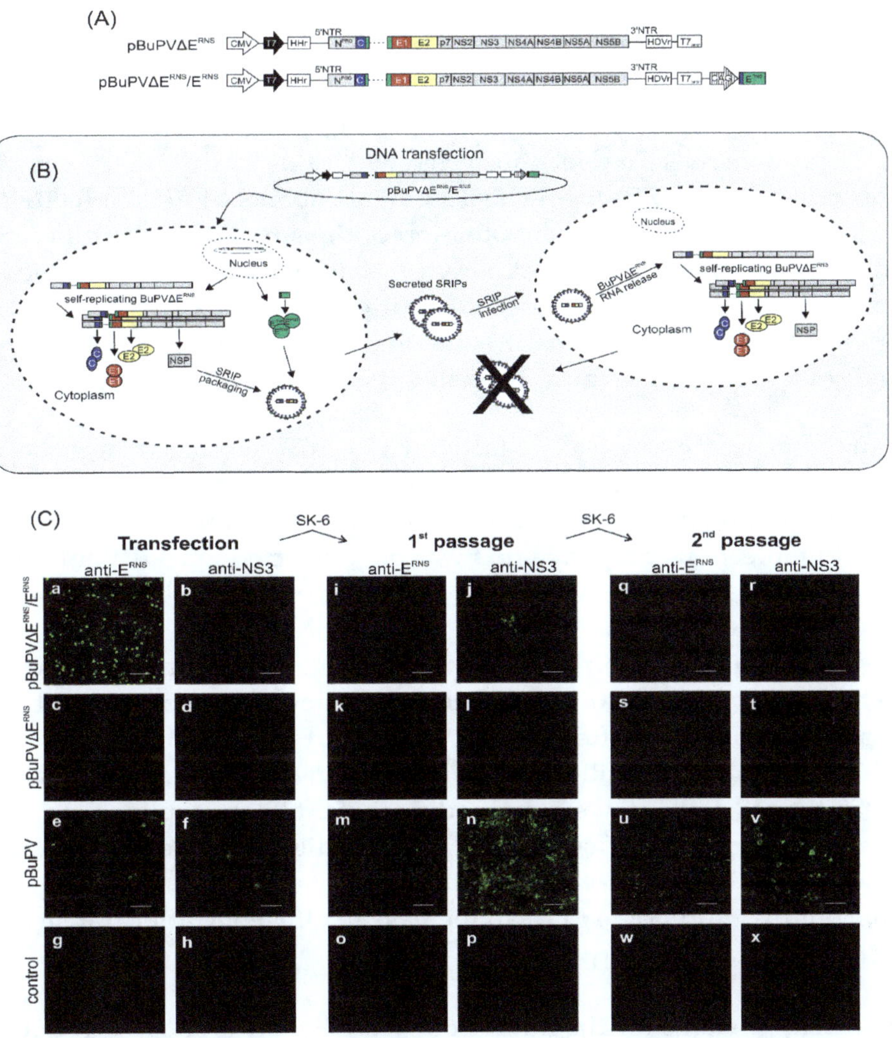

Figure 3. Schematic representation of the plasmids pBuPVΔE^{RNS} and pBuPVΔE^{RNS}/E^{RNS} and production of rBuPV and BuPV-SRIPs. (**A**) The replicon construct pBuPVΔE^{RNS} was generated on the basis of the CMV immediate early promoter containing plasmid pBuPV by partial deletion of the E^{RNS} encoding genomic region (aa 328–483); the split genome plasmid pBuPVΔE^{RNS}/E^{RNS} contains two eukaryotic promoters. The CMV promoter (open arrow) controls transcription of BuPV replicon RNA, BuPVΔE^{RNS}, which expresses the non-structural protein genes and the structural protein genes C, E1, and E2. The CAG promoter (shaded arrow) downstream T7$_{term}$ directs the expression of BuPV-E^{RNS}. Indicated is also the T7 promoter (black arrow), and the hammerhead ribozyme (HHr), and the 3′ hepatitis delta virus ribozyme (HDVr), which are important for the generation of the correct termini of the transcribed replicon RNAs. (**B**) Generation and operation mode of BuPV single round infectious particles (SRIPs) [47]. When cDNA of pBuPVΔE^{RNS}/E^{RNS} is transfected into susceptible cells, RNA-transcription starts in the nucleus under the control of the CMV promoter. The structural proteins C, E1, E2, and the non-structural proteins (NSP) are then expressed in the cytoplasm, while E^{RNS} is expressed by the CAG promoter. The self-replicating, truncated RNAs can be packaged in SRIPs by the four essential structural proteins. The secreted SRIPs are able to infect new cells. The released RNA replicates autonomously in the cytoplasm and allows the expression of the structural proteins C, E1, and E2 but not of E^{RNS}. Therefore, no further SRIPs can be produced and spread again (self-restriction). (**C**) IF analysis of BSR-T7/5 cells transfected with pBuPVΔE^{RNS}, pBuPVΔE^{RNS}/E^{RNS} or pBuPV (a–f) or SK-6 cells infected with supernatants of DNA-transfected cells (1st passage, i–n) or infected with supernatants collected from cells after the first infection (2nd passage, q–v). IF staining using anti-NS3 or anti-E^{RNS} monoclonal antibodies was performed at 72 h p.t. and 72 h p.i., respectively. Non-transfected or uninfected cells were used as control (g–h, o–p, and w–x). Scale bars indicate 100 μm.

When in vitro-transcribed RNA produced from an infectious cDNA clone of BuPV was transfected, the deletion of E^{RNS} still allowed the generation of infectious particles [27]. However, in this study there were no indications of cell-to-cell spread in pBuPVΔE^{RNS} DNA-transfected cells or production of SRIPs in transfection supernatants (Figure 3C, panels c, d, k, and l), while transfection with pBuPV resulted in single NS3 and E^{RNS} positive cells. In cells transfected with pBuPV$\Delta E^{RNS}/E^{RNS}$, amplified BuPVΔE^{RNS} replicon RNA was packaged into BuPV-SRIPs (Figure 3C, panel a). The infectivity of BuPV-SRIPs and rBuPV was also demonstrated after inoculation of the supernatants of the pBuPV$\Delta E^{RNS}/E^{RNS}$ DNA-transfected cells to fresh SK-6 cells (1st passage) as indicated by the IF-detection of NS3 at 72 h p.i. Here, replicon RNA amplified itself since no additional SRIPs were produced; only single cells infected with BuPV-SRIPs were observed by IF staining using the anti-NS3 mab and no positive signals could be detected by E^{RNS} staining (Figure 3C, panels i and j).

In contrast, after one passage, the cells infected with rBuPV produced large foci of BuPV-NS3 and -E^{RNS} protein-positive cells resulting from virus replication and spread (Figure 3C, panel m and n). The supernatants from all investigated clones obtained after infection were again transferred to fresh cells (2nd passage), but infectious progeny virus was only detected in rBuPV infected cells (Figure 3C, panels u, v).

While the newly established DNA-based system is well suited to produce infectious viruses, it unfortunately shows only a very low transfection efficiency, as demonstrated by the IF staining of relatively few positive cells at 72 h after transfection (Figures 2 and 3). A possible explanation for the reduced efficiency might be the still insufficient removal of donor splice sites. As BuPV does not naturally replicate in the cell nucleus, we have modified several donor splice sites, although additional splice sites may have an impact on efficiency [49,50]. In addition, further optimization attempts such as the modification of the CMV promoter or the insertion of a polyA tail were made following other flavivirus systems, but they did not lead to an increase in efficiency after transfection for the newly established BuPV system (data not shown).

However, also SRIP systems for the flavivirus West Nile virus showed reduced efficiency after transfection, but still were able to induce neutralizing antibodies and confer protection in immunized mice and horses [47]. Whether this is the case for the BuPV system as well, needs to be evaluated in vaccination experiments. Nevertheless, since a high transfection efficiency might be important for SRIP systems, further optimization of the BuPV system will be necessary and useful. Roby et al. could increase the SRIP production of their beta-galactosidase expression system by using an elongations factor EF1α promoter for the expression and optimized the codon of the capsid protein [51]. Thus, the replacement of the CMV promoter by another, more efficient promoter in SK-6 cells, e.g., the CAG promoter, might be an option to improve the BuPV system in the future. In addition, it could be explored whether other structures of the system, such as the ribozyme sequences, influence the efficiency as was shown previously [31,52,53].

4. Conclusions

In summary, we established a cDNA clone for the rescue of infectious BuPV using an RNA polymerase II-driven system. The full-length clone pBuPV enables further investigation of the atypical pestivirus BuPV by rapid and cost-effective generation of BuPV mutants. Even though the split-genome strategy has to be optimized due to its very low transfection efficiency in cell culture, it could allow the establishment of a platform for *trans*-complementation of viral proteins with a single plasmid. A more efficient version could be an attractive alternative to conventional complementation approaches and will therefore be a major focus for the future research in this field.

Author Contributions: Conceptualization, E.J.S., N.O., I.R., and M.B.; methodology, A.D. and I.R.; formal analysis, I.R.; investigation, A.D., K.W., and I.R.; writing—original draft preparation, A.D. and I.R.; writing—review and editing, K.W., E.J.S., N.O., and M.B.; visualization, A.D. and K.W.; supervision, K.W., I.R., and M.B. All authors have read and agreed to the published version of the manuscript.

Acknowledgments: We thank Doreen Schulz and Gabriela Adam for excellent technical assistance and Stefan Finke for kindly providing the plasmid pHaHd.

References

1. Simmonds, P.; Becher, P.; Bukh, J.; Gould, E.A.; Meyers, G.; Monath, T.; Muerhoff, S.; Pletnev, A.; Rico-Hesse, R.; Smith, D.B.; et al. ICTV Virus Taxonomy Profile: Flaviviridae. *J. Gen. Virol.* **2017**, *98*, 2–3. [CrossRef] [PubMed]
2. Kirkland, P.D.; Frost, M.J.; Finlaison, D.S.; King, K.R.; Ridpath, J.F.; Gu, X. Identification of a novel virus in pigs—Bungowannah virus: A possible new species of pestivirus. *Virus Res.* **2007**, *129*, 26–34. [CrossRef] [PubMed]
3. McOrist, S.; Thornton, E.; Peake, A.; Walker, R.; Robson, S.; Finlaison, D.; Kirkland, P.; Reece, R.; Ross, A.; Walker, K.; et al. An infectious myocarditis syndrome affecting late-term and neonatal piglets. *Aust. Vet. J.* **2004**, *82*, 509–511. [CrossRef] [PubMed]
4. Abrahante, J.E.; Zhang, J.W.; Rossow, K.; Zimmerman, J.J.; Murtaugh, M.P. Surveillance of Bungowannah pestivirus in the upper Midwestern USA. *Transbound. Emerg. Dis.* **2014**, *61*, 375–377. [CrossRef]
5. Michelitsch, A.; Dalmann, A.; Wernike, K.; Reimann, I.; Beer, M. Seroprevalences of newly discovered porcine pestiviruses in German pig farms. *Vet. Sci.* **2019**, *6*, 86. [CrossRef]
6. Kirkland, P.D.; Frost, M.J.; King, K.R.; Finlaison, D.S.; Hornitzky, C.L.; Gu, X.; Richter, M.; Reimann, I.; Dauber, M.; Schirrmeier, H.; et al. Genetic and antigenic characterization of Bungowannah virus, a novel pestivirus. *Vet. Microbiol.* **2015**, *178*, 252–259. [CrossRef]
7. Richter, M.; König, P.; Reimann, I.; Beer, M. N^{pro} of Bungowannah virus exhibits the same antagonistic function in the IFN induction pathway than that of other classical pestiviruses. *Vet. Microbiol.* **2014**, *168*, 340–347. [CrossRef]
8. Richter, M.; Reimann, I.; Wegelt, A.; Kirkland, P.D.; Beer, M. Complementation studies with the novel "Bungowannah" virus provide new insights in the compatibility of pestivirus proteins. *Virology* **2011**, *418*, 113–122. [CrossRef]
9. Richter, M.; Reimann, I.; Schirrmeier, H.; Kirkland, P.D.; Beer, M. The viral envelope is not sufficient to transfer the unique broad cell tropism of Bungowannah virus to a related pestivirus. *J. Gen. Virol.* **2014**, *95 Pt 10*, 2216–2222. [CrossRef]
10. Liess, B.; Moennig, V. Ruminant pestivirus infection in pigs. *Rev. Sci. Tech.* **1990**, *9*, 151–161. [CrossRef]
11. Fernelius, A.L.; Lambert, G.; Hemness, G.J. Bovine viral diarrhea virus-host cell interactions: Adaptation and growth of virus in cell lines. *Am. J. Vet. Res.* **1969**, *30*, 1561–1572. [PubMed]
12. Ames, T.R. Hosts. In *Bovine Viral Diarrhea Virus: Diagnosis, Management, and Control*; Goyal, S.M., Ridpath, J.F., Eds.; Blackwell Publishing: Oxford, UK, 2005; p. 175.
13. Nettleton, P.F. Pestivirus infections in ruminants other than cattle. *Rev. Sci. Tech.* **1990**, *9*, 131–150. [CrossRef] [PubMed]
14. Løken, T. Ruminant pestivirus infections in animals other than cattle and sheep. *Vet. Clin. N. Am. Food Anim. Pract.* **1995**, *11*, 597–614. [CrossRef]
15. Rasmussen, T.B.; Risager, P.C.; Fahnøe, U.; Friis, M.B.; Belsham, G.J.; Höper, D.; Reimann, I.; Beer, M. Efficient generation of recombinant RNA viruses using targeted recombination-mediated mutagenesis of bacterial artificial chromosomes containing full-length cDNA. *BMC Genom.* **2013**, *14*, 819. [CrossRef] [PubMed]
16. Mischkale, K.; Reimann, I.; Zemke, J.; König, P.; Beer, M. Characterisation of a new infectious full-length cDNA clone of BVDV genotype 2 and generation of virus mutants. *Vet. Microbiol.* **2010**, *142*, 3–12. [CrossRef] [PubMed]
17. Moormann, R.J.; van Gennip, H.G.; Miedema, G.K.; Hulst, M.M.; van Rijn, P.A. Infectious RNA transcribed from an engineered full-length cDNA template of the genome of a pestivirus. *J. Virol.* **1996**, *70*, 763–770. [CrossRef] [PubMed]

18. Ruggli, N.; Tratschin, J.D.; Mittelholzer, C.; Hofmann, M.A. Nucleotide sequence of classical swine fever virus strain Alfort/187 and transcription of infectious RNA from stably cloned full-length cDNA. *J. Virol.* **1996**, *70*, 3478–3487. [CrossRef]
19. Vassilev, V.B.; Collett, M.S.; Donis, R.O. Authentic and chimeric full-length genomic cDNA clones of bovine viral diarrhea virus that yield infectious transcripts. *J. Virol.* **1997**, *71*, 471–478. [CrossRef]
20. Kümmerer, B.M.; Meyers, G. Correlation between point mutations in NS2 and the viability and cytopathogenicity of Bovine viral diarrhea virus strain Oregon analyzed with an infectious cDNA clone. *J. Virol.* **2000**, *74*, 390–400. [CrossRef]
21. Rasmussen, T.B.; Reimann, I.; Uttenthal, A.; Leifer, I.; Depner, K.; Schirrmeier, H.; Beer, M. Generation of recombinant pestiviruses using a full-genome amplification strategy. *Vet. Microbiol.* **2010**, *142*, 13–17. [CrossRef]
22. Buchholz, U.J.; Finke, S.; Conzelmann, K.K. Generation of bovine respiratory syncytial virus (BRSV) from cDNA: BRSV NS2 is not essential for virus replication in tissue culture, and the human RSV leader region acts as a functional BRSV genome promoter. *J. Virol.* **1999**, *73*, 251–259. [CrossRef] [PubMed]
23. Hebsgaard, S.M.; Korning, P.G.; Tolstrup, N.; Engelbrecht, J.; Rouzé, P.; Brunak, S. Splice site prediction in Arabidopsis thaliana pre-mRNA by combining local and global sequence information. *Nucleic Acids Res.* **1996**, *24*, 3439–3452. [CrossRef] [PubMed]
24. Brunak, S.; Engelbrecht, J.; Knudsen, S. Prediction of human mRNA donor and acceptor sites from the DNA sequence. *J. Mol. Biol.* **1991**, *220*, 49–65. [CrossRef]
25. Orbanz, J.; Finke, S. Generation of recombinant European bat lyssavirus type 1 and inter-genotypic compatibility of lyssavirus genotype 1 and 5 antigenome promoters. *Arch. Virol.* **2010**, *155*, 1631–1641. [CrossRef] [PubMed]
26. Nolden, T.; Pfaff, F.; Nemitz, S.; Freuling, C.M.; Höper, D.; Müller, T.; Finke, S. Reverse genetics in high throughput: Rapid generation of complete negative strand RNA virus cDNA clones and recombinant viruses thereof. *Sci. Rep.* **2016**, *6*, 23887. [CrossRef] [PubMed]
27. Dalmann, A.; Reimann, I.; Wernike, K.; Beer, M. Autonomously replicating RNAs of Bungowannah pestivirus: E^{RNS} is not essential for the generation of infectious particles. *J. Virol.* **2020**. [CrossRef] [PubMed]
28. Hoffmann, E.; Neumann, G.; Kawaoka, Y.; Hobom, G.; Webster, R.G. A DNA transfection system for generation of influenza a virus from eight plasmids. *Proc. Natl. Acad. Sci. USA* **2000**, *97*, 6108–6113. [CrossRef]
29. Steel, J.J.; Henderson, B.R.; Lama, S.B.; Olson, K.E.; Geiss, B.J. Infectious alphavirus production from a simple plasmid transfection. *Virol. J.* **2011**, *8*, 356. [CrossRef]
30. Tretyakova, I.; Nickols, B.; Hidajat, R.; Jokinen, J.; Lukashevich, I.S.; Pushko, P. Plasmid DNA initiates replication of yellow fever vaccine in vitro and elicits virus-specific immune response in mice. *Virology* **2014**, *468*, 28–35. [CrossRef]
31. Tan, C.W.; Tee, H.K.; Lee, M.H.; Sam, I.C.; Chan, Y.F. Enterovirus A71 DNA-launched infectious clone as a robust reverse genetic tool. *PLoS ONE* **2016**, *11*, e0162771. [CrossRef]
32. Almazán, F.; González, J.M.; Pénzes, Z.; Izeta, A.; Calvo, E.; Plana-Durán, J.; Enjuanes, L. Engineering the largest RNA virus genome as an infectious bacterial artificial chromosome. *Proc. Natl. Acad. Sci. USA* **2000**, *97*, 5516–5521. [CrossRef] [PubMed]
33. Li, L.; Pang, H.; Wu, R.; Zhang, Y.; Tan, Y.; Pan, Z. Development of a novel single-step reverse genetics system for the generation of classical swine fever virus. *Arch. Virol.* **2016**, *161*, 1831–1838. [CrossRef] [PubMed]
34. Li, C.; Huang, J.; Li, Y.; He, F.; Li, D.; Sun, Y.; Han, W.; Li, S.; Qiu, H.J. Efficient and stable rescue of classical swine fever virus from cloned cDNA using an RNA polymerase II system. *Arch. Virol.* **2013**, *158*, 901–907. [CrossRef] [PubMed]
35. Yamanaka, A.; Moi, M.L.; Takasaki, T.; Kurane, I.; Matsuda, M.; Suzuki, R.; Konishi, E. Utility of Japanese encephalitis virus subgenomic replicon-based single-round infectious particles as antigens in neutralization tests for Zika virus and three other flaviviruses. *J. Virol. Methods* **2017**, *243*, 164–171. [CrossRef] [PubMed]
36. Suzuki, R.; Ishikawa, T.; Konishi, E.; Matsuda, M.; Watashi, K.; Aizaki, H.; Takasaki, T.; Wakita, T. Production of single-round infectious chimeric flaviviruses with DNA-based Japanese encephalitis virus replicon. *J. Gen. Virol.* **2014**, *95 Pt 1*, 60–65. [CrossRef]
37. Yamanaka, A.; Suzuki, R.; Konishi, E. Evaluation of single-round infectious, chimeric dengue type 1 virus as an antigen for dengue functional antibody assays. *Vaccine* **2014**, *32*, 4289–4295. [CrossRef]

38. Li, W.; Ma, L.; Guo, L.P.; Wang, X.L.; Zhang, J.W.; Bu, Z.G.; Hua, R.H. West Nile virus infectious replicon particles generated using a packaging-restricted cell line is a safe reporter system. *Sci. Rep.* **2017**, *7*, 3286. [CrossRef]
39. Khromykh, A.A.; Varnavski, A.N.; Westaway, E.G. Encapsidation of the flavivirus kunjin replicon RNA by using a complementation system providing Kunjin virus structural proteins in trans. *J. Virol.* **1998**, *72*, 5967–5977. [CrossRef]
40. van Gennip, H.G.; Bouma, A.; van Rijn, P.A.; Widjojoatmodjo, M.N.; Moormann, R.J. Experimental non-transmissible marker vaccines for classical swine fever (CSF) by trans-complementation of E^{rns} or E2 of CSFV. *Vaccine* **2002**, *20*, 1544–1556. [CrossRef]
41. Gehrke, R.; Ecker, M.; Aberle, S.W.; Allison, S.L.; Heinz, F.X.; Mandl, C.W. Incorporation of tick-borne encephalitis virus replicons into virus-like particles by a packaging cell line. *J. Virol.* **2003**, *77*, 8924–8933. [CrossRef]
42. Reimann, I.; Meyers, G.; Beer, M. Trans-complementation of autonomously replicating Bovine viral diarrhea virus replicons with deletions in the E2 coding region. *Virology* **2003**, *307*, 213–227. [CrossRef]
43. Scholle, F.; Girard, Y.A.; Zhao, Q.; Higgs, S.; Mason, P.W. trans-Packaged West Nile virus-like particles: Infectious properties in vitro and in infected mosquito vectors. *J. Virol.* **2004**, *78*, 11605–11614. [CrossRef] [PubMed]
44. Widjojoatmodjo, M.N.; van Gennip, H.G.; Bouma, A.; van Rijn, P.A.; Moormann, R.J. Classical swine fever virus E^{rns} deletion mutants: Trans-complementation and potential use as nontransmissible, modified, live-attenuated marker vaccines. *J. Virol.* **2000**, *74*, 2973–2980. [CrossRef] [PubMed]
45. Maurer, R.; Stettler, P.; Ruggli, N.; Hofmann, M.A.; Tratschin, J.D. Oronasal vaccination with classical swine fever virus (CSFV) replicon particles with either partial or complete deletion of the E2 gene induces partial protection against lethal challenge with highly virulent CSFV. *Vaccine* **2005**, *23*, 3318–3328. [CrossRef]
46. Reimann, I.; Semmler, I.; Beer, M. Packaged replicons of bovine viral diarrhea virus are capable of inducing a protective immune response. *Virology* **2007**, *366*, 377–386. [CrossRef]
47. Chang, D.C.; Liu, W.J.; Anraku, I.; Clark, D.C.; Pollitt, C.C.; Suhrbier, A.; Hall, R.A.; Khromykh, A.A. Single-round infectious particles enhance immunogenicity of a DNA vaccine against West Nile virus. *Nat. Biotechnol.* **2008**, *26*, 571–577. [CrossRef]
48. Miyazaki, J.; Takaki, S.; Araki, K.; Tashiro, F.; Tominaga, A.; Takatsu, K.; Yamamura, K. Expression vector system based on the chicken beta-actin promoter directs efficient production of interleukin-5. *Gene* **1989**, *79*, 269–277.
49. Yamshchikov, V.; Mishin, V.; Cominelli, F. A new strategy in design of +RNA virus infectious clones enabling their stable propagation in *E. coli*. *Virology* **2001**, *281*, 272–280. [CrossRef]
50. Shiu, J.S.; Liu, S.T.; Chang, T.J.; Ho, W.C.; Lai, S.S.; Chang, Y.S. The presence of RNA splicing signals in the cDNA construct of the E2 gene of classical swine fever virus affected its expression. *J. Virol. Methods* **1997**, *69*, 223–230. [CrossRef]
51. Roby, J.A.; Bielefeldt-Ohmann, H.; Prow, N.A.; Chang, D.C.; Hall, R.A.; Khromykh, A.A. Increased expression of capsid protein in trans enhances production of single-round infectious particles by West Nile virus DNA vaccine candidate. *J. Gen. Virol.* **2014**, *95 Pt 10*, 2176–2191. [CrossRef]
52. Martin, A.; Staeheli, P.; Schneider, U. RNA polymerase II-controlled expression of antigenomic RNA enhances the rescue efficacies of two different members of the Mononegavirales independently of the site of viral genome replication. *J. Virol.* **2006**, *80*, 5708–5715. [CrossRef] [PubMed]
53. Kanai, Y.; Kawagishi, T.; Nouda, R.; Onishi, M.; Pannacha, P.; Nurdin, J.A.; Nomura, K.; Matsuura, Y.; Kobayashi, T. Development of stable rotavirus reporter expression systems. *J. Virol.* **2019**, *93*. [CrossRef] [PubMed]

Field Experience of Antibody Testing against *Mycoplasma bovis* in Adult Cows in Commercial Danish Dairy Cattle Herds

Mette Bisgaard Petersen [1,*], Lars Pedersen [2], Lone Møller Pedersen [3] and Liza Rosenbaum Nielsen [4]

1 Department of Veterinary Clinical Sciences, University of Copenhagen, Agrovej 5A, 2630 Taastrup, Denmark
2 SEGES, 8200 Aarhus, Denmark; larp@seges.dk
3 Eurofins Milk Testing Denmark, 6600 Vejen, Denmark; lonemollerpedersen@eurofins.dk
4 Department of Animal and Veterinary Sciences, University of Copenhagen, Grønnegårdsvej 8, 1870 Frederiksberg, Denmark; liza@sund.ku.dk
* Correspondence: mbp@sund.ku.dk

Abstract: *Mycoplasma bovis* in cattle is difficult to diagnose. Recently, the ID screen® mycoplasma bovis indirect ELISA (ID screen) was commercially released by IDVet. The objectives of this study were to: (1) gain and share experience of using the ID screen in adult dairy cows under field conditions; (2) determine the correlation between antibody levels in milk and serum and (3) compare the ID screen results with those of the Bio K 302 (BioX 302) ELISA from BioX Diagnostics. Paired serum and milk samples were collected from 270 cows from 12 Danish dairy herds with three categories of *M. bovis* disease history. The ID screen tested nearly all cows positive in all, but the three non-infected herds, while the BioX 302 tested very few cows positive. The ID screen is therefore a much more sensitive test than the BioX 302. However, cows in five exposed herds without signs of ongoing infection and two herds with no history of *M. bovis* infection also tested ID screen positive. Therefore, the performance and interpretation of the test must be investigated under field conditions in best practice test evaluation setups. A concordance correlation coefficient of 0.66 (95% CI: 0.59–0.72) between the ID screen serum and milk results indicates that milk samples can replace serum samples for the ID screen diagnosis of *M. bovis* in adult cows.

Keywords: *Mycoplasma bovis*; diagnosis; control; immune response; ELISA

1. Introduction

Mycoplasma bovis (*M. bovis*) is an emerging bacterium associated with disease in cattle of all ages in many countries around the world [1]. In dairy cows, the usual presentation is mastitis, pneumonia and/or arthritis, while calves typically suffer from pneumonia, otitis media and/or arthritis [2,3]. Diagnosing *M. bovis* is challenging at both animal and herd level. *M. bovis*-associated disease can be diagnosed by using bacterial culture or PCR on body fluids or organ specimens and antibody measurements in serum or milk [3]. However, the fact that *M. bovis* bacteria lead to so many different disease manifestations and varying test responses in different age groups, and the fact that there is not one single diagnostic material that can test for and differentiate between all these disease manifestations makes it difficult to diagnose *M. bovis*-associated disease [4].

Antibody tests are inexpensive and for some purposes, it is an advantage that they can also detect previous (recent) infection. The first and previously only commercially available test for antibodies directed against *M. bovis* was produced by BioX Diagnostics in Belgium. The Bio K 302 ELISA kit (BioX 302) has been reported to have low sensitivity ranging from 0.37–0.50 and specificity ranging from 0.90–0.96 in experimental studies [5–7] and very short-lasting antibody detection in individual cows [8] and calves [9]. Petersen et al. [8] found that the mean antibody level in cows with clinical indication of *M. bovis* was only above the recommended cutoff (37 ODC%) for approximately 60 days after the disease outbreak, which implies that frequent testing would be necessary to detect disease among cows if the BioX 302 were to be used to assess the *M. bovis* status of dairy cows or herds. One explanation could be the large antigenic variation of *M. bovis* and the alterations of membrane surface lipoproteins over time [10]. Studies have compared the BioX 302 to an in-house *M. bovis* ELISA based on a different antigen. The agreement between the results from the two tests was low, and the antibodies detected by the in-house ELISA persisted in serum from cows 1.5 years after the disease outbreak regardless of the current *M. bovis* clinical status [9,11]. Results from one ELISA test can therefore not be extrapolated to other *M. bovis*-detecting ELISAs. The differences in test performance may be influenced by the different antigens used in each ELISA, how immunogenic they are, how long the immune system reacts to the particular protein and how similar the gene of that particular protein is in different *M. bovis* strains.

The ID screen® mycoplasma bovis indirect (ID screen) from IDvet (Grabels, France) is a reasonably new commercially available antibody test. According to the manufacturer, the diagnostic sensitivity and specificity are 95.7% and 100%, respectively [12]. The test has only been evaluated in calves [12], but the age of the animals is very likely to influence the test performance when used under field conditions [13,14]. Therefore, current knowledge about the ID screen test performance may not be valid for adult cows and may vary depending on whether the test material is serum or milk.

Applying the BioX 302 to herd-level testing using bulk tank milk has been evaluated and found useful in estimating the prevalence at a national level when the cutoff was raised to 55 ODC% [15]. However, the challenge is that bulk tank milk primarily reflects *M. bovis* udder infections in the herd [8]. In fact, one study found that the hospital herd was the most indicative group to use for the detection of herd-level *M. bovis* infection based on bulk tank milk tested using the BioX 302 [16]. Danish cattle farmers have experienced many *M. bovis* disease outbreaks characterized by arthritis rather than mastitis as the primary clinical sign [8], and bulk tank milk samples would most likely fail to detect these outbreaks. Use of the BioX 302 on milk samples is non-optimal due to the need for frequent testing to ensure infected herds are detected (e.g., for classification of herds in relation to trade, shows, etc.), and because not all disease manifestations can be detected when measuring antibodies in milk [4,16]. As the ID screen is more sensitive than BioX 302, antibody measurements in milk may be more reliable, potentially making it feasible to use antibody testing of individual and bulk tank milk samples for surveillance or outbreak diagnostics, providing the specificity is sufficiently high. The potential use of ELISA on milk samples to classify or monitor dairy herds for *M. bovis* infection will be of interest in a setting like the Danish dairy industry, since the sampling can be automated via the mandatory milk quality control scheme and bulk tank milk surveillance for other cattle diseases.

The objectives of this study were therefore to: (1) gain and share experience of using the new commercial ELISA ID screen for the detection of antibodies against *M. bovis* in adult dairy cows under field conditions; (2) determine the correlation between the measured antibody levels in milk and serum and (3) compare the ID screen results with the results of the frequently used and commercially available BioX 302 ELISA.

2. Results

Paired serum and milk samples were collected from a total of 270 cows from 12 Danish dairy herds. All nasal swabs and milk samples from lactating cows in the Robust Calves herds (RC-herds) tested negative for the presence of *M. bovis* by PCR. See Table 1 and the Section 4 for a description of the different herds included in the study.

The serum and milk ID screen sample-to-positive percentage (S/P%) was plotted with jittered dots for each of the 12 herds (Figures 1 and 2). All cows had a S/P% below the recommended cutoff in both serum and milk in three herds (herds 1–3). In all other herds, all or nearly all cows had a S/P% above the recommended cutoff.

The serum and milk BioX 302 sample-coefficient (ODC%) was plotted with jittered dots for each of the 12 herds (Figures 3 and 4). All, but 16 cows from seven different herds had serum ODC% values below the recommended cutoff in serum, while all, but 17 cows from nine different herds had milk ODC% values below the recommended cutoff.

Correlation between Serum and Milk S/P%

The concordance correlation coefficient between serum and milk S/P% across the full dataset of paired serum and milk samples was 0.66 (95% CI: 0.59–0.72). The correlation between serum and milk samples within each herd is shown in Figure 5. Correlations are not shown for the BioX 302 due to the low number of positive samples.

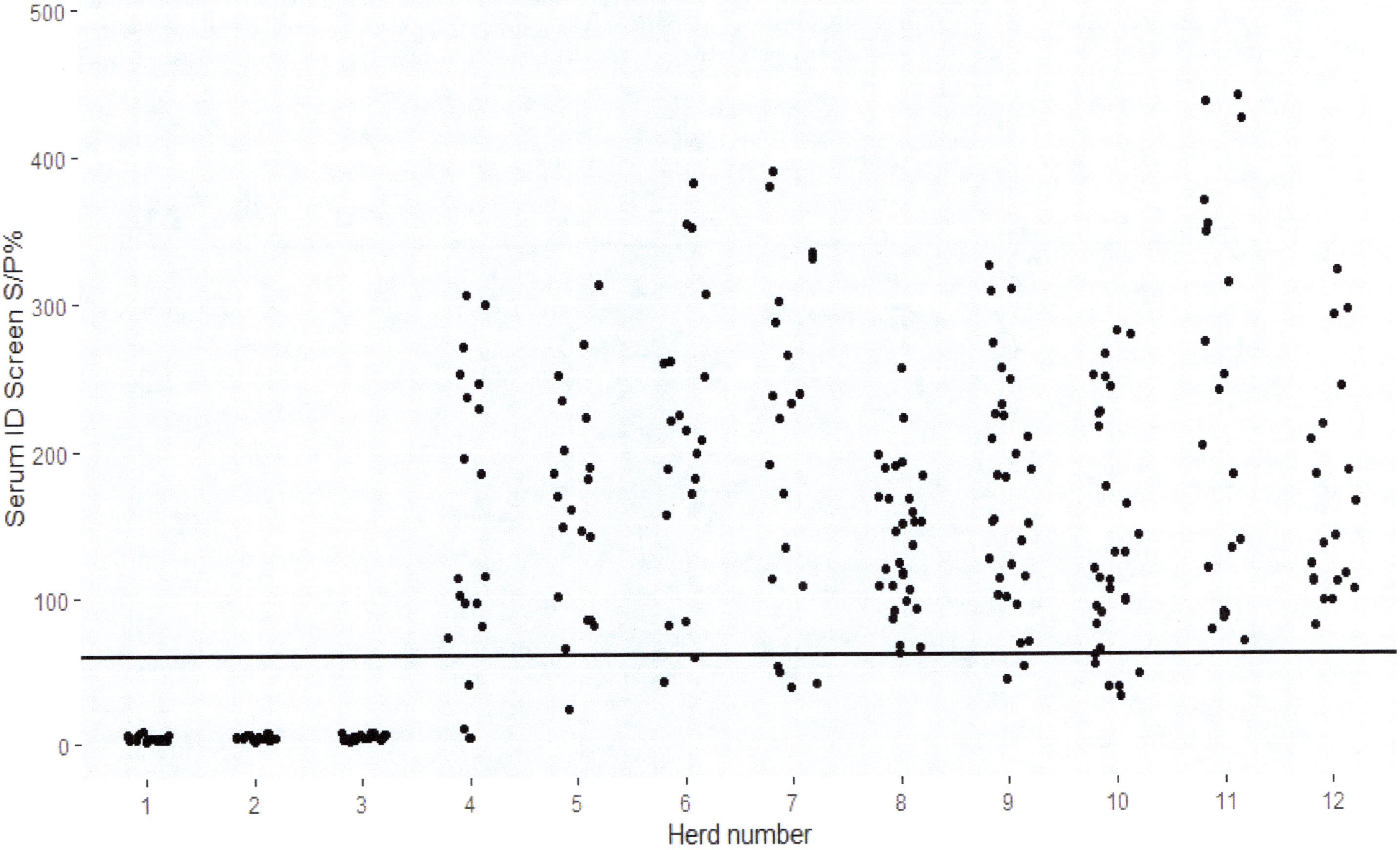

Figure 1. Serum antibody levels against *Mycoplasma bovis* in cows from 12 Danish dairy herds tested with the ID screen® mycoplasma bovis indirect ELISA kit from IDvet. Herds 1–6 and 11–12 had 20 cows tested and herds 8–10 had 30 cows tested. The horizontal black line indicates the manufacturer-recommended cutoff value (sample-to-positive percentage (S/P%) of 60) for serum.

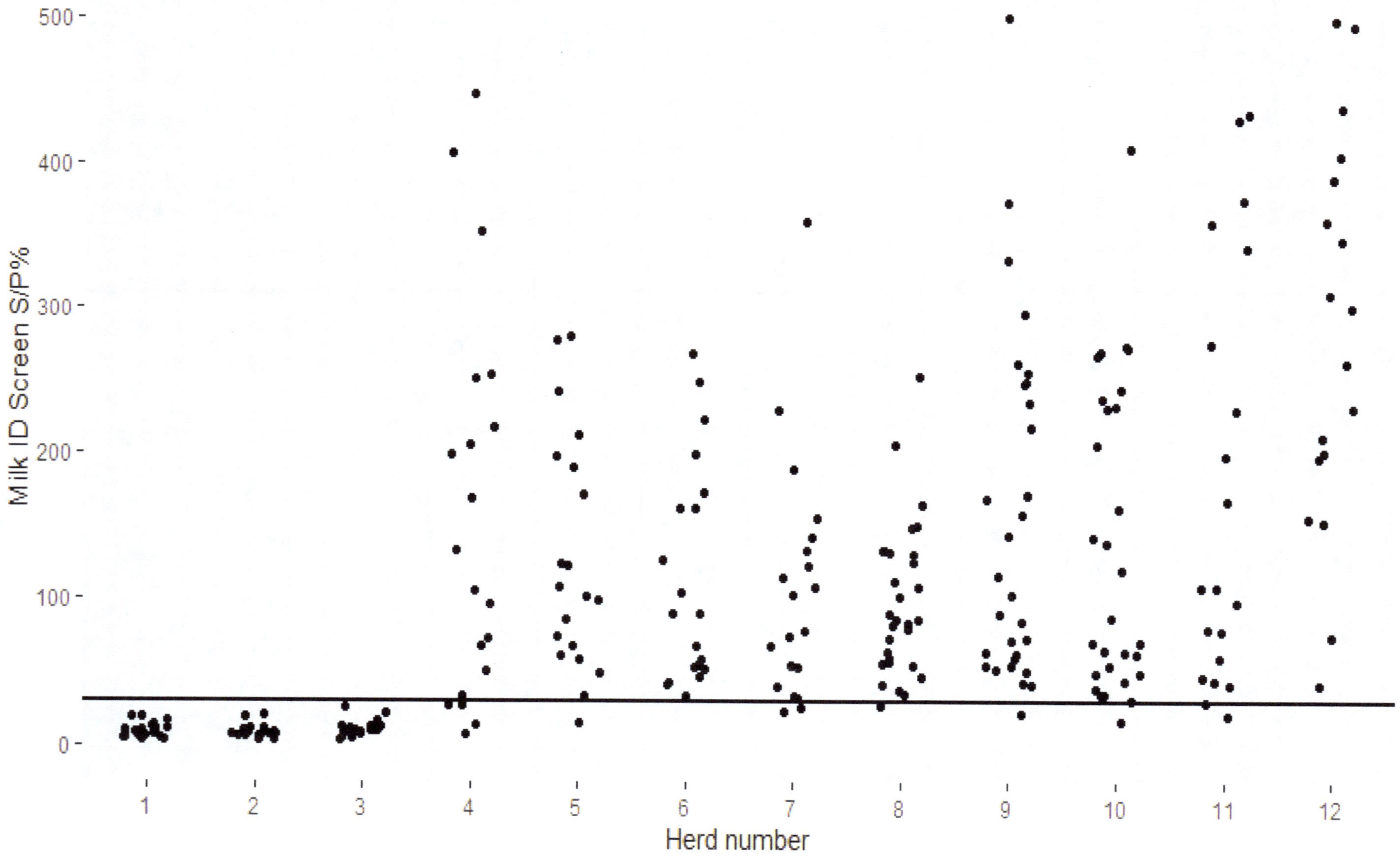

Figure 2. Milk antibody levels against *Mycoplasma bovis* in cows from 12 Danish dairy herds tested with the ID screen® mycoplasma bovis indirect ELISA kit from IDvet. Herds 1–6 and 11–12 had 20 cows tested and Herds 8–10 had 30 cows tested. The horizontal black line indicates the manufacturer-recommended cutoff value (sample-to-positive percentage (S/P%) of 30) for the overnight protocol for milk.

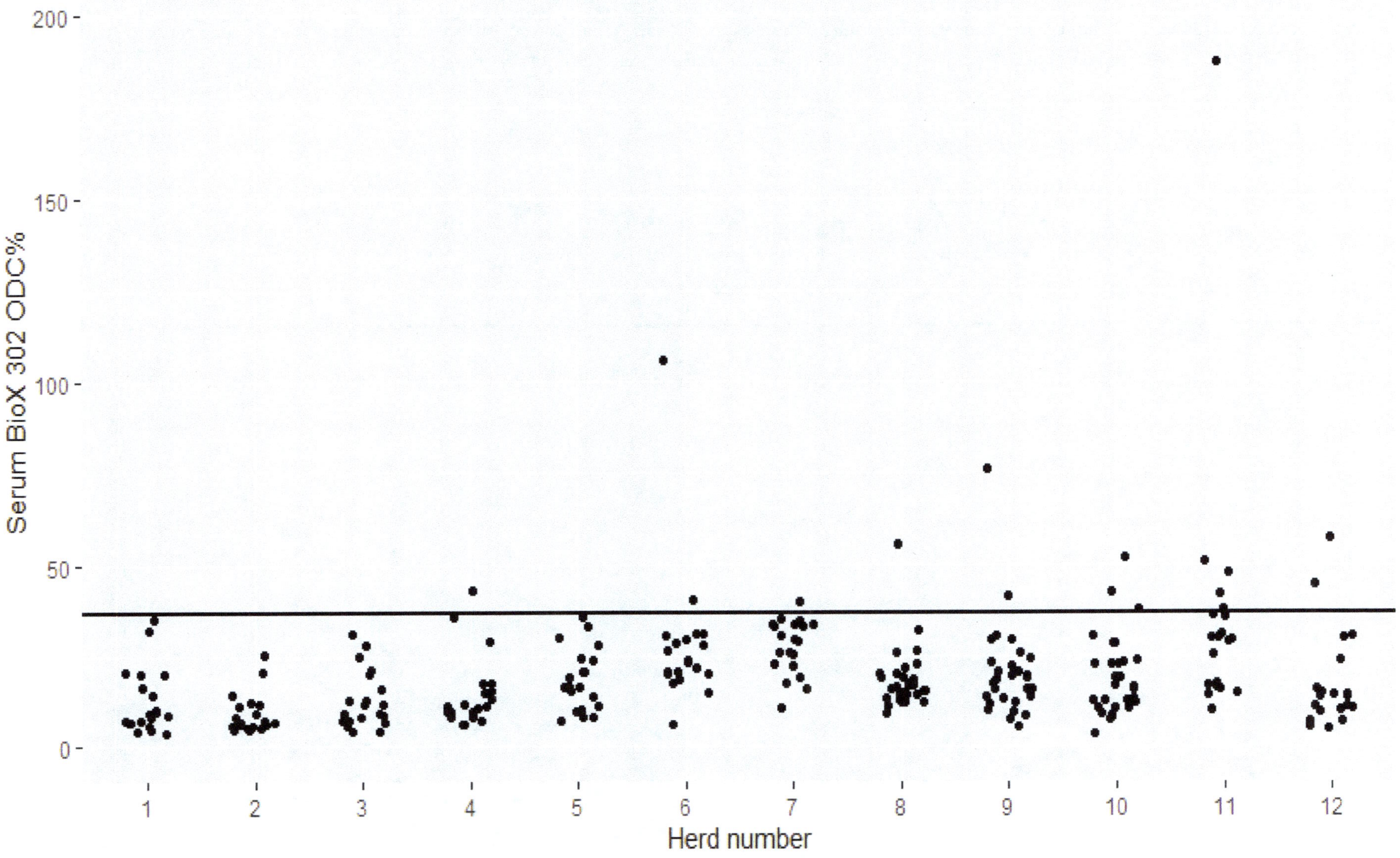

Figure 3. Serum antibody levels against *Mycoplasma bovis* in cows from 12 Danish dairy herds tested with the Bio K 302 ELISA kit from BioX. Herds 1–6 and 11–12 had 20 cows tested and Herds 8–10 had 30 cows tested. The horizontal black line indicates the manufacturer-recommended cutoff value (sample-coefficient (ODC%) of 37).

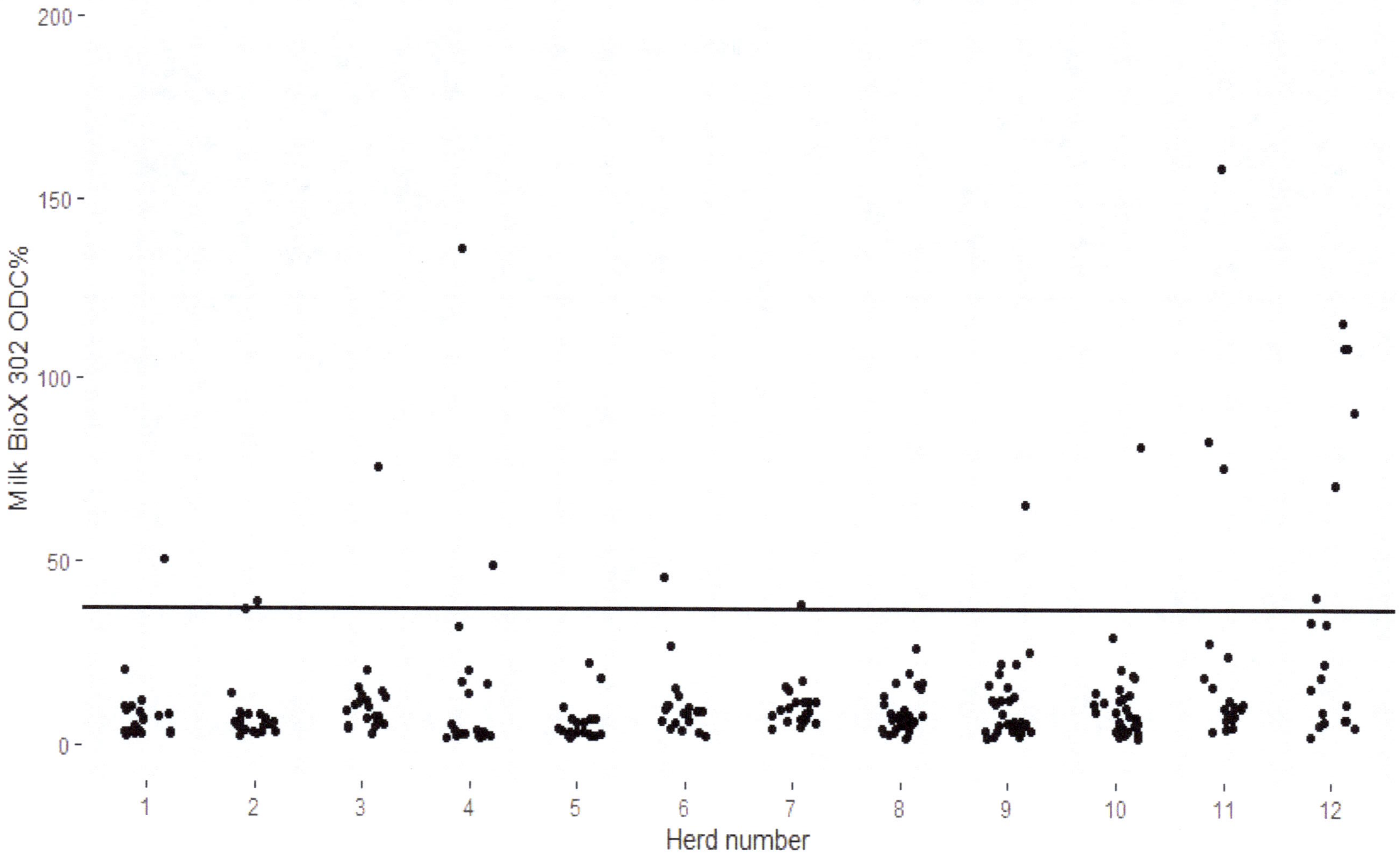

Figure 4. Milk antibody levels against *Mycoplasma bovis* in cows from 12 Danish dairy herds tested with the Bio K 302 ELISA kit from BioX. Herds 1–6 and 11–12 had 20 cows tested and Herds 8–10 had 30 cows tested. The horizontal black line indicates the manufacturer-recommended cutoff value (sample-coefficient (ODC%) of 37).

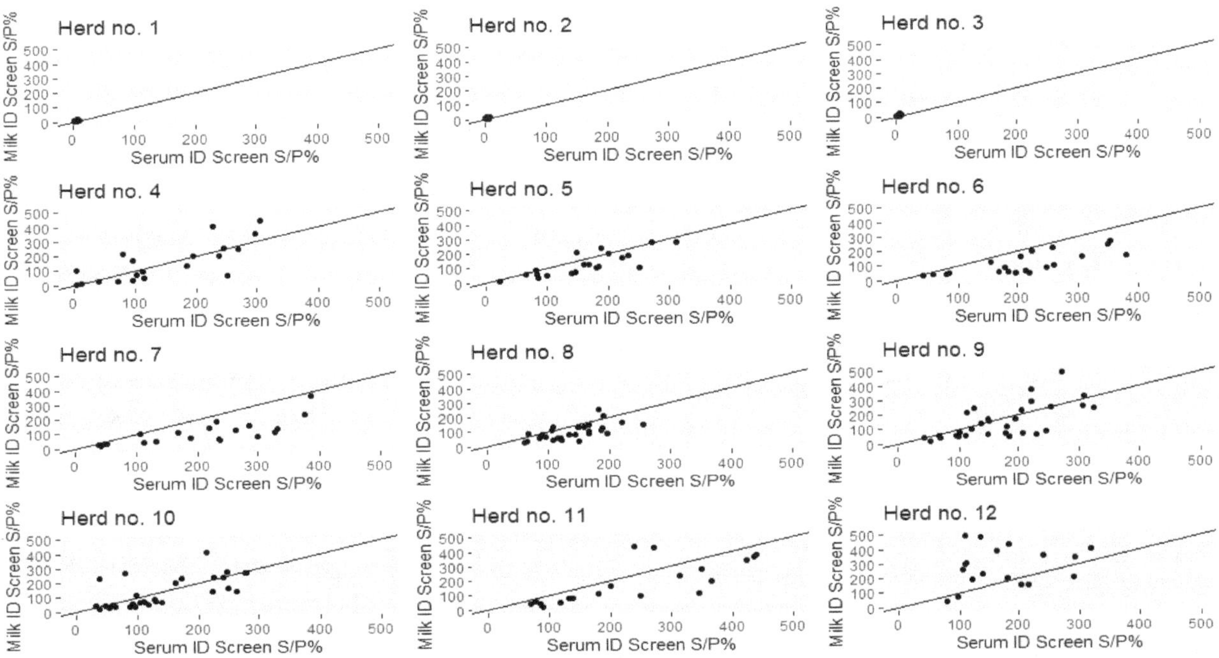

Figure 5. Correlations between paired serum and milk sample-to-positive percentage (S/P%) against *Mycoplasma bovis* using the ID screen® mycoplasma bovis indirect ELISA kit, stratified across 12 Danish dairy herds. The diagonal line indicates perfect agreement between serum and milk values.

3. Discussion

In the present study, we tested milk and serum samples from cows in Danish dairy herds for which we had prior knowledge of the *M. bovis* infection status, in order to gain and share experience of using the ID screen for detecting antibodies against *M. bovis* in adult dairy cows under field conditions and to compare the results with the results of BioX 302. We also determined the correlation between the measured antibody levels in milk and serum for the ID screen across the full dataset of 12 dairy herds and inspected visualizations of the different correlation patterns for the individual herds.

3.1. Field Performance of the ID Screen and BioX 302

Overall, many cows and most of the herds tested positive in both serum and milk when the ID screen was used (Figures 1 and 2). In only three of the 12 herds (Herds 1–3), all samples were negative in both serum and milk. These herds were all previously classified as not infected with *M. bovis*, indicating good concordance between the classification and the test results for these three herds. However, herds 4 and 5 were also classified as not infected, but most both serum and milk samples were positive. This is interesting and there could be several reasons for this, as discussed below.

With regard to the five herds classified as infected with *M. bovis* within the last 5 years (Herds 6–10), nearly all cows tested positive using the ID screen, despite the fact that none of the farmers thought that they had ongoing disease problems related to *M. bovis* at sampling. Four of the herds had an *M. bovis* disease outbreak 4–5 years prior to sampling. Most sampled cows in the three Outbreak-herds had not been born at the time of the disease outbreak. The persistence of antibodies in these herds therefore suggests that the cows were still exposed to *M. bovis*, despite not showing clinical signs around the time of sampling in this study. The two RC-herds classified as infected within the last 5 years both had calves that tested positive for antibodies in both the ID screen and BioX 302, as well as positive PCR samples. In these herds, it is more apparent that the animals were probably exposed to *M. bovis* around the time of sampling. If milk samples and nasal swabs for PCR-testing had been collected from the Outbreak-herds, it cannot be ruled out that some of them would have been positive as well, indicating a recent exposure to *M. bovis* despite there being no sign of disease.

The two herds classified as infected at the time of sampling both had all, but one sample above the cutoff and some of the highest S/P% seen in this study. This makes good sense in terms of the classification, and there was good concordance between the classification and test results in these herds. There was ongoing *M. bovis* infection at least among the calves, where the positive PCR samples were collected. However, none of the PCR tests from nasal swabs or milk samples collected from cows were positive. These were samples from healthy cows, and it cannot be ruled out that if the same samples had been collected from diseased cows, an indication of *M. bovis* infection may have been observed among the cows [4,16].

None of the study herds had ongoing clinical signs of an *M. bovis* disease outbreak. However, the herds still tested positive using the ID screen. All sampled cows were considered to be healthy by the farmer, were housed in the main milking herd and delivered milk to the bulk tank on the day of sampling. Based on this, it is not possible to use the ID screen to differentiate between healthy and diseased cows, but it is likely that the ID screen tests for exposure to *M. bovis*. Cattle can be subclinically infected with *M. bovis* [3], and if the ID screen tests positive in subclinically infected animals, it is potentially a very useful test to use in relation to prevent the spread of infection. However, further studies are needed as this study did not determine the *M. bovis* status of the individual cow, but the herd as a whole.

The ID screen is a sensitive test, as all or nearly all cows in each herd tested either positive or negative. This makes the test good for herd-level control and surveillance purposes, as a small sample of cows would give a good indication of the exposure status of the age group as a whole. However, there may be issues with the diagnostic (field-use) specificity of ID screen, as many of the cows in two out of the five herds classified as not infected within the previous 5 years prior to sampling did test positive. A possible explanation could be that the tested cows in the herds classified as non-infected had been subclinically infected [3] and had therefore never shown any clinical signs. The historical serologic herd classification for this study was based on the BioX 302, which primarily detects clinically ill animals [8,16]. The specificity under field conditions must therefore be investigated further, preferably in field studies based on best practice diagnostic test evaluation [17].

The BioX 302 showed a rather different test pattern. In general, most of the serum and milk samples tested negative. However, there were a small number of positive serum and milk samples in some herds (Figures 3 and 4). The BioX 302 has been shown to have a poor sensitivity [5] and to primarily detect clinically ill animals [8,16]. Taking these findings into account, it is not surprising that the cows in this study generally tested negative when using the BioX 302, as only two herds were classified as having an ongoing *M. bovis* infection. The few positive test results were found in all three herd classifications (not infected, infected within the last 5 years and infected at sampling), and in particular, few positive results were found in milk samples from the non-infected herds (Figures 3 and 4). Herd 4 was classified as not infected but had one positive serum sample and two positive milk samples, one of which was very high in ODC% (140). This could suggest subclinical mastitis in these cows, although they were not positive in PCR on milk. Herds 11 and 12 were classified as having an ongoing *M. bovis* infection, and both of these herds tested positive in a low number of serum and milk samples tested using BioX 302, and this was most pronounced in milk samples. Again, this could suggest subclinical mastitis cases in these herds. Based on the PCR samples from calves (Table 1), it seems that at least this age group was infected with *M. bovis* in herds 11 and 12. It would have been interesting to see the results of the BioX 302 on serum samples from calves—and whether this method would have detected the infection among calves. However, we have previously shown that the BioX 302 did not detect antibodies in calves exposed to *M. bovis* before 3 months of age [9], and all of the samples from the RC-project (Robust Calves project) are from calves under 3 months of age. Previous results have shown that the disease status among calves is not reflected in the bulk tank milk [18], and the findings of this study support that *M. bovis* infection in young stock cannot be measured using the BioX 302 in serum or milk samples from the cows either.

In comparison, there are very large differences in the test patterns between ID screen and BioX 302. Nearly all cows in all, but three non-infected herds were found to be positive when using the ID screen, while in contrast, very few cows tested positive using the BioX 302. As discussed above, the ID screen is a much more sensitive test than the BioX 302 and may be able to detect subclinically infected animals [3], as opposed to the BioX 302, which primarily detects diseased animals [8]. However, nearly all cows tested positive in herds without an ongoing infection, as well as in herds with no history of *M. bovis* infection. This leads to the hypothesis that the ID screen will measure exposure to *M. bovis* rather than colonization and dissemination of the organism in the infected animal. Whatever the reason for the very different test patterns, the interpretation and recommendations for the use of ID screen must be different from that of the BioX 302.

3.2. Correlation between Serum and Milk Samples

The concordance correlation coefficient between serum and milk S/P% was 0.66 (95% CI: 0.59–0.72). In general, the serum values were higher than the milk values, except in herd 12 (Figure 5). This could be explained by different clinical manifestations, e.g., clinical or subclinical mastitis cases could induce mostly high milk S/P% and systemic disease could induce mostly high serum S/P%, as previously shown when using the BioX 302 test [8]. This may also be the case for the ID screen, but to a lesser degree since the cows still test positive in both serum and milk.

The clinical signs present in the Outbreak-herds (herds 8–10) during the *M. bovis* disease outbreak are known as they were part of another *M. bovis* project. Herd 8 had many cows with clinical signs of arthritis and no *M. bovis* PCR-positive milk samples, while herds 9 and 10 experienced a combination of arthritis and mastitis among the cows. Herd 8 had clearly higher S/P% in serum than milk, while herds 9 and 10 had some very high milk values (Figure 5). Even though 4–5 years had passed since the *M. bovis* disease outbreak, the initial clinical expression may still be evident in the ID screen results. If this is the case, it is likely that herd 12 had subclinical mastitis cases.

The observed correlation between ID screen serum and milk values suggests that milk samples may be a promising replacement for serum samples. Strong responses observed in individual cows are also promising signs for the potential use of ID screen on bulk tank milk samples for herd-level diagnosis. This would be advantageous for surveillance and control purposes and for sampling many cows, since milk samples are easier and cheaper to collect than blood samples.

3.3. Uncertainty in Herd Classification

Herd classification is, among other things, based on previous BioX 302 tests and PCR on individual and bulk tank milk samples. The bulk tank milk samples were primarily collected as yearly surveillance tests and are therefore not sampled often enough to ensure the detection of new and mild infections–in the case of an *M. bovis* infection, the detectable response in bulk tank milk can be very short-lived for both BioX 302 and PCR [4,16]. It is possible that some of the herds could have had a previous *M. bovis* infection that was not detected in bulk tank milk by either BioX 302 or PCR, especially if the clinical signs were not severe and the farmer had not collected additional samples.

Herd 2 was classified as not infected despite one positive PCR sample and two positive BioX 302 serum samples, all from calves. The positive PCR test was one out of 209 tested samples. Taking into account that the PCR test is not 100% specific [19], this was judged to be a false positive result. Overall, based on the uncertainties in the diagnostic tests and no other indications of previous or current *M. bovis* infection, we have chosen to classify this herd as not infected.

The farmer from Herd 5 stated that the herd had experienced an *M. bovis* disease outbreak in 2012. It is possible that the ID screen would still be able to detect this exposure, even though seven years had passed since the disease outbreak. However, it is noteworthy that the calves did not test positive in the ID screen, despite calves often being the reservoir of the infection [3]. As discussed above, the BioX 302 is not a sensitive test in young calves, but an in-house ELISA with another antigen (MilA) has been evaluated with good sensitivity in young calves [9], indicating that another ELISA could perform better than the BioX 302 in calves. Based on the ID screen and PCR tests of calves, it seems likely that the young calves were not infected with *M. bovis*, and transmission must therefore occur among older calves in Herd 5. This implies that the milk management and separation of cows from young calves must be adequate in hindering transmission to the young calves. In this herd, the calves were born in a common calving pen and left with the cow for at least 12 h. The calves were then moved to single pens outside, very well separated from the cows. This management may have been sufficient to stop the young calves being exposed, even though there was infection among the cows. In Herd 4, none of the available tests were positive and the farmer stated that the herd had not had an *M. bovis* disease outbreak. This also highlights the difficulties in assessing infection with *M. bovis*. If the positive results of the ID screen are truly a sign of ongoing *M. bovis* infection or exposure within that herd, then it is a very difficult organism to detect. With nearly all cows testing positive in both serum and milk, we find it unlikely that these would be false positive samples. It could be that the ID screen cross-reacts with antibodies against other mycoplasma species. The importance of testing for cross-reactivity with other *Mycoplasma* spp., especially *M. agalactiae*, has been emphasized for other *M. bovis* ELISAs [20], however no such information can be found in the documentation for the ID screen [12,21].

4. Materials and Methods

4.1. Study Herds

Herds were selected for participation based on the availability of prior information about the *M. bovis* status. Information from dairy herds participating in two other research projects as well as knowledge from test results from previously collected samples made it possible to include herds known to have had an *M. bovis* outbreak and herds that had not had an outbreak (Table 1). Nine herds were included due to their participation in a large Danish calf-health research project ('Robust calves project' running from 2018–2021 in which nasal swabs, tracheal washes and blood samples were collected from randomly selected calves across three age groups). These herds are referred to as the RC-herds. The remaining three herds were included because they were known to have had an *M. bovis* disease outbreak with test-positive samples while participating in an *M. bovis* research project 3–4 years prior to the initiation of the present study [8]. These three herds are referred to as the Outbreak-herds.

There was variation among herds in how difficult it was to determine the present and previous *M. bovis* status and additional samples and diagnostic test history were therefore also included from on-farm animal health monitoring activities in order to facilitate the grouping of herds. Details are shown in Table 1.

Previous individual and bulk tank milk *M. bovis* PCR and ELISA results were confirmed from the Danish Cattle Database, which is a national cattle register for all Danish cattle herds. Both national surveillance and diagnostic tests voluntarily conducted on the request of the local veterinarian and farmers are registered here, and we included the available data from 2012–2019. PCR-tested milk samples from which results were available in the Danish Cattle Database were analyzed using the Pathoproof Major-3 or Complete-16 assays (Thermo Scientific, Waltham, MA) or Mastit 4 (DNA Diagnostic, Risskov, Denmark); the ELISA test used was the BioX 302.

Blood samples were collected from many calves in the RC-herds on several occasions during autumn and winter 2019 and 2020 as part of another project. To better characterize potential *M. bovis* infection in these herds, approximately 30 blood samples from seven of these herds were analyzed with the ID screen and BioX 302. During the RC-project, nasal swabs and tracheal washes were also collected from between 129 and 431 calves in each RC-herd (see Table 1 for details), and they were all tested for the presence of *M. bovis* with the Fluidigm PCR test (see Laboratory Analysis for details). No additional diagnostic tests were performed in the three Outbreak-herds.

On the basis of all the information gathered—and considering the fact that the sensitivity and specificity of the BioX 302 ELISA and the Fluidigm PCR tests are not perfect [5,6,19]—all herds were classified as either:

- Not infected—meaning that none (or very few, likely false positives) of the available test results were positive for *M. bovis* and the farmer stated that they had never had clinical signs of *M. bovis*-associated disease or that the clinical signs occurred more than 5 years prior to sampling;
- Infected within the last 5 years—meaning that there were multiple positive diagnostic test results in previously or recently collected samples and/or reporting of clinical signs of *M. bovis* within the last 5 years prior to sampling;
- Infected at sampling—meaning that diagnostic tests indicated an ongoing infection with *M. bovis* among one or more age groups at the time of sampling for the present study.

4.2. Sample Collection

Paired serum and milk samples were collected from cows from the 12 dairy herds during the first quarter of 2019. For all nine RC-herds, paired blood and milk samples were collected from 20 lactating dairy cows, and a nasal swab was collected from the same cows for the detection of *M. bovis*. We aimed to collect samples from primiparous cows, but it was not practically feasible in all herds (Herds 1, 2 and 3), so older cows were also included in the sample collection. The blood samples were collected from the coccygeal vein in plain serum tubes. Prior to milk sampling, the teats were cleaned with ethanol on a tissue, the first milk was discarded and a composite milk sample consisting of milk from all udder quarters was collected from each cow in a bronopol-coated tube to preserve the milk sample. The nasal swabs were taken with a long sterile cotton swab, rubbed gently against the mucosa in one naris until saturated and placed in phosphate-buffered saline until analysis.

All procedures involving animals in this study were conducted in accordance with guidelines from the Danish Ministry of Justice with respect to animal experimentation and care of animals under study (The Danish Ministry of Justice, 2014, LBK no. 474). The Danish Animal Experiments Inspectorate under the Danish Veterinary and Food Administration was consulted for guidance on required permissions and approved the project activities in writing without requiring further formal application or approval processes. Following sampling of the animals, all herd owners were interviewed about their perception and experience with *M. bovis*-associated disease at their farm (summarized in Table 1).

Paired blood and milk samples were collected from 30 cows from the Outbreak-herds. No further tests were done in these herds as they were all known to have had a confirmed outbreak of *M. bovis*-associated disease in 2015–2016.

The number of cows included in each herd was optimized according to the available budget.

The serum and milk samples were analyzed for antibodies against *M. bovis* using the ID screen and the BioX 302. Following antibody analysis, the milk samples were frozen and stored for approximately 6 months and then tested for the presence of *M. bovis* bacterial DNA using the commercial PCR Pathoproof Major-3 assay. The nasal swabs were analyzed for the presence of *M. bovis* using the Fluidigm PCR system.

4.3. Laboratory Analysis

For the ID screen, a S/P% $\geq$ 60 for the serum sample was considered positive and for the milk samples the overnight incubation protocol was used in order to optimize the sensitivity and the samples were considered positive if S/P% $\geq$ 30 [12]. For the BIO K 302, an ODC% $\geq$ 37 was considered positive [22]. The Pathoproof Major-3 assay (Thermo Scientific, Waltham, MA, USA) and the Mastit 4 PCR assay (DNA diagnostic, Risskov, Denmark) were considered positive if the cycle threshold (Ct) value < 37. All these diagnostic tests were performed at Eurofins Milk Testing Denmark, Vejen, Denmark, according to the manufacturer's instructions.

Nasal swabs from cows and calves and tracheal washes from calves were tested for the presence of *M. bovis* using the Fluidigm PCR system at the Technical University of Denmark, Lyngby, Denmark, and a Ct value < 30 was considered positive [19]. Cutoff values and test performance have not yet been established for this test.

Table 1. Overview of the herd type and size, previous *Mycoplasma bovis*-associated disease history, as well as previous diagnostic test results (from 2012–2019) and results of additional samples taken (RC-Calves in 2019–2020) for *Mycoplasma bovis* classification of 12 Danish dairy cattle herds (RC = Robust calves project, N/A = not available, BTM = bulk tank milk).

Herd No.	Herd Type	No. of Cows [a]	PCR—Individual Cows [b] (Positives/n)	ELISA—Individual Cows/ Calves [c] (Positives/n)	BTM PCR [b] (Positives/n)	BTM ELISA [c] (Positives/n)	RC-Calves—ID Screen [d] (Positives/n)	RC-Calves—BioX 302 [c] (Positives/n)	RC-Calves—PCR Test [e] (Positives/n)	*Mycoplasma bovis* Disease Outbreak	*Mycoplasma bovis* Classification
1	RC	150	N/A	N/A	0/21	0/16	0/27	1/27	0/182	No [f]	Not infected
2	RC	190	0/348	N/A	0/14	0/8	0/27	2/27	1/209	No [f]	Not infected
3	RC	350	0/9	0/8	0/9	1/5	0/29	1/29	0/228	Yes (2013) [f]	Not infected
4	RC	220	0/1	N/A	0/10	0/6	0/29	0/29	0/172	No [f]	Not infected
5	RC	200	0/3	N/A	0/11	1/6	1/29	0/30	0/129	Yes (2012) [f]	Not infected
6	RC	700	1/398	N/A	0/9	2/5	16/30	2/30	3/431	No [f]	Infected within the last 5 years
7	RC	600	0/284	N/A	1/23	0/6	24/30	10/30	1/179	Yes (2014–2015) [f]	Infected within the last 5 years
8	Outbreak	190	7/140	85/372	0/34	0/23	N/A	N/A	N/A	Yes (2015–2016) [g]	Infected within the last 5 years
9	Outbreak	430	69/1188	70/282	18/327	1/9	N/A	N/A	N/A	Yes (2015–2016) [g]	Infected within the last 5 years
10	Outbreak	200	21/98	91/303	3/16	1/12	N/A	N/A	N/A	Yes (2015–2016) [g]	Infected within the last 5 years
11	RC	600	10/25	0/3	0/10	1/7	N/A	N/A	11/256	Yes (2014) [f]	Infected at sampling
12	RC	330	4/234	N/A	0/14	0/6	N/A	N/A	9/228	No [f]	Infected at sampling

[a] Average number of cows per year during 2016–2019 [b] Pathoproof Major-3 or Complete-16 assays (Thermo Scientific, Waltham, MA, USA) or Mastit 4 (DNA diagnostic, Risskov, Denmark), test results collected on the farmers' initiatives prior to this study (e.g., for herd health management), positive cycle threshold < 37 [c] BioX 302 (BioX Diagnostics, Rochefort, Belgium), test results collected on the farmers' initiatives prior to this study (e.g., for herd health management), positive ≥ 37 sample coefficient (ODC%) [d] ID screen® mycoplasma bovis indirect (IDvet, Grabels, France), positive ≥ 60 sample-to-positive percentage (S/P%) [e] Fluidigm In-house PCR (Technical University of Denmark), positive cycle threshold < 30. [f] According to the farmer [g] Confirmed test-positive for *M. bovis*.

4.4. Statistical Analysis

The correlation between serum and milk S/P% was calculated as the concordance correlation coefficient [23]. All data management and statistical analyses were carried out in R version 3.2.2 [24] using the packages "dplyr", "ggplot2", "gridExtra" and "DescTools".

5. Conclusions

In the present study, we gained and shared experience of using the ID screen for the detection of antibodies against *M. bovis* in adult dairy cows under field conditions and compared this with the results of the BioX 302 test. When using the ID screen, nearly all cows in all, but three non-infected herds tested positive, while in contrast, very few cows tested positive when using the BioX 302. The ID screen is therefore a much more sensitive test than the BioX 302. However, some herds without ongoing infection, and even some herds with no history of *M. bovis* infection also tested positive. This indicates either lack of specificity (e.g., cross-reactions with other mycoplasma species) or that the ID screen measures exposure to *M. bovis* rather than the colonization and dissemination of the organism in the infected animal. The latter implies that the interpretation and recommendations for using the ID screen should be different from that of BioX 302. A concordance correlation coefficient between the ID screen serum and milk results of 0.66 (95% CI: 0.58–0.72) indicates that easy-to-collect milk samples can replace serum samples for ID screen diagnosis of *M. bovis* in adult cows, and the use of ID screen on bulk tank milk samples for surveillance and control purposes is promising. This, in addition to assessments of the ID screen performance (in particular regarding the specificity) under field conditions can provide new research questions to pursue. We therefore recommend field studies for best practice diagnostic test evaluation of the ID screen.

Author Contributions: Conceptualization, M.B.P., L.P. and L.R.N.; methodology, M.B.P., L.P., L.M.P. and L.R.N.; R-code, M.B.P.; formal analysis, M.B.P.; resources, M.B.P., L.P., L.M.P. and L.R.N.; data curation, M.B.P., L.P., L.M.P. and L.R.N.; writing—original draft preparation, M.B.P.; writing—review & editing, M.B.P., L.P., L.M.P. and L.R.N.; visualization, M.B.P.; supervision, L.P. and L.R.N.; project administration, M.B.P., L.P. and L.R.N.; funding acquisition, M.B.P., L.P., L.M.P. and L.R.N. All authors have read and agreed to the published version of the manuscript.

References

1. Nicholas, R.A.J.; Ayling, R.D. Mycoplasma bovis: Disease, diagnosis, and control. *Res. Vet. Sci.* **2003**, *74*, 105–112. [CrossRef]
2. Maunsell, F.P.; Donovan, G.A. Mycoplasma bovis Infections in young calves. *Vet. Clin. N. Am. Food Anim. Pract.* **2009**, *25*, 139–177. [CrossRef] [PubMed]
3. Maunsell, F.P.; Woolums, A.R.; Francoz, D.; Rosenbusch, R.F.; Step, D.L.; Wilson, D.J.; Janzen, E.D. Mycoplasma bovis Infections in Cattle. *J. Vet. Intern. Med.* **2011**, *25*, 772–783. [CrossRef] [PubMed]
4. Petersen, M.B. Mycoplasma Bovis in Dairy Cattle—Clinical Epidemiology and Antibody Measurements for Decision Making. Ph.D. Thesis, University of Copenhagen, Frederiksberg, Denmark, 15 August 2018.
5. Schibrowski, M.L.; Barnes, T.S.; Wawegama, N.K.; Vance, M.E.; Markham, P.F.; Mansell, P.D.; Marenda, M.S.; Kanci, A.; Perez-Casal, J.; Browning, G.F.; et al. The performance of three immune assays to assess the serological status of cattle experimentally exposed to Mycoplasma bovis. *Vet. Sci.* **2018**, *5*, 27. [CrossRef] [PubMed]
6. Wawegama, N.K.; Markham, P.F.; Kanci, A.; Schibrowski, M.; Oswin, S.; Barnes, T.S.; Firestone, S.M.; Mahony, T.J.; Browning, G.F. Evaluation of an IgG enzyme-linked immunosorbent assay as a serological assay for detection of mycoplasma bovis infection in feedlot cattle. *J. Clin. Microbiol.* **2016**, *54*, 1269–1275. [CrossRef] [PubMed]
7. Andersson, A.M.; Aspán, A.; Wisselink, H.J.; Smid, B.; Ridley, A.; Pelkonen, S.; Autio, T.; Lauritsen, K.T.; Kensø, J.; Gaurivaud, P.; et al. A European inter-laboratory trial to evaluate the performance of three serological methods for diagnosis of Mycoplasma bovis infection in cattle using latent class analysis. *BMC Vet. Res.* **2019**, *15*, 1–10. [CrossRef] [PubMed]

8. Petersen, M.B.; Pedersen, J.; Holm, D.L.; Denwood, M.; Nielsen, L.R. A longitudinal observational study of the dynamics of Mycoplasma bovis antibodies in naturally exposed and diseased dairy cows. *J. Dairy Sci.* **2018**, *101*, 7386–7396. [CrossRef] [PubMed]
9. Petersen, M.B.; Wawegama, N.K.; Denwood, M.; Markham, P.F.; Browning, G.F.; Nielsen, L.R. Mycoplasma bovis antibody dynamics in naturally exposed dairy calves according to two diagnostic tests. *BMC Vet. Res.* **2018**, *14*. [CrossRef]
10. Bürki, S.; Frey, J.; Pilo, P. Virulence, persistence and dissemination of Mycoplasma bovis. *Vet. Microbiol.* **2015**, *179*, 15–22. [CrossRef]
11. Vähänikkilä, N.; Pohjanvirta, T.; Haapala, V.; Simojoki, H.; Soveri, T.; Browning, G.F.; Pelkonen, S.; Wawegama, N.K.; Autio, T. Characterisation of the course of Mycoplasma bovis infection in naturally infected dairy herds. *Vet. Microbiol.* **2019**, *231*, 107–115. [CrossRef] [PubMed]
12. Anonymous. Internal Validation Report ID Screen®Mycoplasma Bovis Indirect. Available online: https://www.id-vet.com/produit/id-screen-mycoplasma-bovis-indirect/ (accessed on 30 June 2020).
13. Howard, C.J.; Gourlay, R.N. Imunne Response Of Calves Following The Inoculation Of Mycoplasma Dispar And Mycoplasma Bovis. *Vet. Microbiol.* **1983**, *8*, 45–56. [CrossRef]
14. Jacobson, R.H. Validation of serological assays for diagnosis of infectious diseases. *Rev. Sci. et Tech. de l'OIE* **1998**, *17*, 469–486. [CrossRef] [PubMed]
15. Nielsen, P.K.; Petersen, M.B.; Nielsen, L.R.; Halasa, T.; Toft, N. Latent class analysis of bulk tank milk PCR and ELISA testing for herd level diagnosis of Mycoplasma bovis. *Prev. Vet. Med.* **2015**, *121*, 338–342. [CrossRef] [PubMed]
16. Parker, A.M.; House, J.K.; Hazelton, M.S.; Bosward, K.L.; Morton, J.M.; Sheehy, P.A. Bulk tank milk antibody ELISA as a biosecurity tool for detecting dairy herds with past exposure to Mycoplasma bovis. *J. Dairy Sci.* **2017**, *100*, 8296–8309. [CrossRef] [PubMed]
17. Anonymous. Standard Operating Procedure for OIE Registration of Diagnostic Kits. Available online: https://www.oie.int/doc/ged/D12069.PDF (accessed on 29 July 2020).
18. Petersen, M.B.; Krogh, K.; Nielsen, L.R. Factors associated with variation in bulk tank milk Mycoplasma bovis antibody-ELISA results in dairy herds. *J. Dairy Sci.* **2016**, *99*, 3815–3823. [CrossRef] [PubMed]
19. Goecke, N.B.; Hjulsager, C.K.; Krog, J.S.; Skovgaard, K.; Larsen, L.E. Development of a high-throughput real-time PCR system for detection of enzootic pathogens in pigs. *J. Vet. Diagn. Investig.* **2020**, *32*, 51–64. [CrossRef] [PubMed]
20. Wawegama, N.K.; Browning, G.F.; Kanci, A.; Marenda, M.S.; Markham, P.F. Development of a recombinant protein-based enzyme-linked immunosorbent assay for diagnosis of mycoplasma bovis infection in cattle. *Clin. Vaccine Immunol.* **2014**, *21*, 196–202. [CrossRef] [PubMed]
21. Anonymous. IDVet Screen Mycoplasma Bovis Indirect Material Safety Data Sheet. Available online: https://www.id-vet.com/produit/id-screen-mycoplasma-bovis-indirect/ (accessed on 30 June 2020).
22. Anonymous. BioX Diagnostics Monoscreen Ab ELISA. Available online: https://www.biox.com/en/bio-k-302-monoscreen-abelisa-mycoplasma-bovis-indirect-monowell-p-250/ (accessed on 30 June 2020).
23. Lin, L.I.-K. A Concordance Correlation Coefficient to Evaluate Reproducibility. *Biometrics* **1989**, *45*, 255. [CrossRef] [PubMed]
24. R Core Team. R: A Language and Environment for Statistical Computing. R Foundation for Statistical Computing: Vienna, Austria,2016. Available online: https://www.R-project.org/ (accessed on 30 June 2020).

12

The Effect of Bovine Viral Diarrhea Virus (BVDV) Strains and the Corresponding Infected-Macrophages' Supernatant on Macrophage Inflammatory Function and Lymphocyte Apoptosis

Karim Abdelsalam [1,2,*], Mrigendra Rajput [1], Gamal Elmowalid [2], Jacob Sobraske [1], Neelu Thakur [1], Hossam Abdallah [2], Ahmed A. H. Ali [2] and Christopher C. L. Chase [1,*]

1 Department of Veterinary and Biomedical Sciences, South Dakota State University, Brookings, SD 57007, USA; mrajput@atu.edu (M.R.); jacob.sobraske@sdstate.edu (J.S.); neelu.thakur@sdstate.edu (N.T.)
2 Faculty of Veterinary Medicine, Zagazig University, Zagazig 44519, Egypt; gelmowalid@yahoo.com (G.E.); bactine_ho@yahoo.com (H.A.); ahhmht35@yahoo.com (A.A.H.A.)
* Correspondence: karim.abdelsalam@sdstate.edu (K.A.); christopher.chase@sdstate.edu (C.C.L.C.)

Abstract: Bovine viral diarrhea virus (BVDV) is an important viral disease of cattle that causes immune dysfunction. Macrophages are the key cells for the initiation of the innate immunity and play an important role in viral pathogenesis. In this in vitro study, we studied the effect of the supernatant of BVDV-infected macrophage on immune dysfunction. We infected bovine monocyte-derived macrophages (MDM) with high or low virulence strains of BVDV. The supernatant recovered from BVDV-infected MDM was used to examine the functional activity and surface marker expression of normal macrophages as well as lymphocyte apoptosis. Supernatants from the highly virulent 1373-infected MDM reduced phagocytosis, bactericidal activity and downregulated MHC II and CD14 expression of macrophages. Supernatants from 1373-infected MDM induced apoptosis in MDBK cells, lymphocytes or BL-3 cells. By protein electrophoresis, several protein bands were unique for high-virulence, 1373-infected MDM supernatant. There was no significant difference in the apoptosis-related cytokine mRNA (IL-1beta, IL-6 and TNF-a) of infected MDM. These data suggest that BVDV has an indirect negative effect on macrophage functions that is strain-specific. Further studies are required to determine the identity and mechanism of action of these virulence factors present in the supernatant of the infected macrophages.

Keywords: bovine viral diarrhea virus; cytopathic BVDV; immunosuppression; lymphocyte apoptosis; monocyte-derived macrophages; non-cytopathic BVDV

---

1. Introduction

Bovine viral diarrhea virus (BVDV) causes immune dysfunction in cattle and other ruminants, resulting in severe economic losses. The immune dysfunction associated with BVDV is believed to be, in part, a consequence of lymphoid depletion that could be mild or severe based on the virulence of the BVDV strains [1–4]. Furthermore, BVDV induces multiple abnormalities to immune cell function and immune mediators that could potentiate viral infection and pathogenesis [5,6]. BVDV infects neutrophils and decreases their microbicidal activity [7]. It also infects alveolar macrophage and decreases the expression of complement Fc receptors and chemokine production, reducing their ability to engulf opsonized pathogens [8].

Although only cytopathogenic (Cp) strains can induce direct apoptosis to peripheral blood mononuclear cells (PBMCs) [9,10], other studies have suggested that Ncp BVDV induces apoptosis in vitro in PBMCs isolated from BVDV-infected animals [11]. Ncp BVDV causes the most severe

BVDV immune dysfunction and is associated with severe lymphoid depletion [2,3,12–15]. Some Ncp BVDV strains have been categorized under a new biotype, lymphocytopathogenic, as they can induce apoptosis in lymphocytes while not effecting epithelial cells [3,16]. In addition, Ncp BVDV has been reported to induce apoptosis in vitro in PBMCs isolated from BVDV-infected animals [11].

Factors associated with Cp BVDV-induced apoptosis include: (i) oxidative stress and (ii) soluble factor(s) produced by monocytes that induced apoptosis in uninfected cells after lipopolysaccharide (LPS) treatment, [9,10,17,18]. However, the exact mechanism by which Ncp/lymphocytopathogenic BVDV induced the apoptotic effect is not well understood. Several studies suggest the role of macrophages in lymphoid depletion and immune dysfunction associated with BVDV. These studies demonstrated the importance of monocytes/macrophage in lymphocyte apoptosis in a mixed population of PBMCs [9,13]. However, the role of apoptotic-associated cytokines, which are important for classic swine fever virus (CSFV)-induced lymphocyte apoptosis, do not appear to be important for BVDV [13]. BVDV and CSFV are classified under the same genus: *Pestivirus*, Family: *Flavivirdae.* It has also been hypothesized that the *Pestivirus'* specific secreted Erns glycoprotein could play a role in the apoptosis mechanism associated with CSFV [19,20].

Immune mediators potentiate viral infection and pathogenesis. CSFV [21], and Cp BVDV [17], prime uninfected cells for activation-induced apoptosis. The mechanism for activation-induced apoptosis is virus-specific, where direct contact between infected and uninfected cells may also be involved in CSFV [21]. CSFV infection of bone marrow hematopoietic cells does not induce apoptosis in the majority of infected cells but does cause apoptosis in the uninfected cells, suggesting an apoptotic role for soluble factors released from infected cells. Cp BVDV induces apoptosis, while Ncp BVDV inhibits apoptosis [9,10,17,18,22,23].

Cp BVDV induces apoptosis in epithlial cellls in cell culture and in PBMCs, making it different from Lymphocytopathogenic BVDV, which can only induce apoptosis in lymphocytes. The soluble factor(s) involved in apoptosis has not been well characterized in any of these studies. Several studies have identified cytokines that prime for apoptosis, including IL-4 [24], TNF-α, IFN-γ [25–27] and IL1beta [28]. However, these cytokines are produced by lymphocytes rather than macrophages [23].

To investigate the indirect effect of different strains of BVDV on macrophage activity and lymphocytes apoptosis, both peripheral blood lymphocytes and a BVDV-free BL-3 cell line were used [3]. The direct apoptotic effect of BVDV was examined by the infection of lymphocytes with different BVDV strains. The indirect effect was investigated by infection of the MDM with one of two different strains of BVDV, followed by treatment of lymphocytes with the irradiated virus-free supernatant from BVDV-infected macrophages [29].

2. Materials and Methods

2.1. Viruses and Cells

Two Ncp strains of BVDV 2 were used in the current study: a high virulent 1373 and, a low virulent 28508-5, in addition to Cp 296C strain as control for apoptosis [30]. All strains were titrated using TCID50 titration assay [31].

BVDV-free Madin Darby bovine kidney MDBK cells (passage 113–135) were grown in minimal essential medium (MEM, Gibco BRL, Grand Island, NY, USA) (pH 7–7.4) supplemented with 10% BVDV-free fetal bovine serum (FBS) (Hyclone Laboratories, Logan, UT, USA), penicillin (100 U/mL) and streptomycin (100 μg/mL). MDBK cells were maintained at 37 °C with 5% CO_2 in humidified incubator and were used for viral titration and propagation as well as apoptosis experiments.

Bovine lymphosarcoma cell line (Bl-3) is a non-adherent, BVDV-free B cell line clone derived from BL-3.1 cell line that was obtained from ATCC, Manassas, VA, USA. BL-3 cell line was cultured as previously described [3] and they were used to examine the direct and indirect apoptotic effect of different BVDV strains.

2.2. *Isolation of Monocytes and Differentiation to Monocyte Derived Macrophage (MDM)*

PBMCs were isolated as previously described [32,33] with modifications. Briefly, the heparinized blood was diluted 1:1 with PBS and overlaid over histopaque 1083 gradient using SepMate™ 50 mL tubes (Stemcell Technologies, Cambridge, MA, USA) and centrifuged at 1200× *g* for 20 min at room temperature (RT). The buffy-coat was then transferred to a clean 50 mL conical tube and washed five times with PBS, followed by centrifugation at 120× *g* for 10 min at RT. The viability of PBMCs was determined by trypan blue exclusion assay according to Strobber [34]. The PBMCs were suspended in RPMI 1640 medium (GE Healthcare, Hyclone Laboratories, Logan, UT, USA) supplemented with 10% FBS, penicillin (100 U/mL) and streptomycin (100 μg/mL) to achieve a final concentration of 1×10^6 cells/mL. The cells were incubated in T175 flasks for 3 h at 37 °C. Then, the adherent monocyte was washed with PBS five times and detached by incubation for 10 min with Accutase™ (eBioscience, San Diego, CA, USA). Detached monocytes were PBS-washed twice to get rid of Accutase. The isolated monocyte cultured in complete RPMI 1640, as described by Elmowalid [29], at a concentration of 10^5 cells/well in 48-well plate, followed by incubation for 5 days at 37 °C. The incubated cells were fed every other day by replacing half of the conditioned media with fresh complete RPMI. At day 5, the MDM were characterized phenotypically as MHCI-, MHCII-, CD11b- and CD14-positive cells.

2.3. *Production and Inactivation of Infected MDM Supernatant*

The MDM were infected with 100 μL of 10^5 TCID50 BVDV strains at MOI of 1 in triplicate as described by Elmowalid [29], with modifications. The infected cells were incubated for 1 h, then washed to remove the excess unbound virus, and 500 μL of complete RPMI 1640 medium was added to each well in a 24-well plate. At least one column of the plate was mock-infected with complete RPMI 1640 medium as a negative control. The infected MDM were incubated for 12, 24 or 48 h at 37 °C in CO_2 incubator. The BVDV-infected macrophage supernatants were collected at 12, 24 and 48 hpi (hours post-infection) and centrifuged at 1000× *g* for 10 min at RT to remove cellular debris. The supernatant was UV-inactivated for 20 min on ice to exclude the direct virus effect [35]. The absence of any infectious viral particles in the treated supernatants was confirmed by inoculation on MDBK cells followed by a 5-day incubation and BVDV specific immune-staining of the inoculated MDBK cells using both immune-peroxidase and immunofluorescence. The positive control was 1373 infected MDBK cells.

2.4. *Phagocytosis*

One mL of virus-free (UV-inactivated) supernatants collected at 24 or 48 hpi from Ncp1373 or 28508-5 BVDV strains or mock-infected MDM were used to treat MDM, cultured on 24-well plates (approximately 5×10^5 cells/well whose viability was >92%), for 24 h. This was followed by washing the treated cells twice with PBS and then exposed to 250 μL containing approximately 2×10^7 of TRITC-labeled *C. albicans* (50 yeast/macrophage) and incubated for 30 min at 37 °C. Finally, the cells were washed twice in cold PBS and re-suspended in 200 μL/well freshly prepared paraformaldehyde (PFA) to be examined under UV-microscopy. The number of yeast/cell counted and the cells were classified into two groups: cells that contained >20 TRITC labeled yeast/cell that indicated normal phagocytic activity and cells that contained <20 TRITC labeled yeast/cell that indicated insufficient phagocytic activity. A total number of 100 MDM containing yeast were counted and the percentage of phagocytic activity was calculated according to the following formula: Phagocytic% = (number of MDM containing >20 yeasts/total number of MDM) × 100.

2.5. *Bactericidal Activity*

MDM were treated with 1 mL/well of UV-inactivated supernatant from MDM infected with 1373, 28508-5 or mock-infected 24 and 48 h supernatant, and incubated for 24 h at 37 °C. The cells were then washed twice in PBS and incubated for 30 min or more (up to 120 min) with 1×10^7 *E. coli* (20 bacteria/macrophage) suspended in RPMI 1640 supplemented with 5% FBS and no antibiotics to allow bacterial phagocytosis. One group of the cells were washed three times with cold PBS 30 post-incubation to stop phagocytosis and to remove excess bacteria (time 0) and were lysed and the lysates were centrifuged at 800× *g* for 10 min and the supernatants were aspirated, while the pellets were suspended in LB broth and stored at 4 °C. The other group of cells were incubated in 5% FBS, and no antibiotics for extra 90 min to allow killing (total 120 min) followed by washing and lysis, as described above. Cell lysates of both 0 and 90 min timepoints were placed in 96-well plates and incubated for 18 h at 37 °C, followed by adding 30 µL/well of of 50 mg/mL 3-(4,5-dimethylthiazol-2-yl)-2,5-diphenyl tetrazolium bromide (MTT, Sigma, St. Louis, MO, USA) and the plates were incubated at 37 °C for another 6–8 h. Optical density was measured at 540 nm wavelengths in ELISA reader (Biotek, ELx808, Winooski, VT, USA). The percentage of killing was calculated by the following formula: Killing% = (absorbance after incubation for 90 min/Absorbance at time 0) × 100.

2.6. Nitric Oxide Production

Nitric oxide (NO) assay was done in 24-well plates. MDM were treated by adding 1 mL/well of UV-treated supernatant from 1373 or by direct infection with 1373 strain of BVDV (MOI of 1) kept with the cells. Mock-infected supernatant or RPMI 1640 media containing 5% FBS were used as a control. The cells were incubated for 24 h at 37 °C. The cells were then stimulated with lipopolysaccharide (25 µg/mL) (LPS, Sigma, St. Louis, MO, USA) for another 24 h. Then, supernatants were collected and nitric oxide (NO) concentration was determined using Griess reagent (Sigma, St. Louis, MO, USA) using Nitrite (NO_2) measurement as an indicator of NO production according to the protocol of Blond et al., 2000: briefly, 100 µL of culture supernatant was added to 100 µL of Griess reagent, made of a 1/1 mixture of 1% (wt/vol) sulfanilamide and 0.5% (wt/vol) *N*-(1-naphthyl)ethylenediamine dihydrochloride (Sigma, St. Louis, MO, USA) in 30% acetic acid, in each well of a 96-well plate. Reactions were performed in triplicate at RT for 10 min. Chromophore absorbance was then measured at 550 nm in a microplate reader (Bio-TEK Instruments model EL 311; OSI, Paris, France). Nitrite concentration was evaluated by comparison with the nitrate standard curve (Sigma, St. Louis, MO, USA). The lower limit of detection for nitrite is 250 nM.

2.7. Immunostaining and Flow Cytometry of CD14 and MHC II

To examine the effect of BVDV direct infection or its supernatant on macrophage surface marker expression, the MDM were either infected or treated with different BVDV-48 h-supernatants: including 1373 and 28508-5 strains. This was in addition to the supernatant from mock-infected MDM. Surface marker expression was investigated 48 hpi, starting with using Accutase^{TM} (eBioscience, San Diego, CA, USA) to detach the MDMs that were washed twice in PBS and plated in a U-bottom-96-well plate by adding100 µL of cells (2×10^5 cell) per well. Cells were then suspended in blocking buffer (50 µL/well) (PBS containing 2% FCS and 0.1% sodium azide) for 20 min at RT. 50 µL/well of mouse anti-bovine CD14, or MHC II (VMRD, Pullman, WA, USA) diluted at 1:200 in PBS was added and the cells incubated for 20 min at 4 °C, followed by washing three times in PBS. Subsequently, the cells were incubated with FITC-conjugated goat anti-mouse Ig G (Ig G whole molecule, ICN/Cappel laboratories, Santa Mesa, CA, USA) diluted at 1:1000 in staining buffer for 20 min in dark at 4 °C, followed by washing three times in PBS. Fifty (50) µL/well of propidium iodide (1 µg/mL) were added directly before analysis to stain the dead cells. Both cell control (without staining) and the FITC control (just FITC staining without the primary anti-bovine antibodies) were included to eliminate nonspecific background. For each sample, mean fluorescent intensity of immune-stained cells was estimated and analyzed on FACScan flow cytometry (Becton Dickinson, Mountain View, CA, USA) using CELL Quest software (BD Biosciences).

2.8. *Examining the Indirect or Direct Effect of BVDV Strains on Peripheral Blood Lymphocyte Population and MDBK*

To examine the indirect effect of BVDV strains, peripheral blood lymphocytes, BL-3 or MDBK were treated with various time-point irradiated supernatants from BVDV-infected macrophages at a dilution of 1:1 and incubated for 12, 24 or 48 h post treatment, as previously described [36]. To examine the direct effect of BVDV strains, peripheral blood lymphocytes or BL3 were infected with BVDV strain at MOI of 1, as described by Ridpath et al. [37]. The effect of the direct infection of lymphocyte with Cp 296C strain was included as a positive apoptosis control.

2.9. *Chromatin Condensation*

The apoptotic effect of the infected MDM supernatant on epithelial cells was investigated by incubating MDBK cells for 12, 24, or 48 h at 37 °C with 1 mL/well of UV-treated supernatant from 1373, or 28508-5 as well as the non-infected supernatant. The cells were then washed twice in PBS, and then stained using 4,6-diamidino-2-phenylindole (DAPI, Sigma, St Louis, MO, USA) according to the protocol of Mi Hyeon et al., 2002. Simply, one volume of pre-staining solution [citric acid (2.1 g), Tween 20 (0.5 mL), and distilled H_2O (100 mL)] was added and the cells were incubated for 5–7 min at RT in the dark. After the incubation, another six volumes of staining solution [(citric acid (2.1 g), DAPI (0.2 mg/mL), 1 mg DNAse, and distilled H_2O (100 mL)] were added for another 5–7 min. Cells were washed three times in PBS and examined under fluorescence microscopy. Two hundred cells (200) were counted and the mean value was calculated. The apoptotic index was the mean of three independent experiments.

2.10. *Annexin V Staining*

Both direct BVDV infection or the indirect effect of its supernatant on bovine lymphocytes and MDBK cells was investigated using the AnnexinV staining kit (eBioscience, San Diego, CA, USA). Briefly the infected or supernatant-treated lymphocytes were washed once with PBS and the cells were re-suspended in 100 µL of 1x binding buffer supplied by the kit. Five µL of FITC conjugated annexin v antibody added to the lymphocytes suspended in 100 µL of binding buffer and incubated for 10 min in the dark. This was followed by washing the cells twice by suspending the cells in 1x binding buffer followed by adding another five µL of propidium iodide to exclude the dead cells. Finally, the cells were re suspended in 200 µL of 1x BD FACSTM lysing solution followed by analysis with BD Accuri^{TM} C6 Plus Flow Cytometer (BD Biosciences, San Jose CA, USA). The result was expressed as % of apoptosis.

2.11. *Protein Electrophoresis*

The BVDV-infected MDM supernatant was fractionated on 10% sodium dodecyl sulphate polyacrylamide gel (SDS-PAGE) according to the protocol of Schagger and von Jagow, 1987. Briefly, 40 µL of the supernatant (around 50 µg) were added to 10 µL of 5x sample buffer (65 mM Tris-HCL, pH 7.0, 2% SDS, 10% glycerol, 5% β mercaptoethanol, and 0.001% bromophenol blue) with heating at 100 °C for 3–5 min. Protein electrophoresis was then done by loading the treated sample (50 µL) on the SDS-PAGE gel at 25 mA current for 45–60 min followed by staining with Coomassie blue overnight (in some experiments for 4 h) with shaking at RT. Finally, the gel was immersed in de-staining buffer (40% methanol and 10% glacial acetic acid) with shaking for 15 min at RT until the protein bands become clear [38].

2.12. *Quantification of Apoptosis-Related Cytokines by qRT-PCR of BVDV-Infected MDMs*

Both the infected and mock-infected MDM were pelleted at 500× *g* for 8 min, then washed twice in PBS. The infected MDM were lysed and nucleic acid (NA) extraction done using RNeasy extraction kit (Qiagen, Valencia, CA, USA). The extracted NA of different samples was normalized to 5 ng/µL using Nanodrop ND-1000 Spectrophotometer (Fisher Scientific, Portsmouth, NH, USA). Nucleic acid extracted from mock-infected MDM with complete RPMI 1640 medium was used as a negative control while NA extracted from MDM treated with Concanavalin A (ConA) or lipopolysaccharide (LPS) (Sigma-Aldrich, St. Louis, MO, USA) was used as a positive control. Around 5 μL of the normalized NA was used for relative quantification of apoptosis-related cytokines; TNF-α, IL-1α, IL-1β and IL-6 for each sample in duplicates using quantitative reverse transcriptase PCR (qRT-PCR) and Power SYBR® Green RNA-to-CtTM 1-Step Kit (Thermo Fisher Scientific, Millersburg PA, USA). Additional cytokines were also measured that include: IFN–α, β and γ, IL-4, 8, 10, and 12. The cytokine primers used were described in Table 1 [39]. The relative expression of mRNA was standardized using beta actin and GAPDH as housekeeping genes. Each qPCR experiment was followed by heat dissociation curve step to exclude nonspecific amplification. qRT-PCR results were analyzed using relative expression software tool (REST©2009 software) [40].

Table 1. The set of primers used for quantifications of apoptosis-related cytokine mRNA.

Cytokine	Forward Primer	Reverse Primer	Annealing Temp °C
TNF-α	AGACCCCAGCACCCAGGACTCG	GGAGATGCCATCTGTGTGAGTG	55
IL-1α	GATGCCTGAGACACCCAA	GAAAGTCAGTGATCGAGGG	53
IL-1β	CAAGGAGAGGAAAGAGACA	TGAGAAGTGCTGATGTACCA	53
IL-6	TCCAGAACGAGTATGAGG	CATCCGAATAGCTCTCAG	52
β-actin	CGCACCACTGGCATTGTC	TCCAAGGCGACGTAGCAG	55
IFN-α	ACACACACCTGGT	GATGACAGCAGAAATGA	52
IFN-β	RTCTGSAGCCAAT	CAGGCACACCTGT	52
IFN-γ	ATAACCAGGTCATTCAAAGG	ATTCTGACTTCTCTTCCGCT	55
IL-8	TGGGCCACACTGTGAAAAT	TCATGGATCTTGCTTCTCAGC	53
IL-10	TGCTGGATGACTTTAAGGG	AGGGCAGAAAGCGATGACA	53
IL-12	GAGGCCTGTTTACCACTGGA	CTCATAGATACTTCTAAGGCACAG	58
IL-4	TGCATTGTTAGCGTCTCCTG	AGGTCTTTCAGCGTACTTGT	56

2.13. *Supernatant Neutralization*

To exclude the apoptotic effect induced due to possible viral secreted proteins, 24 or 48 h supernatants from the BVDV-infected macrophages with 1373 strain were incubated at 37 °C for 1 h with Erns specific 15c5 monoclonal antibody (IDEXX Laboratories, Westbrook, ME, USA) or with BVDV-polyclonal antibody (kindly supplied by Dr. Robert Fulton, Food Animal Research, Oklahoma State University). The mixture of the infected supernatant and antibody was prepared as two parts of infected supernatant incubated with one part of concentrated antibody. Three (3) parts of the supernatant/antibody mixture were added to one part of BL-3 cell line seeded at 1×10^5 cells/well, followed by incubation at 37 °C for 36 h post-treatment.

2.14. *Statistical Analysis*

Data were analyzed using a Student's *t*-test (Microsoft EXCEL, MAC 2011) to assess the significance of the differences between mean values of treated and control samples at each timepoint. Differences were considered significant at $p < 0.05$, however some treatments showed very significant difference with p value of <0.01. Every experiment was achieved using at least three different animals and each experiment was done in triplicates. The variations in results were calculated by standard deviations at each timepoint. For cytokine analysis, REST© 2009 [40], that is based on analysis of variance (AVOVA).

3. Results

3.1. Inactivation of Infected Supernatant

The irradiated supernant-treated MDBK cells had no immune-peroxidase stain for the UV-irradiated supernant (Figure 1A) compared to the positive intracytoplasmic staining of 1373-infected-MDBK non-irradiated control (Figure 1B). There was no fluorescence signal for the irradiated strain (Figure 1C) compared to the non-irradiated infection control (Figure 1D).

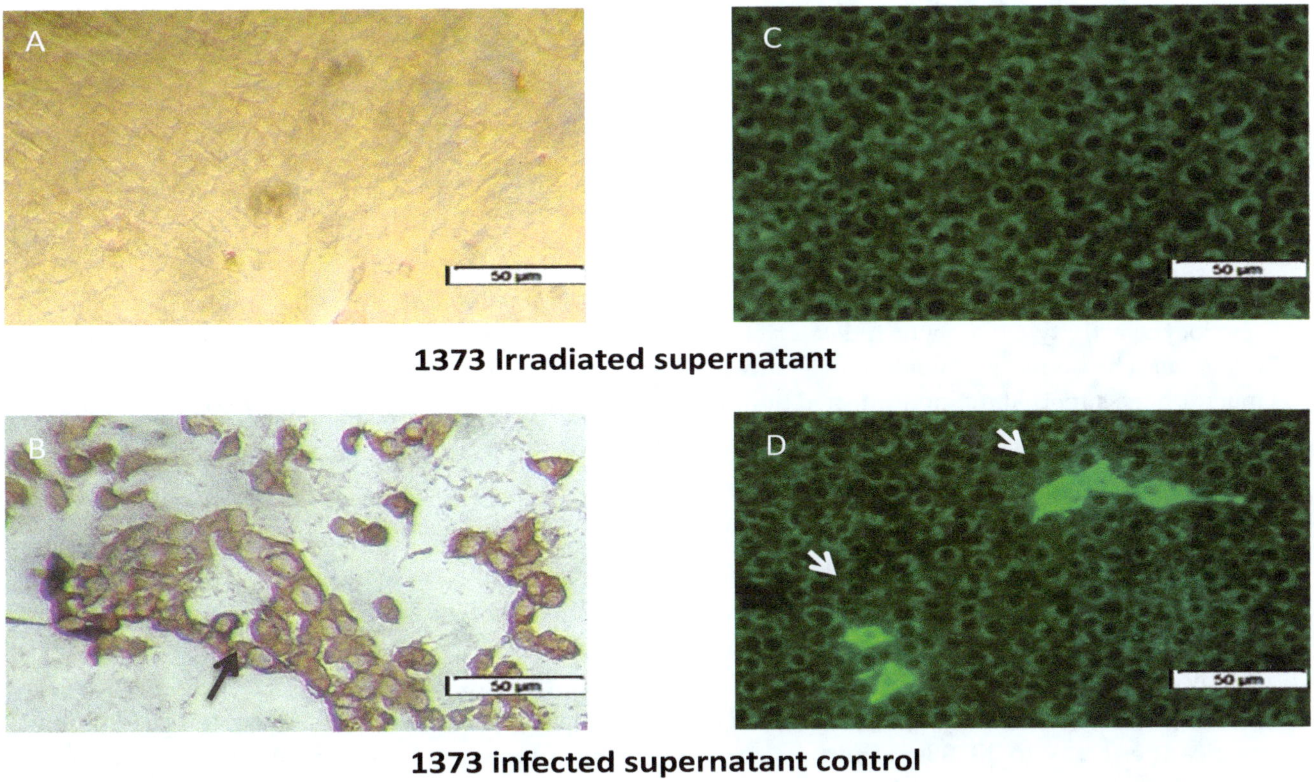

Figure 1. Successful inactivation of 1373-infected monocyte-derived macrophages (MDM) supernatant by UV-irradiation. (**A**,**C**) irradiated 1373-supernatant that show no evidence of intra-cytoplasmic replication by immune-peroxidase (IP) and immune-fluorescence (IF). (**B**,**D**) intra-cytoplasmic replication signal of the infected MDM supernatant, indicated by black and white arrows in the IP and IF assay, respectively (**B**,**D**).

3.2. Effect of Supernatant from BVDV Infected MDM on Macrophage Phagocytic Activity Compared to the Direct BVDV Effect

At 24 h post-treatment, the supernatant from Ncp 1373 significantly reduced MDM phagocytic activity by 38.5%, which continued to decrease to 51% at 48 h post-treatment compared to the supernatant from Ncp 28508-5, which was similar to the mock-infected control at any timepoint (Figure 2). Direct infection of MDM with the highly virulent 1373 strain, but not 28508-5, diminished phagocytic activity of MDM as early as 12 h post-treatment by 27.5% (Figure 2). We also found that heat-treated supernatant from 1373, or 28508-5 BVDV-infected supernatant had no effect on MDM phagocytic ability (data not shown).

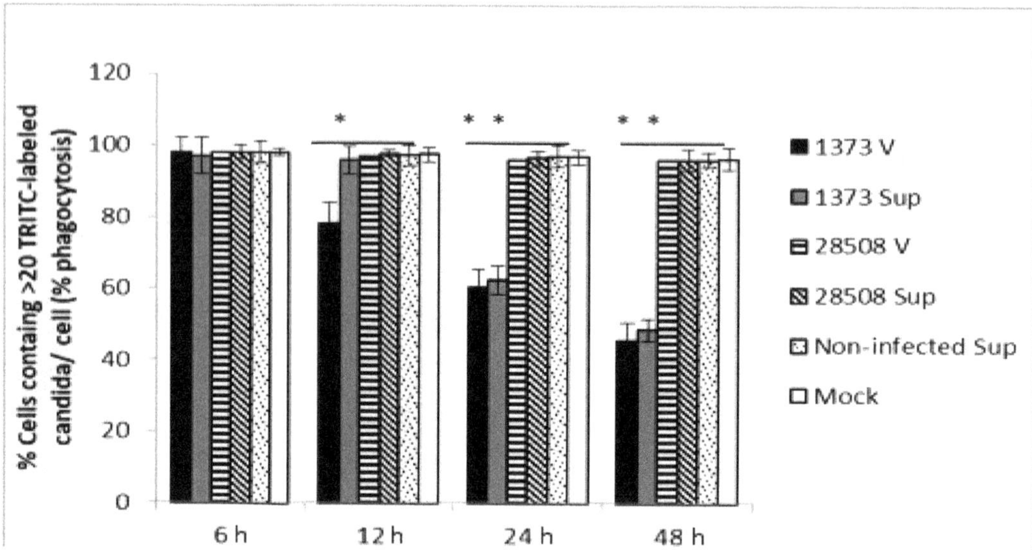

Figure 2. The effect of BVDV strains and the corresponding infected-MDM supernatants on macrophage phagocytic activity. Phagocytic index is defined as the % of MDMs that contains >20 TRITC-labeled *C. albicans*. h: hours post-treatment, V: direct virus infection, no supernatant, Sup: BVDV-infected macrophage supernatant, non-infected Sup: non-infected macrophage supernantant, Mock: culture medium *: $p < 0.05$ (>95% confidence), **: $p < 0.01$ (>99% confidence).

3.3. Effect of Supernatant from BVDV-Infected MDM on Macrophage Bactericidal Activity Compared to the Direct BVDV Effect

No significant effect was observed at 6 or 12 h post-treatment, however, the supernatant from Ncp 1373 strain significantly ($p < 0.05$) reduced MDM bactericidal activity by 37.7% and 51.4% at 24 and 48 h post-treatment, respectively (Figure 3). Direct infection of MDM with 1373 decreased the bactericidal activity by 22%, which began as early as 12 hpi, unlike the late indirect effect. The inhibition of bactericidal activity was time-dependent, and continued to increase to reach 54.7% by 48 hpi. There was no significant effect with 28508-5 strain, its corresponding infected-MDM supernatant, mock-infected, or the non-infected supernatant on bactericidal activity (Figure 3).

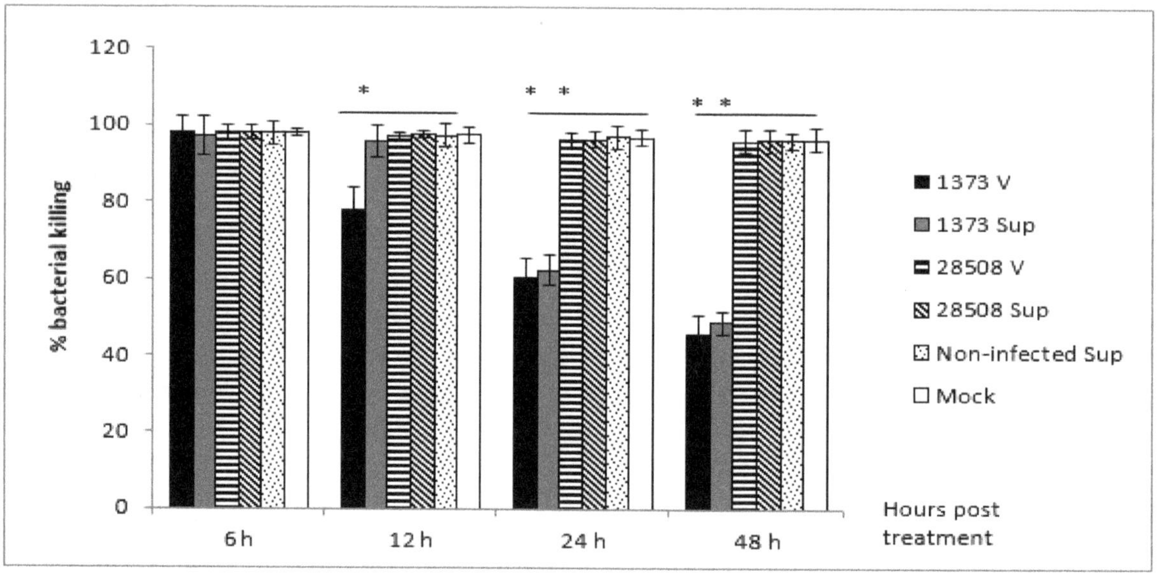

Figure 3. The effect of BVDV strains and the corresponding infected-MDM supernatants on macrophage bactericidal activity for 48 h post-treatment. Sup: supernatant (indirect effect), V: virus (direct effect). *: $p < 0.05$ (>95% confidence), **: $p < 0.01$ (>99% confidence).

3.4. *Effect of Supernatant from BVDV Infected MDM on Macrophage Nitric Oxide Production Compared to the Direct BVDV Effect*

The direct infection of MDM with both BVDV strains significantly increased NO production (158–164 μmol/mL), while neither 1373- nor 28508-5-infected MDM supernatant affected NO production in uninfected MDM (Figure 4). Both supernatant treatments, as well as non-infected supernatant and mock-infected controls, showed low nitric oxide production (93.3 μmol/mL) (Figure 4).

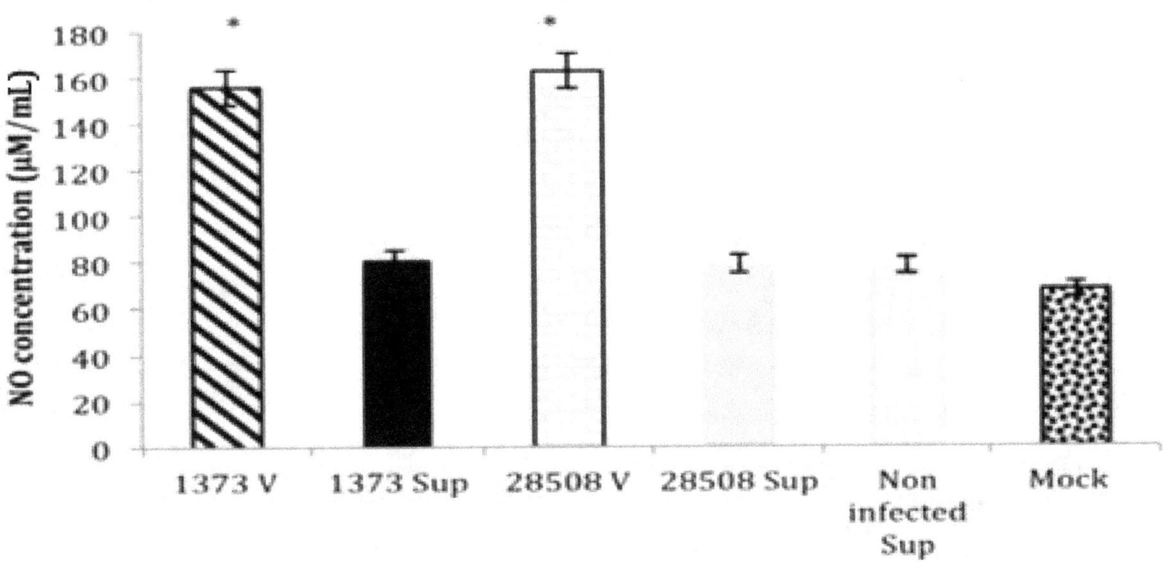

Figure 4. Comparison between the direct effect of BVDV strains and the corresponding infected-MDM supernatants (the indirect effect) on macrophage nitric acid production 24 h post-treatment. Sup: supernatant (indirect effect), V: virus (direct effect). *: $p < 0.05$ (>95% confidence).

3.5. *Effect of Supernatant on MHC II Expression Compared to the Direct BVDV Effect*

At 24 h post-treatment, cells treated with 1373 supernatant had significant reduction in MHC II expression to 61.0% (Figure 5A). At 48 h, MHC II expression was further reduced to 50.0% (Figure 5A) In contrast, 28508-5 or mock-infected supernatant had no significant reduction in MHC II expression and the expression level was greater than 94.0% at 24 or 48 h (Figure 5A).

3.6. *Effect of Supernatant on CD14 Expression Compared to the Direct BVDV Effect*

At 24 h post-treatment, the CD14 expression decreased in MDM infected with Ncp 1373 strain or it's supernatant (Figure 5B). At 36 h post-treatment, CD14 expression further decreased to 44.6% and 49.7% for Ncp 1373 and its supernatant, respectively (Figure 5B). The heat-treated supernatant or supernatant of 28508-5 did not show a significant decrease in the percentage of cells expressing CD14 and the average percentage was over 93% at 24 or 36 h (Figure 5B).

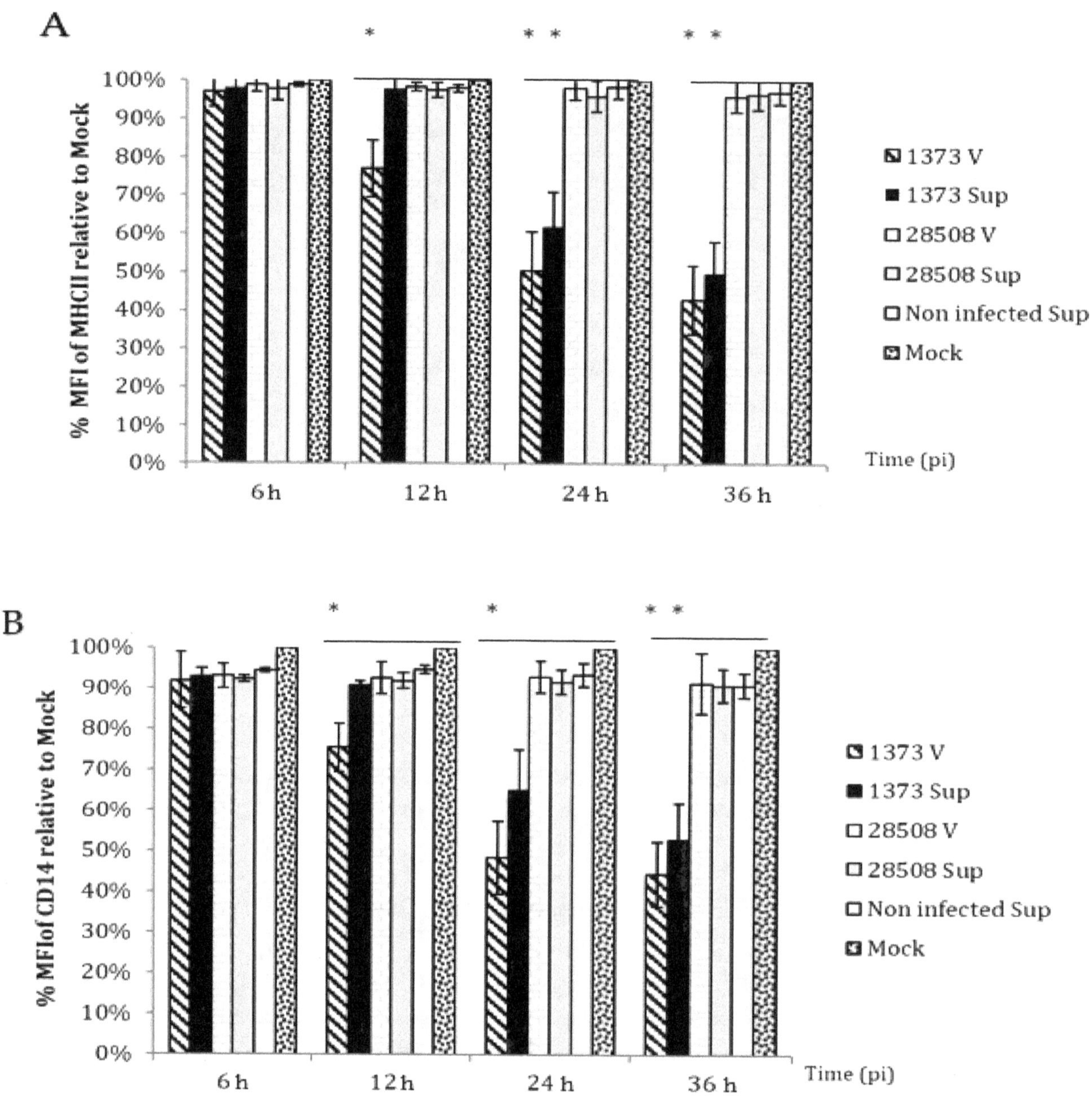

Figure 5. The effect of BVDV strains and the corresponding infected-MDM supernatants (indirect effect) on surface marker expression. (**A**) MHC II and (**B**) CD14 surface marker expression. Sup: supernatant (indirect effect), V: virus (direct effect). *: $p < 0.05$ (>95% confidence), **: $p < 0.01$ (>99% confidence).

3.7. Effect of Supernatant from BVDV Infected Macrophages on MDBK Cells

Chromatin condensation was detected after 24 h in treated MDBK with 1373 supernatant, while no chromatin condensation was detected in MDBK treated with 28508-5 nor non-infected supernatant (Figure 6A). The percentage of apoptotic cells was not significant until 24 h post-infection using Annexin V assay. It increased from 36.3% (24 h post-treatment) to reach 51.3% (48 h post-treatment) in contrast to less than 3% in case of mock-infected or treated MDBK with either 28508-5 or non-infected supernatant (Figure 6B).

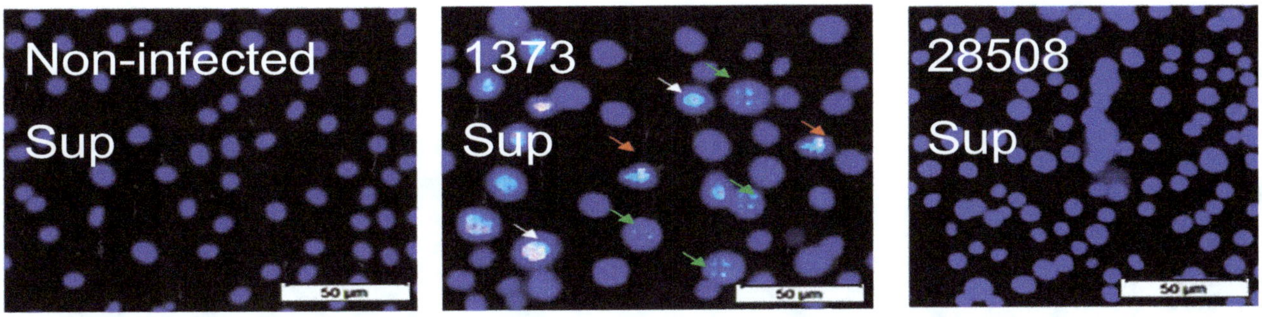

(A)

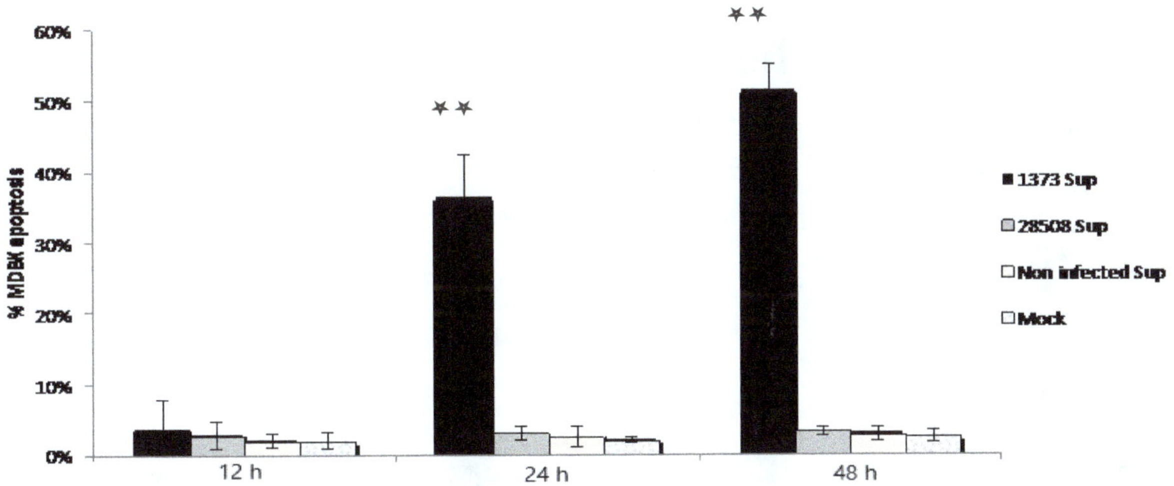

(B)

Figure 6. The indirect (infected MDM 24 h supernatant) effect of different BVDV strains on MDBK apoptosis. (**A**) Chromatin condensation by 1373 strain in contrast to 28508-5 and non-infected supernatant. (**B**) The % of MDBK apoptosis in response to different supernatants. 1373 Sup: BVDV 1373-infected macrophage supernatant, 28508-5 Sup: BVDV 28508-5-infected macrophage supernatant Non-infected Sup: non-infected macrophage supernantant, Mock: culture medium **: $p < 0.01$ (>99% confidence).

3.8. Effect of Supernatant from BVDV-Infected Macrophages on Different Lymphocyte Populations

The 12 h supernatants did not induce apoptosis compared to the mock-infected control (Figure 7). Both 24 and 48 h supernatants of the highly virulent 1373 resulted in an apoptotic effect on either freshly isolated (data not shown) or BL-3 lymphocytes. All supernatants of the low virulent Ncp 28508-5 at different timepoints did not induce apoptotic changes compared to the mock-infected control for either BL-3 lymphocytes or peripheral blood total lymphocyte population (Figure 7A,B).

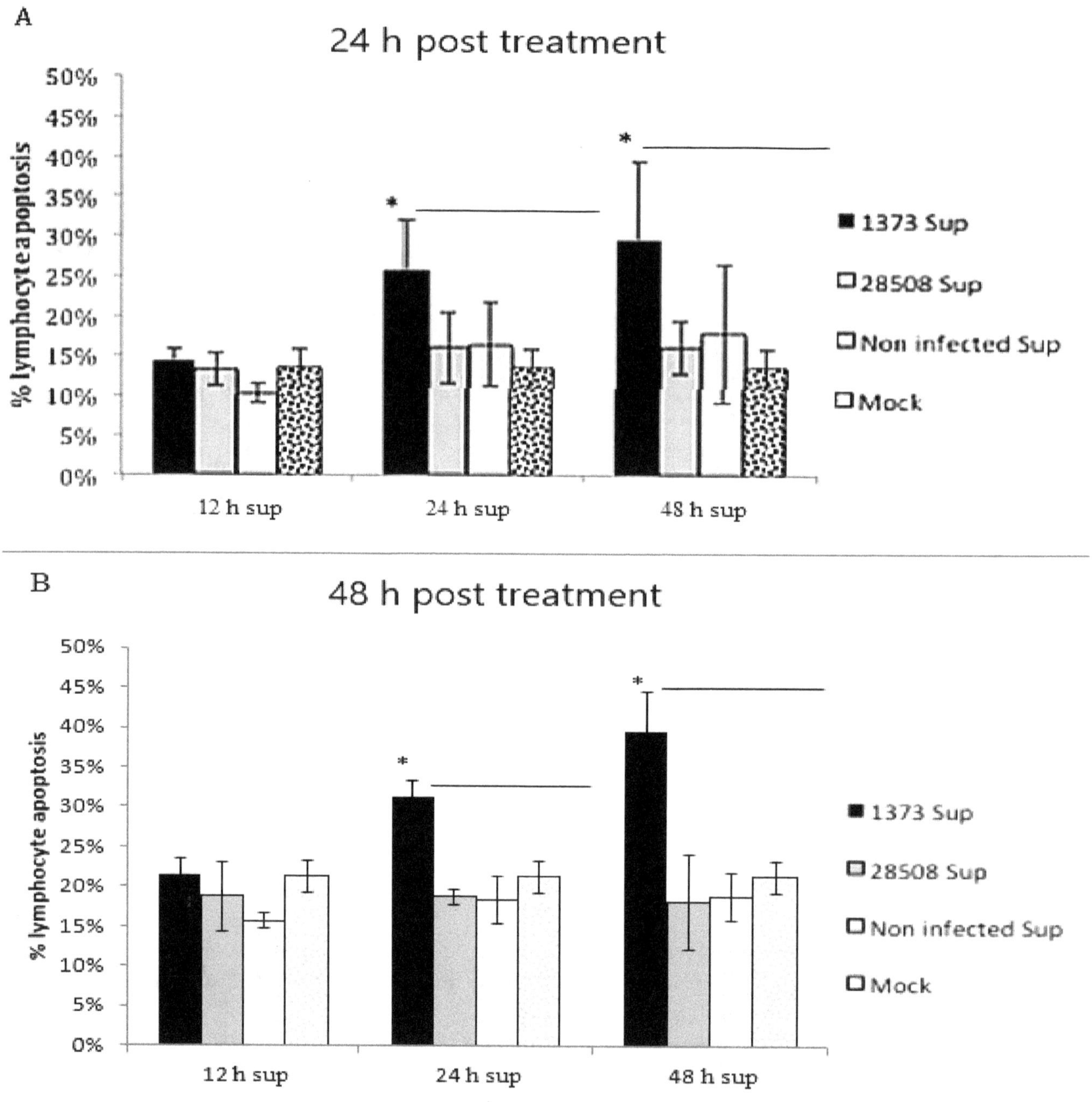

Figure 7. The indirect (infected MDM 12, 24 and 48 h supernatant) and the direct effect of different strains of BVDV on lymphocyte apoptosis. (**A**) The indirect effect 24 h post-treatment (**B**) The indirect effect 48 h post-treatment 1373 Sup: BVDV 1373- infected macrophage supernatant, 28508-5 Sup: BVDV 28508-5-infected macrophage supernatant non-infected Sup: non-infected macrophage supernatant, Mock: culture medium, *: $p < 0.05$ (>95% confidence).

3.9. Effect of Direct Infection of Lymphocyte with BVDV Strains

Only the Cp 296C strain was able to induce significant lymphocyte apoptosis as early as 12 h post-infection compared to the non-infected/mock control and the Ncp BVDV strains (Figure 8A) The direct infection of lymphocytes with 1373 was compared to the indirect effect of this virulent BVDV strain. Interestingly, the direct infection of lymphocytes did not induce significant changes compared to the mock-infected control until 48 h post-infection with 21.8% as the maximum apoptotic effect. The indirect effect of 1373 was tow times greater than the direct infection of lymphocyte at 24 and 48 hpi, with a maximum apoptotic effect of 35% at 48 h post-treatment (Figure 8B).

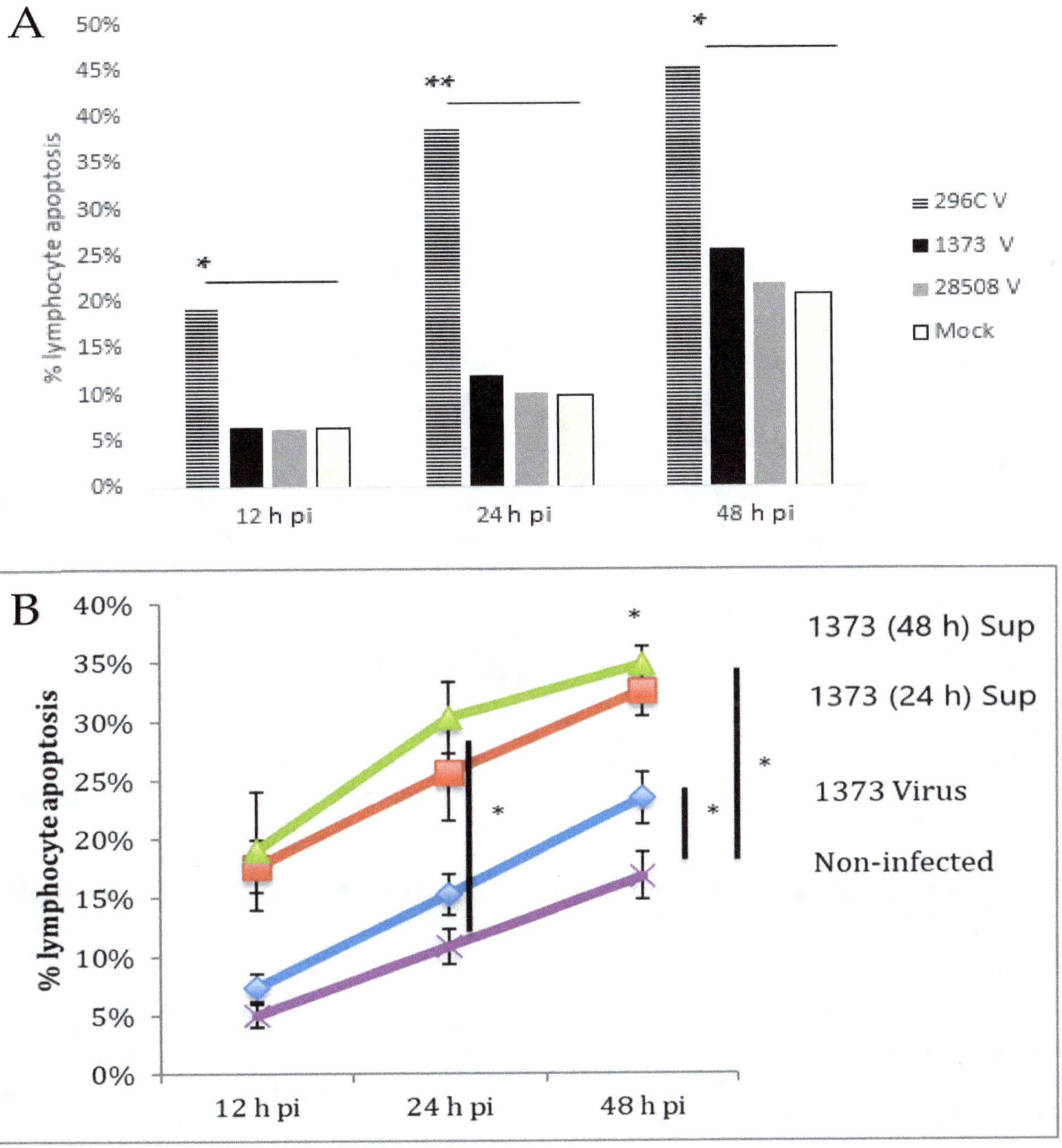

Figure 8. (**A**) The direct effect of BVDV strains on lymphocyte apoptosis (**B**) Comparison between the direct infection and the indirect (infected MDM 24 and 48 h supernatant) effect of the highly virulent 1373 BVDV strain on lymphocyte apoptosis for up to 48 pi. 296C V: direct lymphocyte infection with Cp 296C strain, 1373 V: direct lymphocyte infection with Ncp 1373 strain, 28,508 V: direct lymphocyte apoptosis with Ncp 28508-5 strain, Mock: non-infected lymphocyte, 1373 (48 h) Sup: supernatant from 1373-infected macrophage at 48 h post-treatment, 1373 (24 h) Sup: supernatant from 1373-infected macrophage at 24 h post-treatment, 1373 Virus: direct infection of macrophage with 1373 strain (not supernatant), Non-infected: supernatant from macrophage that was not infected, *: $p < 0.05$ (>95% confidence), **: $p < 0.01$ (>99% confidence).

3.10. Supernatant Protein Analysis

No viral proteins were detected in the supernatants at 6 hpi (Figure 9A), however, faint bands of 40–45 KD started to appear in the 1373-infected MDM supernatant at 12 hpi (Figure 9B). By 24 hpi, bands of 30 and 120 KD were observed in supernatant from Ncp1373. MDM culture infected with 28508-5 showed only one dense band of about 40–45 KD (Figure 9C). At 48 hpi, the band numbers and densities increased in MDM infected with the Ncp 1373. In contrast, only two bands of 40 to 45 KD were observed in supernatant from 28508-5 Ncp BVDV strains by that time (Figure 9D). No bands were observed in supernatant from mock-infected MDM at 6, or 12 h. At 24 or 48 hpi, only one band of 40–45 KD was observed in the mock-infected cells supernatant (Figure 9).

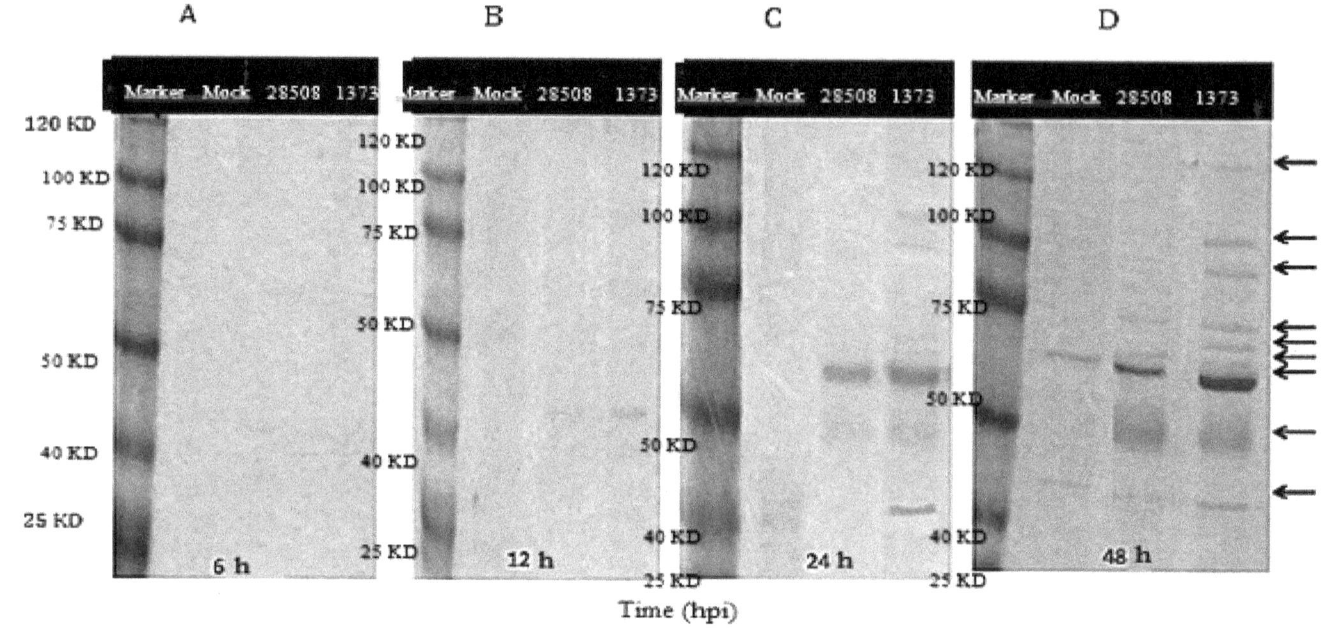

Figure 9. Protein electrophoresis of supernatants from BVDV infected and mock-infected MDM at (**A**) 6 hpi, (**B**) 12 hpi, (**C**) 24 hpi and (**D**) 48 hpi. Marker: protein marker that range from 25 to 120 KD, Mock: non-infected macrophage control, 28508: supernatant from 28508-5-infected macrophage at different timepoints, 1373: supernatant from 1373-infected macrophage at different timepoints, 6, 12, 24, 48 hpi: the corresponding timepoints post treatment of macrophage with supernatant, arrows refer to the different band intensity between strains.

3.11. Role of Cytokines in the Indirect Lymphocyte Apoptosis

Apoptosis-related cytokines including TNF-α, IL-1β and IL-6, did not show significant change at any of the three timepoints compared to mock-infected control. Other cytokines like IFN-γ, IL-10, IFN-α, IFN-β, IL-12, IL-4, IL-8 and TGF-β have also shown no significant difference between groups. The positive control mixture of Concavalin A and LPS upregulated all of the cytokines (data not shown).

3.12. Role of Viral Factors in the Indirect Lymphocyte Apoptosis

There was no significant difference in the percentage of lymphocyte apoptosis between the neutralized supernatant with either mAb or polyclonal Ab and the un-neutralized supernatant (data not shown).

4. Discussion

This study sheds light on the role of macrophages in the pathogenesis of BVDV infection. Phagocytosis is an important immune response of the macrophage and constitutes one of the first defenses against microbial invasion. Successful phagocytic activity leads to the initiation of successful immune response. In this study, supernatant from the highly virulent 1373 strain reduced macrophage phagocytic activity. In a previous study, Ncp BVDV infection of alveolar macrophage decreased expression of complement and Fc receptors and chemokine production, reducing their ability to engulf opsonized pathogens [8]. IL-2 inhibitory substances are produced in BVDV-infected PBMCs cultures that bind to receptors on lymphocytes, macrophages and dendritic cells that activate protein kinase C, resulting in the phosphorylation of proteins and inhibition of basic metabolic activities [41], that may reduce cell movement and the capacity to engulf organisms. A reduction in macrophage phagocytic capacity may be due to the presence of chemokine inhibitory mediators or the decrease in cytokine-induced chemotaxis [42] that lead to the decreased capacity of phagocytic cells for chemotaxis and phagocytosis.

Microbicidal activities are one of the main functions of macrophage to control and clear microbial infection. In vivo experiments suggest that BVDV immunosuppression resulted in subsequent secondary microbial infection. The supernatant from low virulent 28508-5-infected macrophage had no effect on bactericidal activity, while the highly virulent 1373 supernatant decreased the bactericidal activity of macrophages significantly with more than 50% by 48 hpi ($p < 0.05$). Considerable evidence has accumulated that BVDV may be a key component in multiple-etiology diseases [43].

Nitric oxide production was not affected by the supernatant exposure. Direct infection of MDM with highly virulent 1373 strain significantly induced NO production; however, 1373-infected macrophage supernatant (indirect) had no significant effect on NO production in MDM following stimulation with LPS. Another flavivirus, the hepatitis C virus (HCV) ERNS protein and HIV infection was associated with increased NO synthase (NOi) production in mice livers [44,45]. Type I IFN is a potent inducer of NO; however, it is downregulated by Ncp BVDV strains [25,46]. Taking these results together, Ncp BVDV might induce NO production directly through ERNS protein activation to NOi, but not indirectly due to the lack of secreted IFN in the MDM supernatant.

Microbial recognition, processing and presentation to lymphocytes is one of the unique functions of antigen-presenting cells for initiation of immune response. The recognition of pathogens is achieved through surface markers, which initiate the immune response. Our results indicated a significant reduction in surface marker expression of MHC II and CD14, associated with the highly virulent 1373-infected MDM supernatant. MHC II is an important marker for the initiation of immune response and antigen presentation. The current study indicated that the highly virulent 1373 reduced the surface expression of MHC II molecules. A previous study demonstrated that MHC II expression decreased in PBMCs infected with Ncp BVDV [47]. Another study reported that BVDV infection downregulated MHC I and II in monocytes [48]. This is consistent with what we found but in macrophage.

CD14 is important for toll-like receptors and gram-negative recognition and phagocytosis. Our findings indicated that low virulent 28508-5 supernatant had no effect on CD14 expression, while the highly virulent 1373 supernatant significantly decreased CD14 expression. CD14 downregulation was associated with the reduction in the phagocytic activity of neutrophils in HCV patients [49]. In human and mouse models, downregulation of CD14 was associated with suppression of antigen-specific lymphocyte proliferation [50]. Impairment of macrophage inflammatory function is a likely consequence of this surface reduction with subsequent secondary microbial invasion and the immunosuppressive effect of BVDV on the infected animals.

The findings of this study indicate the importance of soluble factors induced in BVDV-infected macrophages in viral pathogenesis. These results demonstrate that only the highly virulent Ncp BVDV strain induced the production of soluble factors capable of impairing macrophage inflammatory functions and surface marker expression as early as 12 h post-infection. These mediators and factors also induced epithelial cell and lymphocyte apoptosis. The release of several BVDV induced-soluble factors release has been reported [8,51–53]. On gel electrophoresis, several proteins ranging from 30 to 120 kDa were produced in 1373-infected MDM supernatants that were either less intense or not present at all in 28508-5-infected MDM supernatant. In a previous study, inflammatory mediators of 40–75 KD play a pivotal role in viral infection and pathogenesis [54].

Another study indicated that PMNC infected with Ncp or Cp released unknown factor(s) in the culture media that could be of cellular or viral origin [52,55]. Previously, secreted Erns viral glycoprotein played an important role in lymphocyte apoptosis induced by BVDV and CSFV [19]. In our study, we found no association of Erns glycoprotein or any other viral factors in the induction of apoptosis. Neither anti-ERNS mAb or a polyclonal BVDV Ab treatment of BVDV-infected MDM supernantant reduced lymphocyte apoptosis. The difference between BVDV and CSFV may be due to the use of a cloned Erns glycoprotein of CSFV that would be expressed at higher levels versus constitutive expression of BVDV Erns in BVDV-infected cells.

In the current study, we found that a supernatant from the highly virulent 1373 infected MDM induced apoptosis in MDBK as early as 24 h post-treatment, while low virulent 28508-5 infected MDM supernatant did not induce apoptosis. Previous work has shown that Ncp 28508-5 BVDV strain did not cause an inflammatory response in vivo, while Ncp 1373 caused inflammation and depletion of lymphocytes [56]. Interestingly, the Ncp 28508-5 strain is much more successful at establishing persistent infection. This lack of an inflammatory response may be one evasion mechanism to avoid the immune response and establish persistent infection in the developing fetus.

Furthermore, we found that the virulence of the BVDV strain is very important in determining the severity of the corresponding lymphoid depletion and subsequent immune suppression. The low virulence of the 28508-5 supernatant failed to induce apoptosis on the freshly isolated lymphocytes, while the highly virulent 1373 supernatant induced significant lymphocyte and somatic cell apoptosis. These results support the association between virulence and the degree of immune suppression that is associated with lymphoid depletion in vivo [1–3,57].

The role of macrophages in lymphocyte apoptosis was investigated in this study. Our results suggested that the supernatant of infected macrophages with only virulent BVDV strains induced lymphocyte apoptosis. These results provide an explanation for the observation that there is an increased number of macrophages in lymph nodes 3 days post-infection prior to lymphoid depletion [13]. Moreover, this indirect effect mediated by macrophages was not significant until 24 h post-infection with virulent BVDV strains, suggesting that rapid treatment strategies may help to limit the infection and would decrease or prevent the severe immune suppression induced by BVDV.

Our data support the results of Pedrera et al., 2009 [13] that did not relate the apoptotic effect to the biotype of the strain but to its virulence. Interestingly, we noted that the highly virulent 1373 strain of BVDV induced a more marked and faster apoptotic effect on lymphocytes indirectly as compared to the direct effect. These results suggest that there is a more severe and rapid immune suppression associated with the highly virulent 1373 that is likely due to the indirect effect mediated by macrophages.

Apoptosis-related cytokines produced by BVDV-infected macrophages did not play a role in lymphocyte apoptosis. There was no significant change in TNF-α, IL-1α, IL-1β or IL-6 transcriptional levels. These results were different from those described for CSFV, where TNF-a was involved in the indirect lymphocyte apoptosis activated by the virus [36]. Although TNF-α induction appears to be included in the mechanism of CSFV-induced lymphocyte apoptosis, this does not appear to be true for BVDV. The lack of TNF-α induced apoptosis is consistent with previous research with BVDV lymphocyte apoptosis [13]. Another study suggested that a role of IFN-γ in inducing apoptosis, unlike our research, was done using monocytes and a different BVDV strain [26].

The BL-3 cell line gave similar results, as seen with the peripheral blood lymphocytes. BL-3 cell findings were consistent with previously reported apoptotic effect of the highly virulent BVDV strains on the BL-3 cell line [30]. The degree of apoptosis induced in the lymphocytes of both peripheral blood or BL-3 cell line was similar. This finding leads us to speculate that B cells are more susceptible than T lymphocytes, but this hypothesis needs to be tested.

Another study suggested the identity of some possible factors that mediate the lymphocyte apoptosis post-BVDV infection, like micro RNA and programmed death-1 (PD-1) [58,59]. Finally, the identification and characterization of these factors and the molecular mechanisms involved in their induction and modes of action will be important goals for future studies.

5. Conclusions

BVDV causes immune dysfunction that leads to vaccination failure and secondary bacterial infection with lymphoid depletion associated with BVDV clinical cases. It was important for our study to focus on immune dysfunction caused by BVDV through investigating the indirect effect of an infected macrophage supernatant of various BVDV strains on macrophage inflammatory function as well as lymphocyte apoptosis, these two cells that are important for clearance of the virus from the body of infected animals. Our data suggested that the immune dysfunction associated with the highly virulent Ncp 1373 strain was mainly due to the indirect effect mediated by macrophage-secreted mediators. These mediators may impair macrophage surface marker expression, which in turn disrupt the general macrophage inflammatory function, including phagocytic and bactericidal activity but not NO production. These soluble factors also enhance lymphocyte apoptosis with subsequent lymphoid depletion associated with BVDV cases. Unlike CSFV, neither TNF-a nor secreted Erns glycoprotein induces BVDV lymphocyte apoptosis. This led us to the hypothesis that host but not virus factors likely mediated the indirect lymphocyte apoptotic effect.

Further investigations of the factors present in the supernatant of the infected macrophages with the highly virulent strains need to be conducted so that we have a better understanding of the disease mechanism. This can lead to finding a way to block these factors that can be used as a therapeutic practice in acutely infected animals to help improve recovery. Understanding these factors better would also help to improve the current control strategies and decrease the risk and the economic losses of BVDV. Future studies that include other BVDV strains need to be conducted to further confirm our findings.

Author Contributions: Conceptualization, K.A., G.E., and C.C.L.C.; writing-original draft preparation, K.A., M.R.; writing-review and editing, K.A., G.E., and A.A.H.A.; visualization N.T., J.S., and H.A. All authors have read and agreed to the published version of the manuscript. K.A. and M.R. have the same contribution as first author.

Acknowledgments: We would like to thank the support from Shollie Falkenberg for providing the BL-3 cell line. Robert Fulton for providing the polyclonal antibodies for BVDV testing. Adam Hoppe help and guidance with using the flow cytometry machine. The Department of Veterinary and Biomedical Sciences/Animal. Disease Research and Diagnostic Laboratory, SDSU, Brookings, SD, USA; SDSU. Functional Genomic Core Facility (FGCF), SDSU.

References

1. Ammari, M.; McCarthy, F.; Nanduri, B.; Pinchuk, G.; Pinchuk, L. Understanding the Pathogenesis of Cytopathic and Noncytopathic Bovine Viral Diarrhea Virus Infection Using Proteomics. In *Proteomic Applications in Biology*; IntechOpen: London, UK, 2012.
2. Bittar, J.H.; Palomares, R.A.; Hurley, D.J.; Hoyos-Jaramillo, A.; Rodriguez, A.; Stoskute, A.; Hamrick, B.; Norton, N.; Adkins, M.; Saliki, J.T.; et al. Immune response and onset of protection from Bovine viral diarrhea virus 2 infection induced by modified-live virus vaccination concurrent with injectable trace minerals administration in newly received beef calves. *Vet. Immunol. Immunopathol.* **2020**, *225*, 110055. [CrossRef] [PubMed]
3. Falkenberg, S.M.; Johnson, C.; Bauermann, F.V.; McGill, J.; Palmer, M.V.; Sacco, R.E.; Ridpath, J.F. Changes observed in the thymus and lymph nodes 14 days after exposure to BVDV field strains of enhanced or typical virulence in neonatal calves. *Vet. Immunol. Immunopathol.* **2014**, *160*, 70–80. [CrossRef] [PubMed]
4. Liebler-Tenorio, E.M.; Ridpath, J.F.; Neill, J.D. Distribution of viral antigen and development of lesions after experimental infection of calves with a BVDV 2 strain of low virulence. *J. Vet. Diagn. Investig.* **2003**, *15*, 221–232. [CrossRef] [PubMed]
5. Potgieter, L.N. Immunology of bovine viral diarrhea virus. *Vet. Clin. N. Am. Food Anim. Pract.* **1995**, *11*, 501–520. [CrossRef]
6. Sopp, P.; Hooper, L.B.; Clarke, M.C.; Howard, C.J.; Brownlie, J. Detection of bovine viral diarrhoea virus p80 protein in subpopulations of bovine leukocytes. *J. Gen. Virol.* **1994**, *75*, 1189–1194. [CrossRef]
7. Roth, J.A.; Kaeberle, M.L. Isolation of neutrophils and eosinophils from the peripheral blood of cattle and comparison of their functional activities. *J. Immunol. Methods* **1981**, *45*, 153–164. [CrossRef]
8. Welsh, M.D.; Adair, B.M.; Foster, J.C. Effect of BVD virus infection on alveolar macrophage functions. *Vet. Immunol. Immunopathol.* **1995**, *46*, 195–210. [CrossRef]

9. Lambot, M.; Hanon, E.; Lecomte, C.; Hamers, C.; Letesson, J.-J.; Pastoret, P.-P. Bovine viral diarrhoea virus induces apoptosis in blood mononuclear cells by a mechanism largely dependent on monocytes. *J. Gen. Virol.* **1998**, *79*, 1745–1749. [CrossRef] [PubMed]
10. Zhang, G.; Aldridge, S.; Clarke, M.C.; McCauley, J.W. Cell death induced by cytopathic bovine viral diarrhoea virus is mediated by apoptosis. *J. Gen. Virol.* **1996**, *77*, 1677–1681. [CrossRef] [PubMed]
11. Risalde, M.A.; Romero-Palomo, F.; Lecchi, C.; Ceciliani, F.; Bazzocchi, C.; Comazzi, S.; Besozzi, M.; Gómez-Villamandos, J.C.; Luzzago, C. BVDV permissiveness and lack of expression of co-stimulatory molecules on PBMCs from calves pre-infected with BVDV. *Comp. Immunol. Microbiol. Infect. Dis.* **2020**, *68*, 101388. [CrossRef] [PubMed]
12. Chase, C.C.; Thakur, N.; Darweesh, M.F.; Morarie-Kane, S.E.; Rajput, M.K. Immune response to bovine viral diarrhea virus—looking at newly defined targets. *Anim. Health Res. Rev.* **2015**, *16*, 4–14. [CrossRef] [PubMed]
13. Pedrera, M.; Gomez-Villamandos, J.C.; Romero-Trevejo, J.L.; Risalde, M.A.; Molina, V.; Sanchez-Cordon, P.J. Apoptosis in lymphoid tissues of calves inoculated with non-cytopathic bovine viral diarrhea virus genotype 1: Activation of effector caspase-3 and role of macrophages. *J. Gen. Virol.* **2009**, *90*, 2650–2659. [CrossRef] [PubMed]
14. Romero–Palomo, F.; Risalde, M.A.; Gómez–Villamandos, J.C. Immunopathologic Changes in the Thymus of Calves Pre–infected with BVDV and Challenged with BHV–1. *Transbound. Emerg. Dis.* **2017**, *64*, 574–584. [CrossRef]
15. Roth, J.A.; Bolin, S.R.; Frank, D.E. Lymphocyte blastogenesis and neutrophil function in cattle persistently infected with bovine viral diarrhea virus. *Am. J. Vet. Res.* **1986**, *47*, 1139–1141.
16. Ridpath, J.F.; Bendfeldt, S.; Neill, J.D.; Liebler-Tenorio, E. Lymphocytopathogenic activity in vitro correlates with high virulence in vivo for BVDV type 2 strains: Criteria for a third biotype of BVDV. *Virus Res.* **2006**, *118*, 62–69. [CrossRef]
17. Adler, B.; Adler, H.; Pfister, H.; Jungi, T.W.; Peterhans, E. Macrophages infected with cytopathic bovine viral diarrhoea virus release a factor(s) capable of priming uninfected macrophages for activation-induced apoptosis. *J. Virol.* **1997**, *71*, 3255–3258. [CrossRef]
18. Schweizer, M.; Peterhans, E. Oxidative stress in cells infected with bovine viral diarrhoea virus: A crucial step in the induction of apoptosis. *J. Gen. Virol.* **1999**, *80*, 1147–1155. [CrossRef] [PubMed]
19. Bruschke, C.J.M.; Hulst, M.M.; Moormann, R.J.M.; Rijn, P.A.V.; Oirschot, J.T.V. Glycoprotein Erns of Pestiviruses Induces Apoptosis in Lymphocytes of Several Species. *J. Virol.* **1997**, *71*, 6692–6696. [CrossRef] [PubMed]
20. Fetzer, C.; Tews, B.A.; Meyers, G. The carboxy-terminal sequence of the pestivirus glycoprotein Erns represents an unusual type of membrane anchor. *J. Virol.* **2005**, *79*, 11901–11913. [CrossRef]
21. Summerfield, A.; Zingle, K.; Inumaru, S.; McCullough, C. Induction of apoptosis in bone marrow neutrophil-lineage by classical swine fever. *J. Gen. Virol.* **2001**, *82*, 1309–1318. [CrossRef]
22. Hoff, H.S.; Donis, R.O. Induction of apoptosis and cleavage of poly (ADP-ribose) polymerase by cytopathic bovine viral diarrhea virus infection. *Virus Res.* **1997**, *49*, 101–113. [CrossRef]
23. Schweizer, M.; Peterhans, E. Noncytopathic bovine viral diarrhea virus inhibits double-stranded RNA-induced apoptosis and interferon synthesis. *J. Virol.* **2001**, *75*, 4692–4698. [CrossRef] [PubMed]
24. Mangan, D.F.; Robertson, B.; Wahl, S.M. IL-4 enhances programmed cell death (apoptosis) in stimulated human monocytes. *J. Immunol.* **1992**, *148*, 1812–1816. [PubMed]
25. Adler, H.; Jungi, T.W.; Pfister, H.; Strasser, M.; Sileghem, M.; Peterhans, E. Cytokine regulation by virus infection: Bovine viral diarrhea virus, a flavivirus, downregulates production of tumor necrosis factor alpha in macrophages in vitro. *J. Virol.* **1996**, *70*, 2650–2653. [CrossRef]
26. Choi, K.S. The effect of bovine viral diarrhea virus on bovine monocyte phenotype. *Iran. J. Vet. Res.* **2017**, *18*, 13.
27. Lopez, B.I.; Santiago, K.G.; Lee, D.; Ha, S.; Seo, K. RNA Sequencing (RNA-Seq) Based Transcriptome Analysis in Immune Response of Holstein Cattle to Killed Vaccine against Bovine Viral Diarrhea Virus Type, I. *Animals* **2020**, *10*, 344. [CrossRef]
28. Aldo, M.A.; Yahel, L.R.; Montserrat, R.H.; Elena, S.S.; Lourdes, A.P.; Alejandro, B.G. The NADL strain of bovine viral diarrhea virus induces the secretion of IL-1β through caspase 1 in bovine macrophages. *Res. Vet. Sci.* **2020**. [CrossRef]

29. Elmowalid, G. Unmasking the Effect of Bovine Viral Diarrhea Virus on Macrophage Inflammatory Functions. Ph.D. Thesis, South Dakota State University, Brookings, SD, USA, 2003.
30. Schaut, R.G.; Ridpath, J.F.; Sacco, R.E. Bovine Viral Diarrhea Virus Type 2 Impairs Macrophage Responsiveness to Toll-Like Receptor Ligation with the Exception of Toll-Like Receptor 7. *PLoS ONE* **2016**, *11*, e0159491. [CrossRef]
31. Reed, L.J.; Muench, H. A simple method of estimating fifty per cent endpoints. *Am. J. Epidemiol.* **1938**, *27*, 493–497. [CrossRef]
32. Mwangi, W.; Brown, W.C.; Splitter, G.A.; Zhuang, Y.; Kegerreis, K.; Palmer, G.H. Enhancement of antigen acquisition by dendritic cells and MHC class II-restricted epitope presentation to CD4+ T cells using VP22 DNA vaccine vectors that promote intercellular spreading. *J. Leukoc. Biol.* **2005**, *78*, 401–411. [CrossRef]
33. Rajput, M.K.; Darweesh, M.F.; Park, K.; Braun, L.J.; Mwangi, W.; Young, A.J.; Chase, C.C. The effect of bovine viral diarrhea virus (BVDV) strains on bovine monocyte-derived dendritic cells (Mo-DC) phenotype and capacity to produce BVDV. *Virol. J.* **2014**, *11*, 1. [CrossRef] [PubMed]
34. Strober, W. Trypan blue exclusion test of cell viability. *Curr. Protoc. Immunol.* **2001**, *111*, A3-B1–A3-B3.
35. Perler, L.; Schweizer, M.; Jungi, T.W.; Peterhans, E. Bovine viral diarrhoea virus and bovine herpesvirus-1 prime uninfected macrophages forlipopolysaccharide-triggered apoptosis by interferon-dependent and-independent pathways. *J. Gen. Virol.* **2000**, *81*, 881–887. [CrossRef] [PubMed]
36. Choi, C.; Hwang, K.K.; Chae, C. Classical swine fever virus induces tumor necrosis factor-alpha and lymphocyte apoptosis. *Arch. Virol.* **2004**, *149*, 875–889. [CrossRef] [PubMed]
37. Ridpath, J.F.; Driskell, E.; Chase, C.C.; Neill, J.D. Characterization and detection of BVDV related reproductive disease in white tail deer. In Proceedings of the 13th International World Association of Veterinary Laboratory Diagnosticians Symposium, Melbourne, Australia, 11–14 November 2007; p. 34.
38. Gels, T.; Schagger, H.; von Jagow, G. Tricine-sodium dodecyl sulfate-polyacrylamide gel electrophoresis for the separation of proteins in the range from 1 to 100 kDa. *Anal. Biochem.* **1987**, *166*, 368–379.
39. Konnai, S.; Usui, T.; Ohashi, K.; Onuma, M. The rapid quantitative analysis of bovine cytokine genes by real-time RT-PCR. *Vet. Microbiol.* **2003**, *94*, 283–294. [CrossRef]
40. Pfaffl, M.W.; Horgan, G.W.; Dempfle, L. Relative expression software tool (REST©) for group-wise comparison and statistical analysis of relative expression results in real-time PCR. *Nucleic Acids Res.* **2002**, *30*, e36. [CrossRef]
41. Hou, L.; Wilkerson, M.; Kapil, S.; Mosie, R.D.; Shuman, W.; Reddy, J.R.; Loughin, T.; Minocha, H.C. The effect of different bovine viral diarrhea virus genotypes and biotypes on the metabolic activity and activation status of bovine peripheral blood mononuclear cells. *Viral Immunol.* **1998**, *11*, 233–244. [CrossRef]
42. Ketelsen, A.T.; Johnson, D.W.; Muscoplat, C.C. Depression of bovine monocyte chemotactic responses by bovine viral diarrhea virus. *Infect. Immun.* **1979**, *25*, 565–568. [CrossRef]
43. Potgieter, L.N.; McCracken, M.D.; Hopkins, F.M.; Walker, R.D.; Guy, J.S. Experimental production of bovine respiratory tract disease with bovine viral diarrhea virus. *Am. J. Vet. Res.* **1984**, *45*, 1582–1585.
44. Blond, D.; Raoul, H.; Le Grand, R.; Dormont, D. Nitric oxide synthesis enhances human immunodeficiency virus replication in primary human macrophages. *J. Virol.* **2000**, *74*, 8904–8912. [CrossRef]
45. Lasarte, J.J.; Sarobe, P.; Boya, P.; Casares, N.; Arribillaga, L.; de Cerio, A.L.D.; Gorraiz, M.; Borrás-Cuesta, F.; Prieto, J. A recombinant adenovirus encoding hepatitis C virus core and E1 proteins protects mice against cytokine–induced liver damage. *Hepatology* **2003**, *37*, 461–470. [CrossRef] [PubMed]
46. Charleston, B.; Hope, J.C.; Carr, B.V.; Howard, C.J. Masking of two in vitro immunological assays for Mycobacterium bovis (BCG) in calves acutely infected with non-cytopathic bovine viral diarrhoea virus. *Vet. Rec.* **2001**, *149*, 481–484. [CrossRef] [PubMed]
47. Archambault, D.; Béliveau, C.; Couture, Y.; Carman, S. Clinical response and immunomodulation following experimental challenge of calves with type 2 noncytopathogenic bovine viral diarrhea virus. *Vet. Res.* **2000**, *31*, 215–227. [CrossRef] [PubMed]
48. Lee, S.R.; Nanduri, B.; Pharr, G.T.; Stokes, J.V.; Pinchuk, L.M. Bovine viral diarrhea virus infection affects the expression of proteins related to professional antigen presentation in bovine monocytes. *Biochim. Et Biophys. Acta (Bba)-Proteins Proteom.* **2009**, *1794*, 14–22. [CrossRef] [PubMed]
49. Jirillo, E.; Greco, B.; Caradonna, L.; Satalino, R.; Pugliese, V.; Cozzolongo, R.; Cuppone, R.; Manghisi, O.G. Evaluation of cellular immune responses and soluble mediators in patients with chronic hepatitis C virus (cHCV) infection. *Immunopharmacol. Immunotoxicol.* **1995**, *17*, 347–364. [CrossRef] [PubMed]

50. Chen, Y.C.; Wang, S.Y.; King, C.C. Bacterial lipopolysaccharide inhibits dengue virus infection of primary human monocytes/macrophages by blockade of virus entry via a CD14-dependent mechanism. *J. Virol.* **1999**, *73*, 2650–2657. [CrossRef]
51. Jensen, J.; Schultz, R.D. Effect of infection by bovine viral diarrhea virus (BVDV) in vitro on interleukin-1 activity of bovine monocytes. *Vet. Immunol. Immunopathol.* **1991**, *29*, 251–265. [CrossRef]
52. Markham, R.J.; Ramnaraine, M.L. Release of immunosuppressive substances from tissue culture cells infected with bovine viral diarrhea virus. *Am. J. Vet. Res.* **1985**, *46*, 879–883.
53. Van Reeth, K.; Adair, B. Macrophages and respiratory viruses. *Pathol.-Biol.* **1997**, *45*, 184–192.
54. Janeway, C.A., Jr.; Travers, P.; Walport, M.; Shlomchik, M.J. *The Complement System and Innate Immunity*; Garland Science: New York, NY, USA, 2001.
55. Darweesh, M.F.; Rajput, M.K.; Braun, L.J.; Rohila, J.S.; Chase, C.C. BVDV Npro protein mediates the BVDV induced immunosuppression through interaction with cellular S100A9 protein. *Microb. Pathog.* **2018**, *121*, 341–349. [CrossRef] [PubMed]
56. Liebler-Tenorio, E.M.; Ridpath, J.F.; Neill, J.D. Distribution of viral antigen and development of lesions after experimental infection with highly virulent bovine viral diarrhea virus type 2 in calves. *Am. J. Vet. Res.* **2002**, *63*, 1575–1584. [CrossRef] [PubMed]
57. Jungmann, A.; Nieper, H.; Müller, H. Apoptosis is induced by infectious bursal disease virus replication in productively infected cells as well as in antigen-negative cells in their vicinity. *J. Gen. Virol.* **2001**, *82*, 1107–1115. [CrossRef] [PubMed]
58. Liu, Y.; Liu, S.; He, B.; Wang, T.; Zhao, S.; Wu, C.; Yue, S.; Zhang, S.; He, M.; Wang, L.; et al. PD-1 blockade inhibits lymphocyte apoptosis and restores proliferation and anti-viral immune functions of lymphocyte after CP and NCP BVDV infection in vitro. *Vet. Microbiol.* **2018**, *226*, 74–80. [CrossRef]
59. Shi, H.; Ni, W.; Sheng, J.; Chen, C. Lentivirus-mediated bta-miR-193a Overexpression Promotes Apoptosis of MDBK Cells by Targeting BAX and Inhibits BVDV Replication. *Kafkas Üniversitesi Vet. Fakültesi Derg.* **2017**, *23*, 587–593.

13

Pestivirus Infections in Semi-Domesticated Eurasian Tundra Reindeer (*Rangifer tarandus tarandus*): A Retrospective Cross-Sectional Serological Study in Finnmark County, Norway

Carlos G. das Neves [1,2,*], Jonas Johansson Wensman [3], Ingebjørg Helena Nymo [1,4], Eystein Skjerve [5], Stefan Alenius [3] and Morten Tryland [4,*]

1 Norwegian Veterinary Institute, N-0106 Oslo/N-9010 Tromsø, Norway; ingebjorg.nymo@vetinst.no
2 Faculty of Health Sciences, UiT The Arctic University of Norway, N-9037 Tromsø, Norway
3 Department of Clinical Sciences, Swedish University of Agricultural Sciences, P.O. Box 7054, SE-75007 Uppsala, Sweden; jonas.wensman@slu.se (J.J.W.); stefan.alenius@slu.se (S.A.)
4 Department of Arctic and Marine Biology, UiT The Arctic University of Norway, N-9037 Tromsø, Norway
5 Centre for Epidemiology and Biostatistics, Faculty of Veterinary Sciences, Norwegian University of Life Sciences, N-0033 Oslo, Norway; eystein.skjerve@nmbu.no
* Correspondence: carlos.dasneves@vetinst.no (C.G.d.N.); morten.tryland@uit.no (M.T.);

Abstract: Members of the Pestivirus genus (family *Flaviviridae*) cause severe and economically important diseases in livestock. Serological studies have revealed the presence of pestiviruses in different cervid species, including wild and semi-domesticated Eurasian tundra reindeer. In this retrospective study, serum samples collected between 2006 and 2008 from 3339 semi-domesticated Eurasian reindeer from Finnmark County, Norway, were tested for anti-pestivirus antibodies using an enzyme linked immunosorbent assay (ELISA) and a subset of these by virus neutralization test (VNT). A seroprevalence of 12.5% was found, varying from 0% to 45% among different herding districts, and 20% in western Finnmark, as compared to 1.7% in eastern Finnmark. Seroprevalence increased with age. Pestivirus-specific RNA was not detected in any of the 225 serum samples tested by real-time RT-PCR. Based on VNT results, using a panel of one bovine viral diarrhea virus (BVDV) strain and two border disease virus (BDV) strains, the virus is most likely a reindeer-specific pestivirus closely related to BDV. A characterization of the causative virus and its pathogenic impact on reindeer populations, as well as its potential to infect other domestic and wild ruminants, should be further investigated.

Keywords: bvdv; epidemiology; reindeer; border disease virus; Norway

1. Introduction

Members of the *Pestivirus* genus, belonging to the family *Flaviviridae*, cause severe and economically important diseases in livestock [1] such as: bovine viral diarrhea virus (BVDV), causing bovine viral diarrhea (BVD) and mucosal disease (MD) in cattle; classical swine fever virus (CSFV)/hog cholera virus, causing classical swine fever in pigs; and border disease virus (BDV), causing border disease (BD) in sheep.

Several serological studies have revealed the presence of pestiviruses in a variety of free-ranging and captive wild cervid species [2,3]. The observed sero-prevalence has varied significantly between studies, geographic regions, cervid species, and proximity to other ruminant species known to harbor e.g., BVDV or BDV [4,5].

A few serological studies have been carried out in different reindeer subspecies and populations across the Arctic region, usually targeting BVDV but allowing for some cross-reactivity with other pestiviruses. In Sweden, several studies in semi-domesticated Eurasian tundra reindeer (*R. t. tarandus*) have revealed a prevalence ranging from 0 to 35% [5–7]. In Norway a study in several wild cervid species identified a prevalence of 4.2% in wild reindeer in southern Norway [8], while a study of 48 carcasses of emaciated semi-domesticated reindeer from Finnmark County, Norway, revealed a prevalence of 33% (BVDV virus neutralization test; VNT) [9]. A study of Svalbard reindeer (*R. t. platyrhynchus*) from the Arctic Archipelago of Svalbard in the 1990s revealed no seropositive animals [10].

Pestiviruses have never been isolated from wild or semi-domesticated reindeer. However, one isolate (Reindeer-1) was obtained from a reindeer that died with signs of severe diarrhea and anorexia at Duisburg Zoo in Germany in 1996 [11]. Phylogenetic studies have revealed that the strain was most closely related to BDV type 2 (BDV-2) strains isolated from German sheep in 1999 and 2000 [11,12].

In an experimental pestivirus infection (BVDV-1) of reindeer [13], the animals displayed clinical signs, such as serous and mucopurulent nasal discharge, bloody diarrhea, laminitis, and coronitis, thus indicating that this species is susceptible to BVDV.

Studies in the early 80s revealed that nearly 30% of the dairy herds in Norway had antibodies to BVDV [14]. An eradication program for cattle was initiated in 1992 with large-scale serological screenings focusing on PI animals and the enforcement of restrictions and culling. In November 2006, Norway was considered free of BVDV [15,16]. BD was identified in both sheep and goats in Norway in the early 1980s, but the disease was associated with BVDV strains rather than BDV strains, which have to our knowledge never been identified in Norway [14,17–20]. Even though the eradication program focused on cattle alone, infections from small ruminants have also not been reported since the 1990s. Studies in goats in Norway in the 1980s revealed low prevalence for pestivirus (3.6%) [21] and only a single PI goat kid was diagnosed [19].

Finnmark County hosts approximately 69% of the semi-domesticated reindeer in Norway, with an estimated population in 2017 of 147,500 reindeer (down from 170,000 reindeer in 2006 and 188,000 in 2008 at the time of sampling). Reindeer are kept under semi-nomadic husbandry conditions, free ranging but herded within well-defined husbandry districts, with seasonal migrations between summer pastures in coastal areas and winter pastures on the inland mountain plateau. Animals are usually gathered at least twice a year for tagging calves, anti-parasitic treatment, sorting, and slaughter.

Reindeer mortality in Finnmark County reached 37% among calves during the years of 2005/2006. Although predators accounted for the majority of mortality, 11% of calf mortalities were of unknown etiology [22]. Fecundity of semi-domesticated reindeer is difficult to evaluate as they usually give birth unattended, while scavengers quickly remove aborted materials. It is therefore difficult to assess the role of abortion or weak-born calves to calf mortality [23].

The goal of this study was to conduct a retrospective cross-sectional serological screening in selected reindeer husbandry districts, to address prevalence and to identify risk factors for becoming infected with pestivirus. It was also anticipated that a study of this nature could help identify which pestivirus species and/or strains are circulating among reindeer in Norway and if reindeer can serve as reservoir hosts for viruses known to cause disease in livestock.

2. Materials and Methods

2.1. Sampling

In this retrospective study we used blood samples collected from reindeer (n = 3339) from 15 summer herding districts at four different slaughterhouses from 2004 to 2008 during the winter slaughtering periods in Finnmark County, Norway. Blood was centrifuged at 3500 rpm for 15 min and sera collected and stored at −20 °C until testing.

2.2. Animal Data

Information on gender, age, and carcass weight was collected from each herding district. Animals were grouped into two age classes: calves (≤1 year) and adults (>1 year).

For each reindeer herding district included in the study, information on total available reindeer pasture area, numbers of adults and calves, and mortality rates were obtained from the 2008 Reindeer Husbandry Authority Report [24]. Animal density, i.e., the number of animals per square kilometer of available reindeer summer pasture (n/km^2), was calculated for each herding district. Districts with animal densities lower than the mean reindeer density for Finnmark (4.6/km^2; range, 1.02–15.93/km^2) were classified as low-density districts, whereas those with a density higher or equal to the mean were classified as high-density districts.

2.3. Enzyme-Linked Immunosorbent Assay (ELISA)

Antibodies to pestivirus were detected using a commercial blocking ELISA (SERELISA® BVD p80 Ab Mono Blocking, Synbiotics, Lyon, France) that detects specific antibodies to a protein highly conserved in sequence between all strains of BVDV and BDV (p80/125 non-structural protein) [25,26]. Competition percentages and cut-off values were calculated according to the manufacturer's instructions for testing small ruminant samples (i.e., sheep and goats). Samples were classified as positive if the competition percentage was greater than 40% and doubtful if it was between 20 and 40%.

To evaluate the kit's performance with reindeer serum samples, we included in addition to the positive and negative bovine control sera supplied by the manufactures, fourteen reindeer sera previously classified as having pestivirus antibodies by VNT [9]. This ELISA kit has previously been used to detect antibodies against pestivirus in red deer (*Cervus elaphus*) [8], and other ruminant pestivirus ELISA kits with the same protein as antigen have been used to test other wild ruminant populations [5].

2.4. Virus Neutralization Test (VNT)

VNT was carried out to investigate to which ruminant virus the reindeer had been exposed. A panel of 30 samples, representative of six different geographical locations (three in eastern and three in western Finnmark), both age groups and both genders were selected. From each herding district, five samples were selected based on the ELISA results: two positive, one doubtful and two negatives. A panel of three different pestivirus strains (BVDV-1 strain NADL; BDV-1 strain 137/4, and BDV-2 strain Reindeer-1) were used to compare the capacity for neutralization of the selected reindeer test sera. Prior to incubation with the virus strains, the sera were heat-inactivated at 56 °C for 30 min. The VNT was performed as described previously by Kautto and co-workers [5]. Samples were considered positive if neutralization was observed in at least one of two wells (replicates) at a dilution ≥ 1:4. BVDV negative serum was used as a negative control. Anti-BVDV polyclonal sera (VLA Weybridge) and ovine antisera raised against BDV-1 strain X818 and BDV-2 strain Reindeer-1 [12] were used as positive controls.

The neutralizing titers were calculated according to the Spearman–Kärber method [27] as the serum dilution necessary to neutralize the virus in 50% of the cell culture wells (effective dose 50%; ED_{50}).

2.5. Real Time Reverse Transcriptase Polymerase Chain Reaction (Real-Time RT-PCR)

A total of 225 reindeer sera from all sampled districts, 15 samples per district, including animals with strong ELISA positive sera, as well as weak positive, doubtful, and negative sera were screened for the presence of pestivirus RNA by real-time reverse transcriptase polymerase chain reaction (real time RT-PCR). Whenever possible the following proportions, 2+1+12, between positive/weak positive, doubtful and negative animals were used when selecting samples per district, resulting in a total of 185 seronegative, 14 doubtful, and 26 seropositive samples being tested by real-time RT-PCR. Total RNA was extracted using QIAamp® Viral RNA Mini Kit (Qiagen, Venlo, The Netherlands) according to the manufacturer's instructions and eluted in a final volume of 40 μL. Reverse transcription was carried out with the iScript™ cDNA synthesis kit (random hexamer primers) from BioRad (Hercules, CA, USA) using the protocol supplied by the manufacturer [5]. For the following real-time PCR, we used the pan-pestivirus primers OPES13A: 5′-GCTAGCCATGCCCTTAGTAGGA -3′ and OPES14A: 5′- ATCAACTCCATGTGCCATTTACAGC -3′ at recommended primer concentrations [28] and the iQ™ SYBR® Green Supermix from BioRad (CA, USA), in a total volume of 20 μL of PCR mix and 5 μL of template (cDNA) [5]. The PCR cycling conditions applied were as follows: primary denaturation at 95 °C for 10 min, and 40 two-step amplification cycles at 95 °C for 15 s and at 60 °C for 1 min. Amplification products were verified for each run using a melting curve analysis of the gradient of temperature between 55 °C and 95 °C, after the final cycle. In addition, the sizes of the amplicons were verified by visualization in 1.5% agarose gel.

2.6. Statistical Analyses

Statistical analysis was carried out using Stata/SE 14 for Windows (Stata Corp., College Station, TX-USA). A non-parametric kernel density estimation of the probability density function for seroprevalence was performed to analyze the distribution of serological status between samples classified as positive, negative, or doubtful and to determine whether different cut-off calculations would have significant effects on results.

Weight was classified into 10 quantiles according to age and seroprevalence in order to assess the relationship between age and carcass weight and to verify that there were no major discrepancies.

Prevalence estimates were established using the survey commands of STATA; where district was the primary sampling unit for the model and data were stratified according to geographical area, carcass weight, and age class. Estimates were corrected using the following sample weighting procedure: 1/(N sampled reindeer/N total reindeer per district).

A multivariable logistic regression model was established using a backwards procedure adding initially all biological and ecological variables (gender, age, weight, geographical area, animal density, and year of sampling) and subsequently removing those with a *p*-value of the likelihood-ratio test >0.05. District was used as a cluster variable in the analyses and sample weighting was performed as for the prevalence estimates. The Hosmer and Lemeshow test for goodness of fit was carried out [29]. A classification table for sensitivity and specificity and a receiving operating characteristic (ROC) curve was calculated to assess the predictive qualities of the model.

ELISA and VNT titer results were categorized as follows: ELISA as positive if ≥ 40%, otherwise negative, and VNT as positive if titer ≥ 1:4, otherwise negative. The agreement between ELISA and VNT results was measured using the Cohen's kappa (κ) test. A threshold of $p = 0.05$ was used when appropriate.

3. Results

3.1. Overall Results

The ELISA classified 418 of the 3339 reindeer samples as positive (12.5%) with an additional 89 samples classified as doubtful. The distribution of the percentage competition values of the ELISA results, using kernel density estimation, is shown in Figure 1. Positive and negative results formed two clearly distinguishable clusters and the positive results were concentrated above a competition percentage of 70%.

The overall seroprevalence by herding district level is shown in Table 1 and Figure 2A (calves) and Figure 2B (adults). Seroprevalence varied from 0% in district 13 to 44.8% in district 34. Table 1 further shows animal densities and the mean carcass weights according to district, which taken together are good indicators of asymmetries in sample composition. Seroprevalence (ELISA) was 1.7% in eastern Finnmark and 20.0% in western Finnmark.

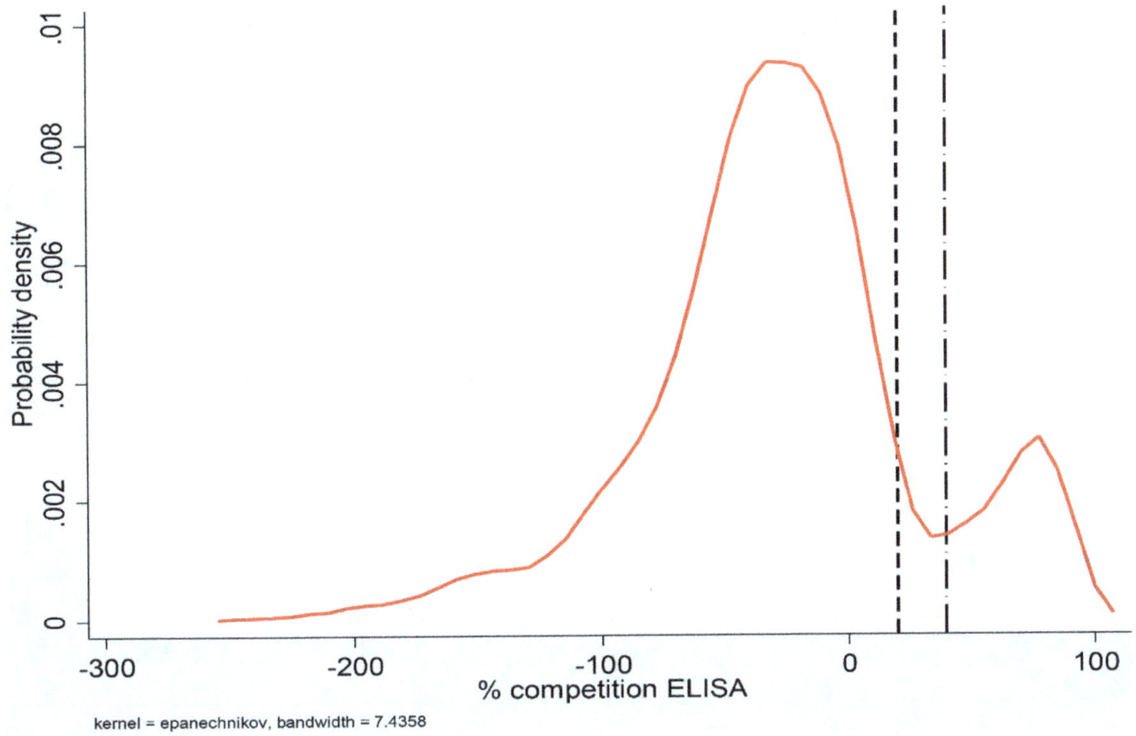

Figure 1. Distribution of percentage competition values for 3339 reindeer sera tested for antibodies against ruminant pestivirus using an ELISA. The density curve represents a kernel estimation of the probability density. The ELISA cut-off values are indicated in the graph by vertical lines; the dashed line (left) indicates a negative cut-off value of 20% and the dash-dot line (right) represents a positive cut-off value of 40%. Percentage competition values between 20% and 40% were considered doubtful.

Table 1. Distribution of ruminant pestivirus seroprevalence according to reindeer herding district in Finnmark County, Norway.

Area	District	Density	Weight	Age	Seroprevalence		
		(n/km²)	Mean	(C/A) [a]	N +/total *(Doubt)* [b]	(%) [c]	95% CI [d]
East	5A	1.0	20.3	90/33	1/185 *(1)*	0.5–1.1	[0–2.6]
	5B	4.2	— [e]	20/53	1/73 *(1)*	1.4–2.7	[0–6.5]
	6	2.1	19.5	110/5	4/119 *(1)*	3.4–4.2	[0.1–7.8]
	7	1.4	24.7	45/23	12/73 *(2)*	16.4–19.2	[7.9–28.3]
	13	4.4	21.8	175/73	0/256 *(2)*	0–0.8	[0–1.9]
	14A	4.3	31.8	10/56	1/66 *(0)*	1.5	[0–4.5]
	16	7.9	24.2	150/426	4/588 *(7)*	0.7–1.9	[0–3.0]
E subtotal		**2.9**	**23.5**	**600/699**	**23/1360 *(14)***	**1.7–2.7**	**[1.0–3.6]**
West	19	4.7		245/38	19/283 *(5)*	6.7–8.5	[3.8–11.7]
	27	14.9	20.9	211/241	74/452 *(13)*	16.4–19.2	[13.0–22.9]
	29	6.0	35.9	1/42	18/43 *(1)*	41.9–44.2	[26.9–59.2]
	33	11.2	23.9	10/145	71/234 *(15)*	30.3–36.8	[24.4–42.9]
	34	11.5	23.7	63/163	162/362 *(25)*	44.8–51.7	[39.6–56.8]
	35	5.5	19.2	194/28	4/224 *(5)*	1.8–4.0	[0–6.6]
	36	3.9	25.9	49/131	5/202 *(0)*	2.5	[0.3–4.6]
	40	15.9	24.5	2/177	42/179 *(11)*	23.5–29.6	[17.2–36.3]
W subtotal		**6.6**	**22.9**	**775/965**	**395/1979 *(75)***	**20.0–23.7**	**[18.2–25.6]**
Total		**4.1**	**23.2**	**1375/1634**	**418/3339 *(89)***	**12.5–15.2**	**[11.4–16.4]**

[a] Age distribution between calves (≤1 year) and adults (>1 year). Information on age was only available for 3009 animals. [b] Bracketed values represent the number of animals classified as doubtful after retesting. [c] Seroprevalence is presented as an interval between % calculated from ELISA positive animals only and % including all doubtful results as positives. [d] Confidence intervals calculated for the maximum interval when animals classified as doubtful were included as if they were positive. [e] No information regarding weight was available for animals sampled in district 5B.

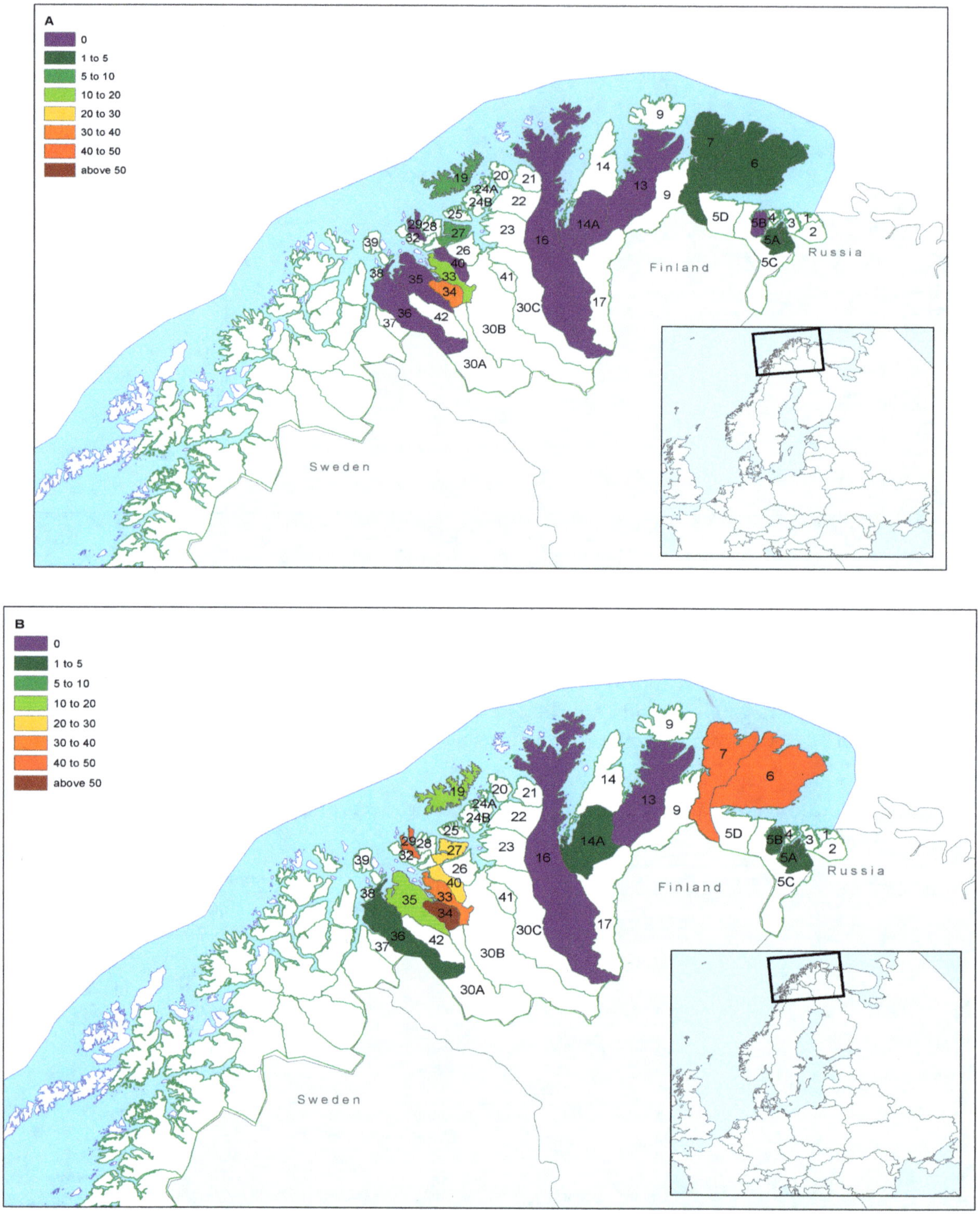

Figure 2. Seroprevalence of pestivirus infection according to herding district and age group (Map (**A**): calves; map (**B**): adults) in Finnmark County, Norway. Tables 1 and 2 provide detailed information on age distribution within districts that should be considered when extrapolating the seroprevalence to the general population in each district. The border between western and eastern Finnmark is between districts 16 and 14A.

Table 2. Distribution of seroprevalence in 10 carcass weight quantiles and classification of age.

	Carcass Weight		Number of Animals			Seroprevalence	
Quantile	Mean (kg)	[Min–Max] (kg)	Calves	Adults	N	%	95% CI
1	13.9	[9.2–15.7]	352	5	22	6.2	[3.7–8.7]
2	16.8	[15.7–17.7]	255	18	13	4.8	[2.2–7.3]
3	18.7	[17.7–19.5]	232	34	13	4.9	[2.3–7.5]
4	20.7	[19.5–21.2]	195	95	18	6.2	[3.4–9.0]
5	22.1	[21.2–22.9]	142	182	36	11.1	[7.7–14.5]
6	23.8	[22.9–24.8]	108	236	47	13.7	[10.0–17.3]
7	25.9	[24.8–27.0]	65	281	55	16.0	[12.1–20.0]
8	27.9	[27.0–29.0]	15	269	59	20.8	[16.0–25.5]
9	30.5	[29.0–32.3]	11	247	41	15.9	[11.4–20.4]
10	38.9	[32.3–69.7]	1	265	45	16.9	[12.4–21.4]

Data from 3008 animals were used since data on weight and age were not available for all animals. Animals were classified as calves (≤1 year old) or adults (>1 year old).

Extrapolation based on the inverse of the number of animals sampled per district divided by the total number of animals in the respective district showed that the samples included in this serosurvey were representative of 111,224 animals, accounting for 66.0% of the total reindeer population in Finnmark County. The overall seroprevalence was 12.5 to 15.2% before extrapolation and 8.2 to 10.2% after extrapolation. The seroprevalence ranged from 1.9 to 2.8% in eastern Finnmark and from 18.1 to 21.2% in western Finnmark.

3.2. *Age Classification and Weight Classes*

Seroprevalence increased from the lowest weight class (quantile 1; seroprevalence = 3.7%) to the highest weight class (quantile 10; seroprevalence = 21.4%). Table 2 shows the relationships between carcass weight and seroprevalence when carcass weight was stratified into 10 quantiles.

3.3. *Factors Affecting Seroprevalence*

Carcass weight was positively correlated with seroprevalence in calves and adults up to 35 kg, irrespective of gender or geographical location (Table 2). No interactions were detected between carcass weight and any of the other variables.

The logistic regression model (Table 3) showed that geographic location, age and gender affected seroprevalence to differing extents. Age (odds ratio = 5.57, CI [2668–11,629]) clearly affected seroprevalence with adult animals having a much higher chance of being seropositive than calves. Geographic location had a minimal effect (odds ratio = 0.084), with animals in western Finnmark having a slightly higher chance of being positive. Concerning gender there seemed to be a slightly higher chance of males being positive than females (odds ratio = 0.472). Differences in seroprevalence between variations in animal density by district or year of sampling were not statistically significant ($p > 0.05$).

Table 3. Logistic regression model for risk factors associated with becoming infected with pestivirus.

Pestivirus Seroprevalence	Odds Ratio	Robust SE	z	P > |z|	95% CI
Region (west to east)	0.084	0.062	−3.36	0.001	[0.020–0.356]
Age (calves to adults)	5.570	2.092	4.57	<0.0001	[2.668–11.629]
Gender (male to female)	0.472	0.167	−2.12	0.034	[0.236–0.944]
Constant	0.093	0.038	−5.82	<0.0001	[0.042–0.207]
No. of observations	3009				

The standard error was adjusted for 15 clusters over districts.
p values < 0.05 were regarded as statistically significant.
Non-significant interactions were removed from the model

None of the additional tests indicated that the model did not fit the data. The Hosmer and Lemeshow goodness of fit test had a chi-square value of 0.46 and a p value of 0.977 (in this instance, the p value is significant if it is greater than 0.05), implying that the model's estimates fitted the data at an acceptable level.

A classification table was compiled to determine the accuracy of the logistic regression model. For a cut-off value of 50% probability ($p = 0.5$), the model correctly predicted the classification of 88.4% of the samples. The area under the ROC curve was 0.81.

3.4. Virus Neutralization Test (VNT)

VNT results are summarized in Table 4, in which the ED_{50} values are presented as the neutralizing titer that corresponded with the respective $\log_2 ED_{50}$. VNT showed that samples negative according to the ELISA were unable to neutralize any of the ruminant pestiviruses, thus being in concordance with the ELISA results for these samples. Doubtful samples had on average low titers for BDV1 and BDV2 and none against BVDV1. All samples that were positive according to the ELISA had higher neutralization titers for BDV1 (average 1:126) and BDV2 (average 1:131) than BVDV1 (average 1:19). Titers against BDV1 and BDV2 were usually very close to each other (within 1 log and non-statistically relevant), with the exception of district 16 where neutralizing titers against BDV1 were not observed.

Table 4. Virus neutralization test of reindeer sera samples for ruminant pestiviruses.

		ELISA	VNT ($\bar{x}$ Titer)		
Region	**District**	**$\bar{x}$ % Compet.**	**BVDV NADL**	**BDV1 137/4**	**BDV2 Reindeer-1**
East	5	64.8	6	68	130
	7	78.4	12	192	96
	16	76.2	6	6	192
West	19	84.2	66	264	132
	34	85.5	6	160	144
	40	79.5	18	128	160
	TOTAL (positives)	**78.1**	**19**	**136**	**142**
	Doubtful (all districts)	33.5	7	33	24
	Negative (all districts)	−68.0	<4	<4	<4

A panel of 30 samples representative of different geographical locations. Both age groups and both genders were selected. From each district, five samples were selected based on the ELISA results: two seropositive, one doubtful, and two seronegative. The neutralizing titers were calculated according to the Spearman–Kärber method as the serum dilution necessary to neutralize the virus in 50% of the wells (effective dose 50%; ED50). Average titers were calculated per district.

Titers against BVDV1 were consistently much lower in every district than those observed for BDV1 and BDV2. No serum sample neutralized BVDV1 at a higher dilution than it neutralized the BDV1 and BDV2.

Statistical analysis of the agreement between ELISA and VNT showed a good correlation between the two tests, where samples with increasing competition ability (ELISA) also had increasing VNT titers. The best correlation between the ELISA and the VNT was found when BDV2 was used in the VNT ($\kappa = 0.580$ for ELISA and BVDV; $\kappa = 0.723$ for ELISA and BDV1; $\kappa = 0.862$ for ELISA and BDV2).

3.5. Realtime RT-PCR

None of the reindeer serum samples selected for real time RT-PCR were positive. Pestivirus positive controls were positive, with an amplicon of the expected size of around 295 base pairs confirmed by electrophoresis.

4. Discussion

The presence of seropositive animals in several districts across eastern and western Finnmark confirmed that a pestivirus is enzootic among semi-domesticated reindeer in Norway. VNT results seem to indicate that the virus is more closely related to BDV than to BVDV1.

Serum samples classified as positive and negative in the ELISA comprised two clearly separated clusters, whereas the probability of a sample being doubtful (i.e., 20–40% competition) was low (Figure 1). Furthermore, all samples classified as negative in the ELISA and subsequently tested in the VNT failed to neutralize the actual virus tested. Thus, we believe that the ELISA cut-off values chosen with this serological kit can be applied when testing reindeer samples. The viral envelope non-structural protein p80 is highly conserved between the different BVDV strains and represents one of the most important markers of cp BVDV [25,26].

The seroprevalence in this study ranged from 0 to 51%, with a mean value of 12 to 15%, and increased with age. This is in line with previous studies, although mean values of prevalence vary considerably between studies. Studies in Sweden identified a prevalence of 35% (5], while previous studies in Norway found a prevalence between 4% [8] and 33% [9]. Differences in analytical methods, geographic regions, and selection criteria for test animals from the herds are some factors that might help explain these differences. It is, however, beyond doubt that pestiviruses are circulating continuously in most tested reindeer populations.

Figure 2B shows two clusters of relatively high prevalence in adults. The cluster around districts 33, 34, and 40 shows a pattern already described for alphaherpesvirus infections [30], in a study that tested the same animals for cervid herpesvirus 2. While these are areas with a higher number of livestock, as compared to districts in eastern Finnmark, the indications that both alphaherpes- and pestiviruses circulating in the reindeer populations are reindeer-specific, suggest that the presence of domestic animals cannot explain the high prevalence in reindeer. Whether this could be the result of husbandry practices, reduced area for the animals to graze (temporary high-density episodes) or presence of other predisposing factors that may increase infection with these two viruses, remains unknown and should be a target for further investigations.

Carcass weight was an important risk factor for seropositivity. The mean weight value for each quantile (Table 2) can be used to correctly interpret seroprevalence at district level (Table 1). Our method of expressing the results as a cross interpretation between weight and seroprevalence avoids misclassification of age. This could have affected the data from 275 animals in this study and resulted in misinterpretation of the results (as shown by some discrepancies in the weight quantiles shown in Table 2, i.e., calves in quantiles 5 to 10 and adults in quantiles 1 to 4).

The strong correlation between seroprevalence and weight/age identified in this study is supported by previous studies [5,8] and supports previous findings of life-long immunity to pestivirus infection. Most likely, the source of infection are PI animals.

Geographic origin (district) and gender seemed to have only a small impact on the risk of infection. We find no compelling argument to explain the slightly higher likelihood of males becoming infected as compared to females, since there is no special difference in the management of males and females that could account for this difference. We thus argue that this association might be the result of a possible bias in the sampling between genders. In fact, several studies of pestivirus infections in wildlife have tried to assess the effect of gender, often obtaining weak or non-significant associations or sometimes-contradictory associations [31].

VNT results indicate that the virus circulating in reindeer is more closely related to BDV1 and BDV2 than BVDV1. Since BVDV was eradicated from domestic animals in Norway in 2006 [15], and BDV has never been reported in Norway [17], the VNT results might therefore indicate the circulation of an unknown virus more closely related to BDV. The relatively low titers against the BDV1 and BDV2 could indicate reduced affinity (i.e., heterologous viruses), but may also suggest a reduction of circulating antibodies over time. The lack of new outbreaks of BVDV1 in cattle in Norway also supports the conclusion that it is unlikely that reindeer would be harboring this virus (as confirmed by low titers in our VNT). Reindeer have sporadic contact with both cattle and small ruminants and one could presume if BVDV1 were circulating in reindeer, it would have been detected during routine screenings of livestock.

Real-time RT-PCR failed to identify any sample positive for viral RNA. Detection of viral RNA is only possible either from PI animals or from transiently infected animals sampled during the period of viremia, which in cervids may last less than 5 days [32]. The lack of detection of PI animals by RT-PCR is not surprising as these animals usually represent a very small fraction of any given host population [33,34]. A study in Sweden including more than 276 reindeer serum samples from districts with high pestivirus seroprevalence also failed to detect viral RNA by real-time RT-PCR [5].

The high seroprevalence in adult animals likely represents continuous episodes of transmission. This requires the presence of PI animals, generated by transplacental infection from a transiently infected mother. Since the fetus must be infected during early pregnancy to become PI, and since this period coincides with the peak of winter when domestic animals are housed, the chance of domestic animals contributing to the maintenance of the infection cycle in reindeer is small or non-existent [5]. This is further supported by the absence of pestivirus infections in domestic ruminants in Norway.

Infections known to be involved in abortion or reduced survival of newborns, such as herpes or pestivirus infections, should be further studied to gain a better understanding of factors affecting mortality and reproductive success. The identification of abortion related to pestiviruses or the mortality of young animals due to mucosal disease—both often described in cattle associated with BVDV [35]—is however difficult, given that aborted calves and dead animals are quickly removed by scavengers.

Another important factor that remains unknown at this point is the potential pathogenicity of a reindeer-specific pestivirus to other ruminant species (wild or domesticated). PI sheep with BDV1 have been shown to transmit the virus to seronegative calves and adult cattle [36,37]. Given the relatively high seroprevalence among reindeer and the possibility of contact with cattle, goats or sheep, it might be that this transmission potential is reduced, or that the virus in question produces mild or no clinical signs in other species.

In conclusion, the present results confirm the circulation of a hitherto unknown pestivirus in the semi-domesticated reindeer population of northern Norway that seems to be serologically closely related to the BDV genotype group 2. Characterization of the causative virus, its infection biology and pathogenic impact in the reindeer populations, as well as its potential to infect other domestic and wild ruminants, should be further investigated.

Author Contributions: Data curation, C.G.d.N. and E.S.; Formal analysis, C.G.d.N.; Funding acquisition, M.T. and C.G.d.N.; Investigation, C.G.d.N., I.H.N., J.J.W. and M.T.; Methodology, C.G.d.N., J.J.W., I.H.N., S.A., and M.T.; Project administration, M.T.; Validation, C.G.d.N., E.S., J.J.W. and S.A.; Writing—original draft, C.G.d.N.; Writing—review and editing, C.G.d.N., J.J.W., I.H.N., E.S., S.A., and M.T. All authors have read and agreed to the published version of the manuscript.

Acknowledgments: For irreplaceable help in the field, we acknowledge veterinary students Therese Berger, Anett K. Larsen, Trine Marhaug, Veronique Poulain, Matthieu Roger, and Gina Petrovich, and guest researcher Frederico Morandi. We thank the staff at the Karasjok, Kautokeino and Šuoššjávri slaughterhouses for their help and hospitality. We also acknowledge the help from Eva M. Breines and Ellinor Hareide in our laboratory in Tromsø, and Irene Dergel, Maj Hjort, and Lena Renström at National Veterinary Institute, Uppsala, Sweden, for laboratory assistance. Finally, we are very thankful to Sophie Ellen Scotter for language corrections.

References

1. Murphy, F.A.; Gibbs, E.P.; Horzinek, M.C.; Studdert, M.J. Laboratory Diagnosis of Viral Diseases. In *Veterinary Virology*, 3rd ed.; Murphy, F.A., Gibbs, E.P.J., Horzinek, M.C., Studdert, M.J., Eds.; Academic Press: London, UK, 1999; pp. 193–224.
2. Vilcek, S.; Nettleton, P.F. Pestiviruses in wild animals. *Vet. Microbiol.* **2006**, *116*, 1–12. [CrossRef] [PubMed]
3. Ridpath, J.F.; Neill, J.D. Challenges in Identifying and Determining the Impacts of Infection with Pestiviruses on the Herd Health of Free Ranging Cervid Populations. *Front. Microbiol.* **2016**, *7*, 921. [CrossRef] [PubMed]
4. Larska, M. Pestivirus infection in reindeer. *Front. Microbiol.* **2015**, *6*, 1187. [CrossRef] [PubMed]
5. Kautto, A.H.; Alenius, S.; Mossing, T.; Becher, P.; Belak, S.; Larska, M. Pestivirus and alphaherpesvirus infections in Swedish reindeer (*Rangifer tarandus tarandus* L.). *Vet. Microbiol.* **2012**, *156*, 64–71. [CrossRef] [PubMed]
6. Rehbinder, C.; Nordkvist, M. A suspected virus infection of the oral mucosa in Swedish reindeer (*Rangifer tarandus*). *Rangifer* **1985**, *5*, 22–31. [CrossRef]
7. Rehbinder, C.; Belak, K.; Nordkvist, M. A serological, retrospective study in reindeer on five different viruses. *Rangifer* **1992**, *12*, 191–195. [CrossRef]
8. Lillehaug, A.; Vikoren, T.; Larsen, I.L.; Akerstedt, J.; Tharaldsen, J.; Handeland, K. Antibodies to ruminant alpha-herpesviruses and pestiviruses in Norwegian cervids. *J. Wildl. Dis.* **2003**, *39*, 779–786. [CrossRef]
9. Tryland, M.; Mørk, T.; Ryeng, K.A.; Sørensen, K.K. Evidence of parapox-, alphaherpes- and pestivirus infections in carcasses of semi-domesticated reindeer (*Rangifer tarandus tarandus*) from Finnmark, Norway. *Rangifer* **2005**, *25*, 75–83. [CrossRef]
10. Stuen, S.; Krogsrud, J.; Hyllseth, B.; Tyler, N.J.C. Serosurvey of three virus infections in reindeer in northern Norway and Svalbard. *Rangifer* **1993**, *13*, 215–219. [CrossRef]
11. Becher, P.; Orlich, M.; Kosmidou, A.; Konig, M.; Baroth, M.; Thiel, H.J. Genetic diversity of pestiviruses: Identification of novel groups and implications for classification. *Virology* **1999**, *262*, 64–71. [CrossRef]
12. Avalos-Ramirez, R.; Orlich, M.; Thiel, H.J.; Becher, P. Evidence for the presence of two novel pestivirus species. *Virology* **2001**, *286*, 456–465. [CrossRef] [PubMed]
13. Morton, J.; Evermann, J.F.; Dieterich, R.A. Experimental infection of reindeer with bovine viral diarrhea virus. *Rangifer* **1990**, *10*, 75–77. [CrossRef]
14. Loken, T.; Krogsrud, J.; Larsen, I.L. Pestivirus infections in Norway. Serological investigations in cattle, sheep and pigs. *Acta Vet. Scand.* **1991**, *32*, 27–34. [PubMed]
15. Kampen, A.H.; Åkerstedt, J.; Gudmundsson, S.; Hopp, P.; Grøneng, G.; Nyberg, O. *The Surveillance and Control Programme for Bovine Virus Diarrhoea (BVD) in Norway*; Norwegian Veterinary Institute: Oslo, Norway, 2007; pp. 65–71.
16. Loken, T.; Nyberg, O. Eradication of BVDV in cattle: The Norwegian project. *Vet. Rec.* **2013**, *172*, 661. [CrossRef] [PubMed]
17. Loken, T. Pestivirus infections in ruminants in Norway. *Revue Sci. Tech.-Off. Int. Épizoot.* **1992**, *11*, 895–899. [CrossRef]
18. Loken, T.; Barlow, R.M. Border disease in Norway. *Acta Vet. Scand.* **1981**, *22*, 137–139.
19. Loken, T.; Bjerkas, I.; Hyllseth, B. Border disease in goats in Norway. *Res. Vet. Sci.* **1982**, *33*, 103–131. [CrossRef]
20. Loken, T.; Hyllseth, B.; Larsen, H.J. Border disease in Norway. Serological examination of affected sheep flocks. *Acta Vet. Scand.* **1982**, *23*, 46–52.
21. Loken, T. Pestivirus infections in Norway. Epidemiological studies in goats. *J. Comp. Pathol.* **1990**, *103*, 1–10. [CrossRef]
22. *Ressursregnskap for Reindriftsnaeringen*; Reindriftsforvaltningen/Norwegian Reindeer Husbandry Authority: Alta, Norway. Available online: https://docplayer.me/49637426-Ressursregnskap-for-reindriftsnaeringen-r-e-i-n-d-r-i-f-t-s-f-o-r-v-a-l-t-n-i-n-g-e-n-j-u-n-i.html (accessed on 26 December 2019).

23. Tveraa, T.; Fauchald, P.; Henaug, C.; Yoccoz, N.G. An examination of a compensatory relationship between food limitation and predation in semi-domesticated reindeer. *Oecologia* **2003**, *137*, 370–376. [CrossRef]
24. *Ressursregnskap for Reindriftsnaeringen*; Reindriftsforvaltningen/Norwegian Reindeer Husbandry Authority: Alta, Norway, 2008. Available online: https://www.landbruksdirektoratet.no/no/reindriften/for-siidaandeler/publikasjoner?index=0 (accessed on 26 December 2019).
25. Collett, M.S. Molecular genetics of pestiviruses. *Comp. Immunol. Microbiol. Infect. Dis.* **1992**, *15*, 145–154. [CrossRef]
26. Deregt, D.; Masri, S.A.; Cho, H.J.; Bielefeldt, O.H. Monoclonal antibodies to the p80/125 gp53 proteins of bovine viral diarrhea virus: Their potential use as diagnostic reagents. *Can. J. Vet. Res.* **1990**, *54*, 343–348. [PubMed]
27. Thrusfield, M. Serological epidemiology. In *Veterinary Epidemiology*; Thrusfield, M., Ed.; Butterworths: London, UK, 1986; pp. 175–186.
28. Elvander, M.; Baule, C.; Persson, M.; Egyed, L.; Ballagi-Pordany, A.; Belak, S.; Alenius, S. An experimental study of a concurrent primary infection with bovine respiratory syncytial virus (BRSV) and bovine viral diarrhoea virus (BVDV) in calves. *Acta Vet. Scand.* **1998**, *39*, 251–264. [PubMed]
29. Hosmer, D.W.; Lemeshow, S. *Applied Logistic Regression*; John Wiley &Sons, Inc.: New York, NY, USA, 1989.
30. das Neves, C.G.; Thiry, J.; Skjerve, E.; Yoccoz, N.G.; Rimstad, E.; Thiry, E.; Tryland, M. Alphaherpesvirus infections in semidomesticated reindeer: A cross-sectional serological study. *Vet. Microbiol.* **2009**, *139*, 262–269. [CrossRef] [PubMed]
31. Pioz, M.; Loison, A.; Gibert, P.; Dubray, D.; Menaut, P.; Le Tallec, B.; Artois, M.; Gilot-Fromont, E. Transmission of a pestivirus infection in a population of Pyrenean chamois. *Vet. Microbiol.* **2007**, *119*, 19–30. [CrossRef]
32. Ridpath, J.F.; Mark, C.S.; Chase, C.C.; Ridpath, A.C.; Neill, J.D. Febrile response and decrease in circulating lymphocytes following acute infection of white-tailed deer fawns with either a BVDV1 or a BVDV2 strain. *J. Wildl. Dis.* **2007**, *43*, 653–659. [CrossRef]
33. Hessman, B.E.; Fulton, R.W.; Sjeklocha, D.B.; Murphy, T.A.; Ridpath, J.F.; Payton, M.E. Evaluation of economic effects and the health and performance of the general cattle population after exposure to cattle persistently infected with bovine viral diarrhea virus in a starter feedlot. *Am. J. Vet. Res.* **2009**, *70*, 73–85. [CrossRef]
34. Loneragan, G.H.; Thomson, D.U.; Montgomery, D.L.; Mason, G.L.; Larson, R.L. Prevalence, outcome, and health consequences associated with persistent infection with bovine viral diarrhea virus in feedlot cattle. *J. Am. Vet. Med. Assoc.* **2005**, *226*, 595–601. [CrossRef]
35. Schweizer, M.; Peterhans, E. Pestiviruses. *Annu. Rev. Anim. Biosci.* **2014**, *2*, 141–163. [CrossRef]
36. Braun, U.; Bachofen, C.; Buchi, R.; Hassig, M.; Peterhans, E. Infection of cattle with Border disease virus by sheep on communal alpine pastures. *Schweiz. Arch. Tierheilkd.* **2013**, *155*, 123–128. [CrossRef]
37. Braun, U.; Reichle, S.F.; Reichert, C.; Hassig, M.; Stalder, H.P.; Bachofen, C.; Peterhans, E. Sheep persistently infected with Border disease readily transmit virus to calves seronegative to BVD virus. *Vet. Microbiol.* **2014**, *168*, 98–104. [CrossRef] [PubMed]

14

Mycoplasma bovis Infections—Occurrence, Diagnosis and Control

Katarzyna Dudek [1,*], Robin A. J. Nicholas [2], Ewelina Szacawa [1] and Dariusz Bednarek [1]

1 Department of Cattle and Sheep Diseases, National Veterinary Research Institute, 57 Partyzantów Avenue, 24100 Pulawy, Poland; ewelina.szacawa@piwet.pulawy.pl (E.S.); dbednarek@piwet.pulawy.pl (D.B.)
2 The Oaks, Nutshell Lane, Farnham, Surrey GU9 0HG, UK; robin.a.j.nicholas@gmail.com
* Correspondence: katarzyna.dudek@piwet.pulawy.pl

Abstract: *Mycoplasma bovis* is a cause of bronchopneumonia, mastitis and arthritis but may also affect other main organs in cattle such us the eye, ear or brain. Despite its non-zoonotic character, *M. bovis* infections are responsible for substantial economic health and welfare problems worldwide. *M. bovis* has spread worldwide, including to countries for a long time considered free of the pathogen. Control of *M. bovis* infections is hampered by a lack of effective vaccines and treatments due to increasing trends in antimicrobial resistance. This review summarizes the latest data on the epizootic situation of *M. bovis* infections and new sources/routes of transmission of the infection, and discusses the progress in diagnostics. The review includes various recommendations and suggestions which could be applied to infection control programs.

Keywords: *Mycoplasma bovis*; cattle; disease; prevalence; control

1. Introduction

In 2017, New Zealand became the last of the major cattle-rearing countries to be infected with *Mycoplasma bovis* [1]. Finland had also remained free until relatively recently but became infected via imported cattle in 2012 [2]. Undoubtedly, *M. bovis* is now the most important mycoplasma of livestock being a primary cause of mastitis, arthritis, keratoconjunctivitis and other disorders as well as a major player in the bovine respiratory disease complex (BRD) [3]. Previously *Mycoplasma mycoides* subsp. *mycoides*, the aetiological agent of the World Organisation for Animal Health (OIE)-listed contagious bovine pleuropneumonia, had this dubious distinction but this mycoplasma is now confined to countries in sub Saharan Africa.

Mycoplasma bovis was first reported in the USA in 1961 from a case of bovine mastitis then was probably exported in cattle of high genetic quality to Israel [3]. It then spread around the world, reaching the UK and the rest of Europe in the mid1970s (Figure 1). International trade in cattle and cattle products like semen has enabled its silent spread to all continents where cattle are kept. The date of isolation in a particular country, of course, is not necessarily the date of introduction even in the USA as mycoplasmas were very much an unknown quantity and their fastidious nature made isolation and detection an extremely difficult task. Indeed, it has only been in the last two decades with the introduction of DNA amplification techniques that detection and identification have become routine in many parts of the world. However, not all countries have veterinary diagnostic laboratories which can identify these organisms.

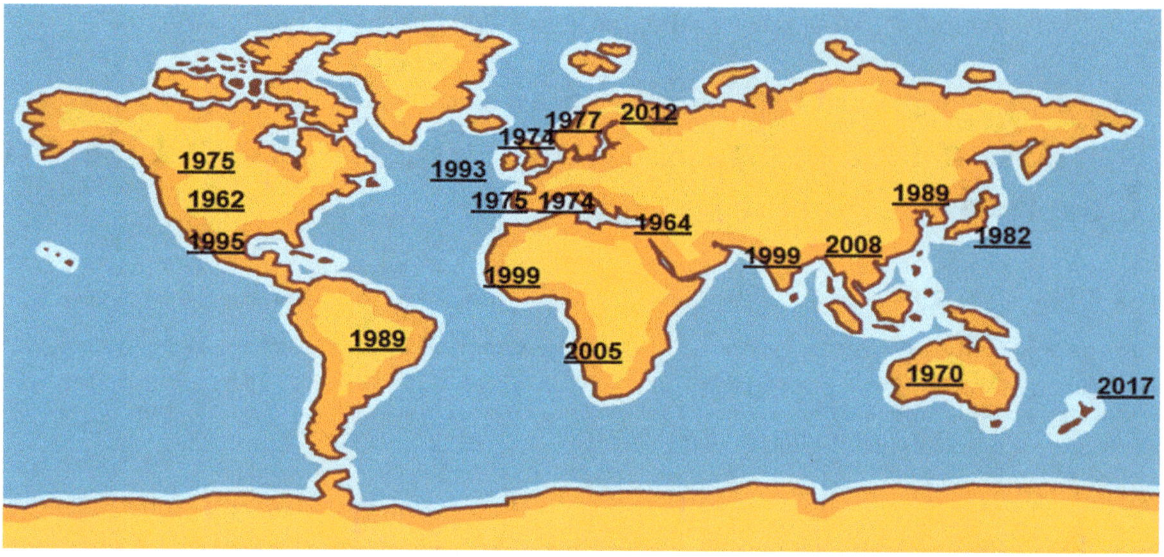

Figure 1. First detections of *Mycoplasma bovis* around the world.

Initially the importance of *M. bovis*, particularly in BRD, was underestimated because of the promotion of more established and easier detectable organisms like the bacteria *Mannheimia haemolytica*, *Histophilus somni* and *Pasteurella multocida* and viruses, namely bovine respiratory syncytial disease, parainfluenza-3 virus, bovine herpesviruses, coronaviruses and bovine viral diarrhoea virus. The presence of *M. bovis* in healthy cattle, although at a much lower levels than infected ones, delayed recognition of its pathogenicity. Once the importance of environmental factors such as weather, variation in strain virulence and its interaction with the BRD pathogens were known, studies quickly demonstrated its widespread prevalence in pneumonic calves and, later, older cattle.

Despite attempts going back nearly half a century, control of *M. bovis* diseases is still problematic because of a lack of an effective commercial vaccine. Many have been marketed, particularly in the USA, but little data exist to assess their immunogenicity and protective properties [4]. To be valuable they are required to be part of multivalent vaccines incorporating the causative bacteria and viruses currently available for BRD. Presently, no vaccine is available for mycoplasma mastitis, a major problem in large dairy herds of North America where they are often untreatable. Indeed, the major trend in the last two decades has been the alarming decrease in susceptibility of *M. bovis* to the commonly used antimicrobials including the fluoroquinolones [5].

This review summarizes the latest data on the epizootic situation of *M. bovis* infections and new sources/routes of transmission of the infection and discusses the progress in diagnostics. The review also covers aspects related to *M. bovis* infection control, collecting various recommendations and suggestions which could be applied in the infection control programs.

2. *Mycoplasma bovis*: Key Facts

Mycoplasma bovis (*M. bovis*) is most often considered to cause caseonecrotic pneumonia, mastitis and arthritis [6,7]. However, cases of infectious keratoconjunctivitis, suppurative otitis media, meningitis, decubital abscesses, endocarditis and reproductive disorders have been associated with *M. bovis* [7–10]. Most importantly *M. bovis* is one of the causes of BRD with other aetiological agents, both bacterial and viral [11,12].

M. bovis is one of 13 species of mycoplasmas diagnosed in cattle; however, not all of them cause serious diseases, and some may even constitute normal flora of the bovine respiratory tract. For example, the most important mycoplasma in bovine severe respiratory diseases is the previously mentioned *Mycoplasma mycoides* subsp. *mycoides*. *Mycoplasma bovigenitalium* is generally associated with bovine reproductive disorders, while *Mycoplasma bovoculi* has been isolated from infectious keratoconjunctivitis in cattle [3]. *M. bovis* infections are non-zoonotic; however, substantial economic and cattle health and welfare impacts are felt worldwide [3]. *M. bovis* affects all age groups of cattle (prewean, postwean, neonate and adult) and all cattle sectors such as beef, milk or rearing [3]. *M. bovis* can persist in a herd for very long periods of time, with the possibility of pathogen shedding by the infected animals for a few weeks to several months [13,14]. The evolutionary absence of a cell wall in principle makes *M. bovis* resistant to penicillins and cephalosporins [3,4]. Moreover, in vitro studies on *M. bovis* field isolates show increasing trends in antimicrobial resistance, including tetracyclines and even newer generation macrolides considered effective against *M. bovis* infections [5,15–18]. *M. bovis* infections are usually characterized by chronic course and are difficult to treat successfully [3]. One recent in vivo study has shown an efficacy of treatment of the *M. bovis* pneumonia in calves using enrofloxacin given alone, unlike the combination therapy with co-administration of flunixin meglumine, a nonsteroidal anti-inflammatory drug or pegbovigrastim (immunostimulator), which rather exacerbated the disease. However, it should be remembered that fluoroquinolones, although effective in this case, should be used as antimicrobials of last resort [19]. Some experimental *M. bovis* vaccines have been shown to be immunogenic and protective; however, currently no commercial vaccines are available in Europe with only some autogenous vaccines in use in the United States and Great Britain [20–22].

3. Current Reports on the Epizootic Situation of *M. bovis*

It was previously reported that *M. bovis* has the ability to spread worldwide to countries for a long time considered free of the pathogen because of the widespread international trade in cattle [2,23,24]. The first case of *M. bovis* infection in Finland was recorded relatively recently in 2012 in pneumonic calves. In 2012–2015, 0.26% of Finnish dairy farms were *M. bovis* infected [2]. To date, it is estimated that only 0.8% of Finnish dairy herds were infected with *M. bovis* between 2012 and 2018 [23]. A two-year survey included 19 Finnish dairy farms previously free of *M. bovis* showed mastitis caused by *M. bovis* in over 89% of all farms tested; however, only a few clinical mastitis cases were seen. In the remaining two farms, no *M. bovis* mastitis cases were detected during the study period; calf pneumonia caused by *M. bovis* were, however, observed. In this study, the results may indicate a rather subclinical course of mastitis due to *M. bovis* infection. Additional data including *M. bovis* antibody detection using the MilA ELISA showed the majority of cows were positive for *M. bovis* throughout the study period, regardless of the infection status of the farm. It confirms that *M. bovis* may circulate for long time in the herd [23].

The detection of *M bovis* in New Zealand was remarkable for several reasons. First, New Zealand was probably the last major cattle-rearing nation to become infected; secondly, it does not import cattle, the main route of cross border infection, and had not done so for nearly a decade; and thirdly, New Zealand took the unprecedented decision to eradicate the organism from its cattle industry despite the fact the clinical disease was overwhelmingly mild. *M. bovis* was first detected in a dairy herd at the Bay of Plenty on the South Island in 2017. Since this isolation, up until June 2020, just over 1800 farms have been affected, involving the slaughter of nearly 160,000 cattle at a cost of NZ$203 million (about 116 million euros). With just over 250 farms still affected, complete eradication looks feasible but challenging and would be a first amongst cattle rearing countries. The origins of the outbreaks have still not been definitively traced but whole genome sequencing of 171 isolates from 30 infected herds indicated that the current outbreak was probably caused by recent entry of *M. bovis*, perhaps 1–2 years before detection, from a single source either as a single entry of a single *M. bovis* clone or, potentially, up to three entries of three very closely related *M. bovis* clones from the same source [25]; this suggests that there were probably several simultaneous outbreaks strongly implicating infected imported semen. Indeed *M. bovis* DNA was detected by PCR in one batch of semen but unfortunately could not be isolated. While analyses to date have not identified the source, the most closely related international isolates that have been characterised are European in origin [25].

Interesting information can be gathered by estimating on-farm/within-herd prevalence of *M. bovis* infections [26,27]. Such a repeated cross-sectional six-month study on *M. bovis* intramammary infections was conducted between 2017 and 2018 in four Estonian dairy herds with previously confirmed *M. bovis* positive status. The qPCR results of examination of pooled cow composite milk samples in the four endemically infected herds showed a differential and relatively low within-herd prevalence, which ranged between 0.4% and 12.3%. For the author, this could be a result of the different infection phases, *M. bovis* strain differentiation, intermittent shedding of the pathogen by the infected cows or low concentration of *M. bovis* in the examined milk samples. Similar prevalence (3.7–11%) was observed in clinical cases of mastitis due to *M. bovis* during a six-month study period in the four dairy herds. Additional evaluation of pooled cow colostrum samples during the same study period also showed low prevalence of *M. bovis* in the study herds ranging between 1.7% and 4.7% [26].

Within-herd prevalence of *M. bovis* DNA in cow colostrum samples was also estimated in 2016–2017 in seventeen Belgian herds with a recent infection of *M. bovis*. This survey was performed on dairy, beef and mixed-dairy farms with *M. bovis* positive status diagnosed less than one month before sample collection. The herds were additionally divided into two groups, depending on whether the infection was confirmed only in calves or in both calves and adult animals. The results showed only seven colostrum samples positive for *M. bovis* DNA originated from four herds, which was 1.9% of the total number of samples tested. In the positive farms on-farm/within-herd prevalence ranged between 2.8% and 30.0%, whereas the average within-herd prevalence estimated for all seventeen herds tested was 3.2%. According to the author, the reason for such low average within-herd prevalence of *M. bovis* DNA obtained in this survey was probably a result of differentiation in the infection phases in the periparturient cows or false positive results of real-time PCR assays used in *M. bovis* DNA detection particularly due to the possibility of ongoing co-infections with other *Mycoplasma* species [27]. In 2009, it was reported that 1.5% of all herd tested had bulk tank milk samples positive for *M. bovis* confirmed by culturing and PCR [28].

Data collected in Great Britain between 2006 and 2017 including diagnoses of respiratory disease, mastitis and arthritis due to *M. bovis* infections demonstrated a significant proportion of pneumonia (86.4%), which showed an increasing trend since 2014. The highest number of pneumonia incidents was diagnosed in 2017 (over 120 diagnoses), reaching 7.5% of all diagnosable submissions. For comparison, the annual cases of arthritis and mastitis for all the examined years were less than 30 per year, with a slight predominance for mycoplasma mastitis. In this survey the incidents of *M. bovis* pneumonia were diagnosed mainly in the postwean age group of calves. However, since 2012, the number of pneumonia diagnoses in the preweaning calves was comparable. The smallest number of *M. bovis* pneumonia cases was diagnosed in the neonate age group of calves. Seasonal data collected from 2006 to 2017 showed the largest number of respiratory diagnoses due to *M. bovis* were in the colder seasons, i.e., between October and March, which could be caused not only by temperature fluctuations, but also by closer contact of animals in the herd during housing [20,24]. Temperature fluctuations are probably related to stress accompanied by elevated blood corticosteroid concentrations, which may consequently predispose calves to *M. bovis* infection, as confirmed in both in vivo and in vitro studies using dexamethasone [29–31]. In the remaining months, i.e., from July to September, and from April to June, the respiratory submissions were comparable, although slightly higher in the spring months. Additional examinations also showed a higher incidence of *M. bovis* respiratory disease in the beef sector of cattle (almost 42%). Another slightly less affected cattle sector was dairy with 32.8% of *M. bovis* respiratory submissions [20]. A previous study performed in Great Britain between 1990 and 2000 showed that over 50% of a total of 1413 cattle isolates tested were *M. bovis*, mostly originating from pneumonia cases. *M. bovis* was also isolated from mastitis cases, joint fluid, eyes and sporadically from sheath washings, urogenital tract and heart blood [32].

The problem of subclinical intramammary infections with *M. bovis* as a consequence of recent clinical mastitis outbreaks in four Australian dairy herds was discussed in the study of Hazelton et al., which concluded that an early diagnosis of such cases may consequently prevent the future spread of *M. bovis* in the herd [13]. The apparent cow-level prevalence of *M. bovis* intramammary infections in these herds was determined immediately after cessation of outbreaks. Before the herd sampling between 2014 and 2016 all clinically affected cows due to *M. bovis* were culled. From a total of 2232 cows located in the main milking group of each herd from which 88 initial pooled milk samples were collected, only two *M. bovis* PCR positive cows were detected, which constituted less than 1% of average apparent cow-level prevalence of subclinical intramammary *M. bovis* infection. Additional tests performed individually on 15 cows located in the hospital group of each herd and *M. bovis* suspected gave five positive PCR results. *M. bovis* DNA was also detected by PCR in bulk tank milk collected from two study herds. However, in 6 out of 1813 cows from three study herds, *M. bovis* was isolated using microbiological culture. Five positive culture results were detected in cows located in the hospital group and *M. bovis* suspected, whereas the remaining one was from the main milking group, both within the same herd. For information, the culture positive cow in the main milking group had also positive *M. bovis* PCR result. In addition, *M. bovis* was isolated from bulk tank milk sampled from one study herd; however, it was not the same herd from which *M. bovis* culture positive cows were detected. To estimate *M. bovis* seroprevalence in the four study herds, a total of 199 sera were collected from 50 cows located in the main milking group of each herd, with the exception of one herd from which 49 results were estimated. The results showed the average *M. bovis* seroprevalence of 38%, which varied from 16% to 76%. It is also worth mentioning that in two of the four herds tested, several months after the herd sampling, new clinical cases or positive results in the hospital group bulk tank were reported, both confirmed by *M. bovis* PCR [13].

4. Disease Course and Source of *M. bovis* Infection

M. bovis infections occur with various clinical manifestations, such as pneumonia, mastitis, arthritis, otitis, keratoconjunctivitis, meningitis, endocarditis and others, the most important of which are summarized in Table 1. The clinical picture of respiratory disease diagnosed as *M. bovis* is not usually characteristic and often does not differ from clinical signs caused by infections with other bovine respiratory tract pathogens, especially in the presence of co-infections [20]. The study on feedlot beef calves showed that *M. bovis* was isolated from all diagnosed pneumonia categories, such as caseonecrotic bronchopneumonia, both caseonecrotic and fibrinosuppurative bronchopneumonia or fibrinosuppurative bronchopneumonia alone. In this study distinct synergism in pneumonia cases between *M. bovis* and *Pasteurellaceae* family pathogens, especially for *M. haemolytica*, was demonstrated. Both pathogens were identified in focal coagulative necrosis lesions within lung tissues [33].

In cases of keratoconjunctivitis as well as brain disorders, *M. bovis* infections, which are often overlooked in the differential diagnosis of these diseases, should be taken into account (Table 1).

As recently reported, both clinical and subclinical courses of mastitis due to *M. bovis* infection were detected [13,23]. However, the possibility of subclinical intramammary infections with *M. bovis* as a consequence of the recent clinical mastitis outbreaks should be considered as previously presented in the Section 3 in the study of Hazelton et al. [13].

It was first recognized that *M. bovis*-positive semen used in artificial insemination was a cause of mastitis outbreak in two naive dairy herds, despite high biosecurity and good farming practice carried out on these farms [2]. Out of the total of ten bulls used to inseminate cows with *M. bovis* mastitis diagnosed, only one of them appeared to be the *M. bovis* carrier. Additionally, only one of the cows from each herd that were inseminated with the contaminated processed semen from the same bull developed mastitis. In both study herds, the infection not only transmitted to other cows that were not inseminated with *M. bovis*-positive semen, but also to calves. The core-genome multilocus sequence typing (cgMLST) analysis of *M. bovis* strains isolated from the mastitis cases and the bull semen clustered together [2].

Table 1. Examples of clinical manifestations of *M. bovis* infections. The sequence presented is consistent with the frequency of each clinical manifestation from the most to the least frequently diagnosed cases in cattle.

Course of *M. bovis* Infection	Type of Research (Experimental/Survey)	Cattle Sector	Main Clinical Signs/Lesions/Subclinical	Methods Used for the Infection Confirmation/Presence	Reference
pneumonia	survey	beef	caseonecrotic bronchopneumonia; fibrinosuppurative bronchopneumonia	IHC; PCR	[33]
	experimental	dairy-cross	nasal discharge; coughing; caseonecrotic pneumonia	ELISA for *M. bovis* antigen detection; IHC; ELISA for specific antibody detection	[19]
mastitis	survey	dairy	clinical mastitis; subclinical mastitis	culture; real-time PCR; two different ELISAs for specific antibody detection (MilA IgG ELISA; BioX ELISA)	[23]
	survey		clinical mastitis; subclinical mastitis	culture; PCR; ELISA for specific antibody detection	[13]
arthritis	survey	beef	arthritis; tenosynovitis	culture; passive hemagglutination test	[33]
	experimental	dairy	joint swelling; lameness/fibrinosuppurative synovitis and tenosynovitis; thrombus presence	culture; indirect hemagglutination test	[34]
otitis	survey	dairy	ear droop; otic exudate	ELISA for specific antibody detection; DGGE	[35]
	survey	beef	ear droop; exudative otitis media; facial paralysis; occasionally nasal exudate; nystagmus, head tilt, ataxia/suppurative lesions in the middle ear; lung consolidation (most cases); cerebellar meningitis (some cases)	culturing; immune-peroxidase test; PCR; IHC; transmission electron microscopy	[7]
kerato-conjunctivitis	survey	beef	"pink eye" signs	culture; RAPD; PCR-RFLP; DNA sequencing	[8]
brain disorders	survey	dairy	head tilt; central nervous system signs/purulent meningitis	ELISA for specific antibody detection	[36]
			lethargy, blindness; teeth grinding/cerebral hemisphere necrosis	enrichment and capture ELISA	
endocarditis	survey	beef	no clinical signs; caseated lesions in the heart	culture; *uvrC* gene PCR; loop-mediated isothermal amplification assay; IHC	[10]

The role of airborne transmission of *M. bovis* is unclear with little experimental evidence supporting this route of infection [37,38]. In response to exposure of calves to aerosolized *M. bovis*, respiratory disease was induced. In the infected calves, specific *M. bovis* lung lesions confirmed by necropsy and histological examinations were observed despite the lack of clinical signs. However, re-isolation of *M. bovis* from the upper trachea in most infected calves was additional confirmation of this infection route [37].

Recent reports on *M. bovis* indicated colostrum as a possible source of infection based on positive results for *M. bovis* DNA [26,27]. Additionally, in one of these studies, herd-specific *M. bovis* strains were isolated from cows with clinical mastitis and calves affected with respiratory disease showing possible transmission of the pathogen between dairy cows and calves via contaminated milk. However, in this study other routes of *M. bovis* infection transmission like direct/indirect contact between animals within the study herds, animal handling or air-borne route cannot be excluded [26]. The most important sources of *M. bovis* infection/routes of *M. bovis* infection transmission are summarized in Table 2. Other no less important sources/routes of *M. bovis* infection transmission not included in the Table 2 such as nose-to-nose contact between animals or fomites (e.g., farm-personnel's contaminated hands, equipment), although difficult to directly prove or document, should also be considered [26,39,40].

Within the host, *M. bovis* disseminates by the haematogenous route, which may result in subsequent lesions in organs other than those initially affected. In one such study all diagnosed cases of arthritis in feedlot beef calves were accompanied by lung lesions, which accounted for nearly 50% of all diagnosed *M. bovis*-related pneumonias. The arthritis cases were probably of pulmonary origin [33]. In post-mortem findings in *M. bovis* affected calves, both meningitis and otitis media/interna were diagnosed. In other calf necropsy examinations, necrosis within the brain and fibrinous heart lesions due to *M. bovis* infection were evident [36]. The ability of *M. bovis* to spread within different organs of the same host was previously confirmed [7]. In the majority of calves diagnosed with suppurative otitis media severe lung lesions were observed. In some of them cerebellar meningitis was also diagnosed. Additionally, in some calves, *M. bovis* antigen was identified in the temporal bone, liver and kidney [7].

Table 2. Examples of sources of *M. bovis* infection/routes of *M. bovis* infection transmission.

Source of Infection/Route of Infection Transmission	Type of Research (Experimental/Survey)	Cattle Sector	Number of Herd/Farms Tested	Methods Used for the Infection Confirmation/Detection	Reference
colostrum	survey	dairy	4	qPCR	[26]
	survey	dairy, beef and dairy-mixed	17	real-time PCR	[27]
milk	survey	dairy	4	qPCR; culturing; core-genome multilocus sequence typing (cgMLST)	[26]
semen	survey	dairy	2	culturing; real-time PCR; WGS; cgMLST analysis	[2]
air-borne	experimental	dairy-cross	not applicable	culturing; *polC* PCR; MilA IgG ELISA; *post mortem* examination; histopathological examination	[37]
intrauterine	survey	dairy	not described	culturing; IHC; ISH	[41]

5. Currently Used Diagnostic Methods

The clinical signs of infections in cattle associated with *M. bovis* are non-specific; for that reason, sensitive, accurate and rapid testing of animals is needed for reliable diagnosis. Culturing of *M. bovis* is a gold standard method but is time-consuming and requires specific conditions. Different kinds of media are widely used in experimental studies and in confirmation of infection caused by *M. bovis*, and include Hayflick's [42], modified PPLO [43] and Eaton's [44]. Mycoplasmas are fastidious, slow growing and can be easily overgrown by other bacteria. During the last few years various tests have been used for the detection of *M. bovis* infections in cattle (Table 3).

Table 3. The characteristics of recently developed methods for *M. bovis* detection in various specimens from cattle.

Assay/Target	Samples	Limit of Detection	Sensitivity	Specificity	Reference
real-time PCR/*uvr*C	lung samples (n = 30); milk samples (n = 21)	100 fg DNA; 40 genome copies/reaction; 250 CFU/mL	10^3-fold more sensitive than conventional PCR	100% (evaluated for 6 *Mycoplasma* spp. and 6 species of bacteria)	[45]
qPCR/*uvr*C	deep nasopharyngeal swabs (n = 208)	1.61×10^2 CFU/mL	100%	87.27%	[46]
qPCR/*gltX*	milk samples from individual quarters (n = 9); bulk tank milk samples (n = 59)	10–100 genome equivalents/reaction; 1×10^4–1×10^5 cells/mL	100%	94.4% (evaluated for 3 *Mycoplasma* spp.)	[47]

real-time multiplex PCR
*M. bovis/uvr*C
*M. californicum/rpo*B
M. bovigenitalium/16S–23S rRNA
	swab samples (n = 95);
	semen samples (n = 44);
	individual milk samples (n = 114);
	bulk tank milk samples (n = 221)
		1.3×10^2 –1.3×10^7 CFU/mL	not applicable	100%
				(evaluated for 10 *Mycoplasma* spp. and 11 species of bacteria)
					[48]

multiplex qPCR Pneumo 4B/*M. bovis* *M. haemolytica* *P. multocida* *H. somni*	tracheal aspirate samples (n = 176)	10 genome copies; 1.1–3.3 $\log_{10}$ CFU/0.5 mL	0.96	0.71 (evaluated for 6 *Mycoplasma* spp. and 66 species of bacteria)	[49]
multiplex qPCR Mastit 4/*M. bovis* *Staphylococcus aureus* *Streptococcus agalactiae* *Streptococcus uberis*	milk samples	-	-	-	[26]
real-time multiplex RPA/*M. bovis/uvrC* *M. haemolytica/nmaA*	deep nasopharyngeal swabs (n = 100)	40 genome copies/reaction	-	98.0 (evaluated for 10 *Mycoplasma* spp. and 35 species of bacteria)	[50]
real-time multiplex PCR PathoProof™ Mastitis Major 4.2/*M. bovis* *Staphylococcus aureus* *Streptococcus agalactiae* *Streptococcus uberis*	milk samples	-	-	-	[13]

Table 3. *Cont.*

Assay/Target	Samples	Limit of Detection	Sensitivity	Specificity	Reference
real-time PCR VetMAX™ *M. bovis*	tissue samples, bronchoalveolar lavage fluid samples, synovial fluid, milk samples	10 genome copies/reaction	100%	100% (evaluated for 50 other bacteria species, including *M. agalactiae*, *Streptococcus uberis* and *Streptococcus dysgalactiae*	[27]
LAMP/*uvr*C, *gyr*B	milk samples from 95 dairy farms	5×10^1 CFU/mL	96.8%–100%	94.7%–100% (evaluated for 2 *Mycoplasma* spp. and 4 species of bacteria)	[51]
LAMP/*opp*D	milk samples from individual quarters (n = 9); bulk tank milk samples (n = 59)	10 genome equivalents/reaction; 1×10^4 cells/mL	87.5%	82.4% (evaluated for 3 *Mycoplasma* spp.)	[47]
PURE-LAMP not applicable	bulk tank milk samples (n = 12); mature milk samples (n = 73); colostrum/transitional milk samples (n = 74); mastitis milk samples (n = 122)	$>10^2$ CFU/mL of milk	57.0%–97.0%	100% (evaluated for 5 *Mycoplasma* spp.)	[52]
RPA-LFD/*uvr*C, *opp*D-*opp*F	nasal swab samples (n = 288); fresh lung samples (n = 80); joint fluid samples (n = 32); bulk tank milk samples (n = 42)	20 genome copies/reaction	99.0%	95.61% (evaluated for 10 *Mycoplasma* spp. and 13 species of bacteria)	[53]
MALDI-TOF MS	culture-enriched bronchoalveolar lavage fluid samples (n = 104)	not applicable	86.6%	86.4%	[54]

5.1. Real-Time PCR Assays for *M. bovis* Detection

Detection of *M. bovis* by real-time PCR preceded by culture enrichment of the samples improves detection when DNA is present at low concentrations. Furthermore, a selective broth-enrichment step increases the probability of *Mycoplasma* recovery when compared to direct plating on agar [55]. In the real-time PCR assay [45], milk samples from dairies and lung tissue samples were culture-enriched in PPLO broth for 24 h before analysis. In another qPCR for *M. bovis* testing [46], the nasopharyngeal swabs were cultured for 3–5 days before the analysis. The molecular methods are optimized for the detection of *M. bovis* in nasopharyngeal swabs and milk samples, but they can be optimized to be used for the detection of *M. bovis* in different specimens [2,26,27,48,49]. In 2020, a qPCR was developed for the detection of *M. bovis* in tracheal aspirate samples derived from calves [49]. In research on *M. bovis* intramammary infection, the presence of this pathogen in colostrum and additionally in milk from clinical cases was assessed with qPCR [26]. It is also possible to detect *M. bovis* in processed semen [2,48]. The real-time PCR assays are characterised often by a low limit of detection (LOD) and specificity near to 100% [45–48]. Taking into consideration that the number of mycoplasmas that are shed during the infection is about $>1 \times 10^6$ CFU/mL in milk [4] and the LOD for real-time PCR for *M. bovis* detection in milk is 1.3×10^2 CFU/mL [48], the probability of the detection of infected cow in a herd is high. To assess the best sensitivity, the real-time PCR assays for *M. bovis* detection are usually used after an enrichment procedure of the samples. Additionally, centrifugation of the milk and plating the resuspended pellet of bacteria improves detection of mycoplasmas with culture. After such treatment, it was four times more likely to detect of a positive sample when compared to traditional culture regarding very small concentrations [56]. The combination of culture of viable bacteria and qPCR results enables the most accurate confirmation of active infection in animals.

5.2. Fast and Cost-Effective Assays for *M. bovis* Detection

Another approach for *M. bovis* detection is to design a simple and cost-effective assay run at a single temperature without the need of using specific equipment, which will be useful to process in developing countries. LAMP is recently of interest because it enables results to be received quickly, and the reaction is normally completed in less than 2 h; furthermore, there is no need to have expensive laboratory equipment, as it is performed at a single temperature [57]. LAMP gives better results than qPCR when performed on purified DNA but is susceptible to contamination. Two assays, namely LAMP and qPCR developed for *M. bovis* detection in milk samples from individual cow quarters and bulk tank milk samples, accurately detected *M. bovis* isolates but gave false positive results for one *Mycoplasma bovigenitalium* isolate [47]. Another method called isothermal DNA amplification assay, a technique based on recombinase polymerase amplification (RPA) with lateral flow dipstick (LFD), allows one to obtain the result in 30 min and is dedicated for *M. bovis* DNA extracted directly from clinical samples i.e., nasal swabs, lungs tissue samples, joint fluids and bulk tank milk samples; no cross-reactions were observed with other *Mycoplasma* species [53]. Usually, LAMP assays are more sensitive than end-point PCRs, for example high sensitivity and specificity for all milk sample types was obtained with the use of LAMP combined with a procedure for ultra-rapid extraction (PURE-LAMP), in which various sample types i.e., bulk tank milk, mature milk, colostrum/transitional milk and mastitis milk were examined [52]. Similar parameters were obtained in LAMP for the examination of *M. bovis* in milk from mastitis cases [51].

5.3. Immunohistochemistry and In-Situ Hybridization

Although molecular methods are advantageous, they can only provide the data on *M. bovis* DNA, and there is lacking information about the presence of viable bacteria. Immunohistochemistry (IHC) and in-situ hybridization (ISH) are types of techniques which have the advantage that they are able to detect the localization of *M. bovis* antigen or DNA, respectively, in the examined tissue of the infected animals [12,19,41,58,59]. The IHC used in the study on calves experimentally infected with

M. bovis allows one to detect *M. bovis* antigen in the bronchiolar epithelial cells in the lung tissue with histopathological changes that are characteristic for bronchiolitis [19]. Results of another experiment proved that *M. bovis* antigen was detected on the surface and inside the cytoplasm of bronchiolar epithelial cells in the pneumonic foci and in the cytoplasm of phagocytes at the margin of bronchiolar exudates [58]. In the study on aborted foetus and neonatal calf that were infected with *M. bovis*, its antigen was found with the use of IHC in the brain, liver, lungs and placenta of aborted foetus, and ISH showed the presence of its DNA i.e., in lungs and placenta of the examined animals [41]. The research on long-term survival of *M. bovis* in tissues of infected calves showed the persistence of this pathogen in necrotic lung lesions several weeks after the infection with the use of both methods [59]. It is also possible to examine the pulmonary samples of calves with BRD. IHC was used to detect the *M. bovis* antigen intralesional in different areas of the lungs [12]. However, while these techniques allow one to obtain significant information, they are also expensive and labour intensive and require trained staff.

5.4. A Matrix-Assisted Laser Desorption/Ionization Time-of-Flight Mass Spectrometry for M. bovis Detection

The matrix-assisted laser desorption/ionization time-of-flight mass spectrometry (MALDI-TOF MS) procedure has been applied to *M. bovis* detection. It was optimised for the detection of *M. bovis* isolates and found to be a suitable test for routine diagnostics in cattle, especially those from BRD cases. The protocol enables the identification of *M. bovis* from bronchoalveolar lavage fluid (BALF) after enrichment in culture. The higher number of positive samples was obtained after 72 h of enrichment. The main advantage of MALDI-TOF MS is that it only detects viable bacteria, which indicates that cattle have active rather than historic infections [54].

5.5. Molecular Typing

The analysis of *M. bovis* isolates with typing and sequencing methods can give additional information about their relationships and evolution. The multilocus sequence typing (MLST) analysis was proved to be suitable for molecular typing of *M. bovis* and the assessment of geographical relatedness of isolates. The MLST scheme based on eleven housekeeping genes was evaluated. Three genes, *dnaN*, *metS* and *hsp70*, were taken for the sequence analysis and the remaining eight genes, i.e., *adk*, *efp*, *gmk*, *gyrB*, *polC*, *rpoB*, *tpiA* and *uvrC* were not chosen for the further analysis. It allows the acquiring of information on sequence variation, its type of distribution and disappearance of some sequence types [60]. A later study [61] assessed two MLST schemes for *M. bovis* isolate typing. The comparison of the performance of the two MLST schemes and additional identification of a new reference scheme capable of full typing of the examined isolates was made. The PubMLST reference method contains *adh-1*, *gltX*, *gspA*, *gyrA*, *gyrB*, *pta-2*, *tdk* and *tkt* locus; it is thought to be discriminatory and informative enough, but in this study, *adh-1*, one of the typing loci of *M. bovis* isolates, was missed. According to this reference scheme, the *adh-1* locus should be retired from the analysis. This approach was not beneficial for the study because the discrimination index received with the use of the six remaining PubMLST loci failed to reach the benchmark recommended for a reference method, and the addition of a seventh locus had to be made. The alternative scheme contains seven loci: *aptA*, *dnaA*, *metS*, *recA*, *rpoD*, *tkt* and *tufA*. The comparisons of examined *M. bovis* genome sequences identified the *dnaA* locus from the alternative scheme as the optimal replacement for *adh-1*.

Another approach for epidemiological studies is the use of whole genome sequencing (WGS) to evaluate the molecular epidemiology and genomic diversity of *M. bovis* isolates as well as their genetic relationship. The single nucleotide polymorphism (SNP) analysis can be used to assess the intraspecies relationship and the presence of a dominant genotype that can be associated with one type of disease. This study is relevant to better understand the global epidemiology of this important pathogen and to assess control strategies [62]. Comparison of the *M. bovis* sequences can be used in assessing the genetic diversity of the strains [63] or to get the information about gene virulence [64].

WGS was used in New Zealand to track the outbreaks first identified in 2017. In all, 171 isolates from 30 infected herds have so far been sequenced, and results indicate that the current outbreak was probably caused by recent entry of the mycoplasma, perhaps 1–2 years before detection, from a single source either as a single border crossing of a single clone or, potentially, up to three border crossings of three very closely related clones from the same source (TAG 2019) probably in germplasm imported from Europe.

5.6. Serological Approaches

Serological diagnosis based on detection of specific antibodies to *M. bovis* is suitable and practical for the assessment of prevalence and epidemiological studies of herds [39]. Although serological testing is a reliable method for identification of infected animals, specific antibodies do not appear until 10 to 14 days after the infection but remain elevated for several months [65]. Various indirect ELISAs are used for anti-*M. bovis* antibody detection in cattle herds. The BIO K302 ELISA (BioX Diagnostics) was applied for evaluation of antibody response to *M. bovis* in serum and milk samples [13,66,67]. A study conducted in Belgium [67] showed that the ELISA is able to detect *M. bovis* specific antibodies in bulk tank milk up to 12 months after the outbreak of the disease. Researchers [66] examined bulk milk tank samples for all Danish herds with this ELISA and concluded that the cut-off value should be increased from 37%, as suggested for animal-level diagnosis, to 50%, to obtain more adequate sensitivity and specificity for bulk tank milk analysis. On the other hand, as a result of a European inter-laboratory comparison conducted on 180 serum samples, the sensitivity and specificity of BIO K302 ELISA was determined to be 49.1% and 89.6%, respectively [68]. However, in 2020 it was confirmed that this ELISA was suitable for the serological evaluation of anti-*M. bovis* antibodies in longitudinal studies. Despite the low number of apparent clinical mastitis cases, it was useful in evaluation of *M. bovis* seroprevalence in dairy herds, which was on average 38% (16–76%), as mentioned before [13].

Another indirect ELISA, made in-house and based on a fragment of a recombinant mycoplasma immunogenic lipase A (MilA), was developed [69]. This assay can be also useful for bulk tank milk sample analysis. The results of the presence of anti-*M. bovis* antibodies in bulk tank milk were positively correlated with the antibody detection in sera of the examined animals. Additionally, there was made a comparison between BIO K 260 (BioX Diagnostics) and the MilA ELISA [23], and the latter test gave a higher number of positive samples for *M. bovis*, and they were more convergent with those obtained with culture or real-time PCR. The obtained sensitivity and specificity for this test was 94.3% and 94.4%, respectively. Additionally, it was shown that the MilA ELISA is also suitable for testing the presence of anti-*M. bovis* antibodies in the early stages of calf life (from the 3rd week of life) [70].

5.7. Interlaboratory Trials of Diagnostic Tests

M. bovis causes serious health problems in cattle herds almost all over the world, but its detection is not harmonised as yet and relies on different diagnostic methods, often in-house molecular techniques based on a variety of target genes and various different DNA extraction methods. There was conducted a European interlaboratory comparison of the diagnostic utility of the molecular tests for *M. bovis* detection [71]. Six laboratories from different countries were included in the study. Five different DNA extraction methods from bacterial culture and BALF samples were used. The molecular tests were made with the use of seven different PCR assays based on *polC*, *oppD*, *uvrC* and V4-V4 16S rRNA target genes. The comparison revealed that although the research used various assays, they had comparable diagnostic utility for *M. bovis* detection in cattle. The analytical specificity of the different PCR methods was comparable for all of the laboratories, except one, where *M. agalactiae* was detected because of the use of 16S rRNA target gene. The LOD was from 10 to 10^3 for the real-time, and from 10^3 to 10^6 CFU/mL for the end-point assays. According to the authors, this difference was acceptable. Cultures correctly detected the presence of *M. bovis* in bronchoalveolar lavage fluid samples and were consistent with PCR results. The recent comparison of diagnostic methods used in the different veterinary laboratories fortunately showed consensus.

5.8. Mixed Infections

Other *Mycoplasma* spp. can also be associated with *M. bovis* infections in cattle. In BRD cases, most often *M. dispar*, *M. canis* and *M. arginini* are implicated [3,72]. In mastitis mycoplasmatica and reproductive disorders, *M. bovigenitalium*, *M. californicum* and *M. alkalescens* can also participate [73,74]. A test based on PCR with the 16SrRNA target gene and separation of the PCR products using denaturing gradient gel electrophoresis (PCR–DGGE) enabled the differentiation of 13 *Mycoplasma* spp. of bovine origin in mixed infections [75]. Traditionally, culture is used for the confirmation of BRD infections, but the incubation period for each examined bacterial pathogens is different and samples inoculated onto agar plates are often overgrown with other, fast growing bacteria. For that reason, the multiplex real-time PCRs used by the laboratories [49,50,76] are the most suitable for simultaneous direct detection of *M. bovis* and other pathogens involved in BRD, such as *P. multocida*, *M. haemolytica* and *H. somni*, in contrast to methods not dedicated for different pathogen identification in mixed infections such as one-target PCR, traditional culture or MALDI-TOF MS [77]. When using one target PCR, there is no information about the involvement of other pathogens in the disease, different bacteria have various growth requirements and slow growing bacteria can be easily overgrown by others, and MALDI-TOF MS is not able properly detect all organisms from polymicrobial samples.

Various diagnostics methods for fast and accurate detection of *M. bovis* in various sample types and typing methods for identification and analysis of its strains in the last few years have been developed for evaluation of the disease course. Methods should be chosen according to the purpose of the survey, for herd-level testing or for individuals, or should be considered in terms of its usage for the specimen. The use of a combination of molecular, serological and culture-based methods is necessary for reliable diagnosis of diseases caused by this pathogen in cattle.

6. Control—Recommendations for *M. bovis* Control Programs

Due to the lack of efficient vaccines against *M. bovis* and increasing trends in antimicrobial resistance of *M. bovis* field isolates, it is important to provide consistent, possibly unified rules for effective control and/or eradication of *M. bovis* infections. However, in many ways, preventing the spread of *M bovis* into healthy herds is relatively easy, as the screening of small numbers of cattle from source herds by serological tests, such as ELISA, can ensure that herds remain free of disease; this was successfully achieved in the Republic of Ireland when the national herd free of *M. bovis* was restocked following the BSE crisis [78]. Whether the Irish national herd is still free is unknown. However, few countries have active eradication plans for *M. bovis*, and because of its presence in all cattle-rearing countries, it is not subject to OIE regulations; indeed, it is very difficult for countries to impose trade restrictions when they themselves are infected. Israel has attempted to identify countries that export infected livestock into their country by mass screening between 2010–2011 and found cattle from Lithuania, Hungary and Australia to be highly seropositive [79].

Undoubtedly the most ambitious and unique plan for the complete eradication of *M. bovis* was made in New Zealand where infection was first recognised in 2017. The decision was made to cull infected and contact cattle when the number of infected farms was low but now remains increasingly challenging though still feasible according to Technical Advisory Group in 2019 [25] because of the high number of infected farms traced subsequently. To date over 2000 infected farms have been traced, although most without clinical or gross pathological signs. Detecting infected farms proved difficult at first because of the use of relatively insensitive diagnostic tests, but now serological ELISA testing bulk tank milk is being used in parallel with real-time PCRs. This has increased confidence that eradication can be achieved, although the process is likely to take at least 5 years or maybe longer.

In Finland, there is a voluntary *M. bovis* control program (Animal Health ETT) for cattle farms since 2013, which four years later associated 75% of all dairy farms [2,23].

Pasteurisation or heat treatment is one of proposals to eliminate the risk of *M. bovis* shedding via colostrum or raw milk. Another alternative may be to avoid pooling of colostrum within endemically infected farms, discarding colostrum originating from *M. bovis* affected cows, or colostrum purchasing as replacer [27]. As previously documented, a commercial on-farm pasteurizer was able to destroy *Mycoplasma* spp. tested in 71.7 °C for 15 s, including *M. bovis*. Additional data showed an average 25% reduction in total immunoglobulin concentration in colostrum after 30 min pasteurization, from 22% at the low temperature range (63.9–66.7 °C) to 27% at high temperatures (68.3–70.8 °C) [80]. However, heat treatment of colostrum may affect cytokine absorption and immune response in neonatal calves. A reduction in the circulating IL-1β in dairy calves fed colostrum heat-treated to 60 °C for 60 min was demonstrated, although without affecting other immune parameters tested such as IFN-γ or IgG concentrations [81].

The generally recommended rule to control subclinical intramammary infections due to *M. bovis* is sampling of cows with high somatic cell counts (SCC) in milk; however, as was shown in some studies, cows with no clinical signs of mastitis and low SCCs (<200,000 cells/mL) can be *M. bovis* positive [13,82]. However, these differences may be a result of the disease stage. The study of Kauf et al. [83] showed that infusion of a mastitic *M. bovis* strain in one quarter of ten first-lactation cows with milk SCCs of <200,000 cells/mL caused initial increase in mean milk SCCs within 66 h post infusion. During the study period, the SCC counts fluctuated, with a peak value of 119.82×10^6 cells/mL at 90 h following the infusion; however, they persisted at a higher level than the control until the end of the study at 240 h post infection [83].

It was recommended that clinically affected *M. bovis* cows should be separated and moved from the main milking group to hospital or another group to prevent the infection spread in the herd. According to the author's opinion, cows within main milking group should be constantly monitored via bulk tank milk testing [13]. However, there was evidence of *M. bovis* mastitis incidence and transmission in the hospital pen following the introduction of cows with *M. bovis* clinical mastitis from three different milking pens, which should not be underestimated [84]. Bulk tank milk testing seems to be effective due to previously reported mycoplasma shedding via milk of cows with mastitis at above 1×10^6 CFU/mL [4]. It was suggested that if a positive result is obtained in bulk tank milk testing, it is a good strategy to follow up with pooled milk samples from five cows to identify the individuals [85]. However, SCC screening in bulk tank milk for *M. bovis* infection control does not appear to be effective [13]. An important suggestion for programs designed for *M. bovis* mastitis control is milk testing of newly introduced animals into the lactating herd. Additionally, using antibiotics to treat *M. bovis* mastitis should be discouraged [4].

One recommendation for *M. bovis* control programs is to combine regular monitoring of mastitic cows and pneumonia calves with bulk tank milk testing and longitudinal screening of young stock in herds [23].

Another option in the prevention/eradication of *M. bovis* infections is farm sanitization using effective disinfectants. Only a few studies on disinfectant efficacy in inactivating *M. bovis* has been undertaken. The most recent study estimated the efficacy of different dilutions of citric acid and sodium hypochlorite against *M. bovis*. The results showed that the acceptance criterion for an effective disinfectant of 10^6 fold reduction in the *M. bovis* viability was met for 0.5% citric acid and 1% sodium hypochlorite in the presence of organic material. However, in the absence of organic material, a 10^6 fold reduction in the *M. bovis* viability was observed for 0.25% citric acid and 0.04% sodium hypochlorite [86]. In another study, the efficacy of five different classes of teat dips were tested against *M. bovis* in the context of their use in maintaining pre- and post-milking hygiene and preventing *M. bovis* mastitis. All of them showed germicidal activity against *M. bovis*, but the iodine-based formulation was the most effective in this study [87].

To reduce the risk of *M. bovis* shedding in semen, it is worth paying more attention to the type and volume of antibiotics added to seminal extenders, because currently used mixtures have a more bacteriostatic rather than bactericidal effect on *M. bovis*. According to the author, the antibiotic combination in seminal extenders should be re-evaluated or alternatively *M. bovis* testing in processed semen should be performed [2].

Above all, it is important to recognize the subclinically infected cattle, which can be facilitated by regular monitoring/screening of different age groups of animals using various methods to prevent uncontrolled *M. bovis* shedding [23].

In summary, *M. bovis* infections are difficult to control/eradicate most of all due to the intracellular nature of the pathogen and biofilm production, which effectively hamper disease treatment. Additionally, increasing trends in antimicrobial resistance of field *M. bovis* isolates reduce the effectiveness of the therapy used routinely for *M. bovis* infections. The high genetic and antigenic variability of field *M. bovis* strains makes them easier to avoid the host immune response. In addition, the general chronic nature of the disease facilitates the spread of the mycoplasma in the herd. Additionally, the lack of effective vaccines makes the eradication of *M. bovis* infections very difficult from cattle population. The relentless and silent spread of *M. bovis* into the infection-free areas is also a feature of this disease. Therefore, regular monitoring/screening of different age groups of animals should be applied, especially for early detection of subclinical carriers in cattle herds; work is also required to develop effective vaccines to provide suitable control of *M. bovis* infections. Finally, there is also an urgent need to develop uniform recommendations that will be included in the programs designed for *M. bovis* infection control.

Author Contributions: Conceptualization, K.D.; writing—original draft preparation, K.D., R.A.J.N., E.S.; writing—review and editing, D.B. All authors have read and agreed to the published version of the manuscript.

References

1. Ministry for Primary Industries. First Case of Mycoplasma Bovis Found in Bay of Plenty. 2017. Available online: https://www.tvnz.co.nz/one-news/new-zealand/first-case-mycoplasma-bovis-found-in-bay-plenty (accessed on 20 June 2020).
2. Haapala, V.; Pohjanvirta, T.; Vähänikkilä, N.; Halkilahti, J.; Simonen, H.; Pelkonen, S.; Soveri, T.; Simojoki, H.; Autio, T. Semen as a source of *Mycoplasma bovis* mastitis in dairy herds. *Vet. Microbiol.* **2018**, *216*, 60–66. [CrossRef] [PubMed]
3. Nicholas, R.; Ayling, R.; McAuliffe, L. *Mycoplasma Diseases of Ruminants*, 1st ed.; CABI Publishing: Oxford, UK, 2008.
4. Nicholas, R.A.J.; Fox, L.K.; Lysnyansky, I. Mycoplasma mastitis in cattle: To cull or not to cull. *Vet. J.* **2016**, *216*, 142–147. [CrossRef] [PubMed]
5. Klein, U.; de Jong, A.; Youala, M.; El Garch, F.; Stevenin, C.; Moyaert, H.; Rose, M.; Catania, S.; Gyuranecz, M.; Pridmore, A.; et al. New antimicrobial susceptibility data from monitoring of *Mycoplasma bovis* isolated in Europe. *Vet. Microbiol.* **2019**, *238*, 108432. [CrossRef] [PubMed]
6. Houlihan, M.G.; Veenstra, B.; Christian, M.K.; Nicholas, R.; Ayling, R. Mastitis and arthritis in two dairy herds caused by *Mycoplasma bovis*. *Vet. Rec.* **2007**, *160*, 126–127. [CrossRef]
7. Maeda, T.; Shibahara, T.; Kimura, K.; Wada, Y.; Sato, K.; Imada, Y.; Ishikawa, Y.; Kadota, K. *Mycoplasma bovis*-associated suppurative otitis media and pneumonia in bull calves. *J. Comp. Pathol.* **2003**, *129*, 100–110. [CrossRef]
8. Alberti, A.; Filippa Addis, M.; Chessa, B.; Cubeddu, T.; Profiti, M.; Rosati, S.; Ruiu, A.; Pittau, M. Molecular and antigenic characterization of a *Mycoplasma bovis* strain causing an outbreak of infectious keratoconjunctivitis. *J. Vet. Diagn. Invest.* **2006**, *18*, 41–51. [CrossRef]
9. Kinde, H.; Daft, B.M.; Walker, R.L.; Charlton, B.R.; Petty, R. *Mycoplasma bovis* associated with decubital abscesses in Holstein calves. *J. Vet. Diagn. Invest.* **1993**, *5*, 194–197. [CrossRef]
10. Kanda, T.; Tanaka, S.; Suwanruengsri, M.; Sukmawinata, E.; Uemura, R.; Yamaguchi, R.; Sueyoshi, M. Bovine Endocarditis Associated with *Mycoplasma bovis*. *J. Comp. Pathol.* **2019**, *171*, 53–58. [CrossRef]
11. Pardon, B.; Callens, J.; Maris, J.; Allais, L.; Van Praet, W.; Deprez, P.; Ribbens, S. Pathogen-specific risk factors in acute outbreaks of respiratory disease in calves. *J. Dairy Sci.* **2020**, *103*, 2556–2566. [CrossRef]

12. Oliveira, T.E.S.; Pelaquim, I.F.; Flores, E.F.; Massi, R.P.; Valdiviezo, M.J.J.; Pretto-Giordano, L.G.; Alfieri, A.A.; Saut, J.P.E.; Headley, S.A. *Mycoplasma bovis* and viral agents associated with the development of bovine respiratory disease in adult dairy cows. *Transbound. Emerg. Dis.* **2019**, *67*, 82–93. [CrossRef]
13. Hazelton, M.S.; Morton, J.M.; Parker, A.M.; Sheehy, P.A.; Bosward, K.L.; Malmo, J.; House, J.K. Whole dairy herd sampling to detect subclinical intramammary *Mycoplasma bovis* infection after clinical mastitis outbreaks. *Vet. Microbiol.* **2020**, *244*, 108662. [CrossRef] [PubMed]
14. Punyapornwithaya, V.; Fox, L.K.; Hancock, D.D.; Gay, J.M.; Alldredge, J.R. Association between an outbreak strain causing mycoplasma bovis mastitis and its asymptomatic carriage in the herd: A case study from Idaho, USA. *Prev. Vet. Med.* **2010**, *93*, 66–70. [CrossRef] [PubMed]
15. Ayling, R.D.; Rosales, R.S.; Barden, G.; Gosney, F.L. Changes in antimicrobial susceptibility of *Mycoplasma bovis* isolates from Great Britain. *Vet. Rec.* **2014**, *175*, 486. [CrossRef] [PubMed]
16. Gautier-Bouchardon, A.V.; Ferré, S.; Le Grand, D.; Paoli, A.; Gay, E.; Poumarat, F. Overall decrease in the susceptibility of *Mycoplasma bovis* to antimicrobials over the past 30 years in France. *PLoS ONE* **2014**, *9*, e87672. [CrossRef]
17. Sulyok, K.M.; Kreizinger, Z.; Fekete, L.; Hrivnák, V.; Magyar, T.; Jánosi, S.; Schweitzer, N.; Turcsányi, I.; Makrai, L.; Erdélyi, K.; et al. Antibiotic susceptibility profiles of *Mycoplasma bovis* strains isolated from cattle in Hungary, Central Europe. *BMC Vet. Res.* **2014**, *10*, 256. [CrossRef]
18. Ayling, R.D.; Baker, S.E.; Peek, M.L.; Simon, A.J.; Nicholas, R.A.J. Comparison of in vitro activity of danofloxacin, florfenicol, oxytetracycline, spectinomycin and tilmicosin against recent field isolates of *Mycoplasma bovis*. *Vet. Rec.* **2000**, *146*, 745–747. [CrossRef]
19. Dudek, K.; Bednarek, D.; Ayling, R.D.; Kycko, A.; Reichert, M. Preliminary study on the effects of enrofloxacin, flunixin meglumine and pegbovigrastim on *Mycoplasma bovis* pneumonia. *BMC Vet. Res.* **2019**, *15*, 371. [CrossRef]
20. Ridley, A.; Hateley, G. *Mycoplasma bovis* investigations in cattle. *Vet. Rec.* **2018**, *183*, 256–258.
21. Dudek, K.; Bednarek, D.; Ayling, R.D.; Kycko, A.; Szacawa, E.; Karpińska, T.A. An experimental vaccine composed of two adjuvants gives protection against *Mycoplasma bovis* in calves. *Vaccine* **2016**, *34*, 3051–3058. [CrossRef]
22. Nicholas, R.A.; Ayling, R.D.; Stipkovits, L.P. An experimental vaccine for calf pneumonia caused by *Mycoplasma bovis*: Clinical, cultural, serological and pathological findings. *Vaccine* **2002**, *20*, 3569–3575. [CrossRef]
23. Vähänikkilä, N.; Pohjanvirta, T.; Haapala, V.; Simojoki, H.; Soveri, T.; Browning, G.F.; Pelkonen, S.; Wawegama, N.K.; Autio, T. Characterisation of the course of *Mycoplasma bovis* infection in naturally infected dairy herds. *Vet. Microbiol.* **2019**, *231*, 107–115. [CrossRef] [PubMed]
24. Nicholas, R.A. Bovine mycoplasmosis: Silent and deadly. *Vet. Rec.* **2011**, *168*, 459–462. [CrossRef] [PubMed]
25. Technical Advisory Group (TAG) Report. 2019. Available online: https://www.mpi.govt.nz/dmsdocument/37754-report-of-the-mycoplasma-bovis-technical-advisory-group-tag-in-response-to-the-terms-of-reference-june-2019-18-october-2019 (accessed on 5 August 2020).
26. Timonen, A.A.E.; Autio, T.; Pohjanvirta, T.; Häkkinen, L.; Katholm, J.; Petersen, A.; Mõtus, K.; Kalmus, P. Dynamics of the within-herd prevalence of *Mycoplasma bovis* intramammary infection in endemically infected dairy herds. *Vet. Microbiol.* **2020**, *242*, 108608. [CrossRef] [PubMed]
27. Gille, L.; Evrard, J.; Callens, J.; Supré, K.; Grégoire, F.; Boyen, F.; Haesebrouck, F.; Deprez, P.; Pardon, B. The presence of *Mycoplasma bovis* in colostrum. *Vet. Res.* **2020**, *51*, 54. [CrossRef]
28. Passchyn, P.; Piepers, S.; De Meulemeester, L.; Boyen, F.; Haesebrouck, F.; De Vliegher, S. Between-herd prevalence of *Mycoplasma bovis* in bulk milk in Flanders, Belgium. *Res. Vet. Sci.* **2012**, *92*, 219–220. [CrossRef]
29. Stott, G.H.; Wiersma, F.; Menefee, B.E.; Radwanski, F.R. Influence of environment on passive immunity in calves. *J. Dairy Sci.* **1976**, *59*, 1306–1311. [CrossRef]
30. Alabdullah, H.; Schneider, C.; Fox, L. Effect of dexamethasone administration on shedding of *Mycoplasma bovis* in calves. In Proceedings of the Third International Symposium on Mastitis and Milk Quality, St. Louis, MO, USA, 22–24 September 2011.
31. Alabdullah, H.A.; Fox, L.K.; Gay, J.M.; Barrington, G.M.; Mealey, R.H. Effects of dexamethasone and *Mycoplasma bovis* on bovine neutrophil function *in vitro*. *Vet. Immunol. Immunopathol.* **2015**, *164*, 67–73. [CrossRef]
32. Ayling, R.D.; Bashiruddin, S.E.; Nicholas, R.A.J. *Mycoplasma* species and related organisms isolated from ruminants in Britain between 1990 and 2000. *Vet. Rec.* **2004**, *155*, 413–416. [CrossRef]

33. Gagea, M.I.; Bateman, K.G.; Shanahan, R.A.; van Dreumel, T.; McEwen, B.J.; Carman, S.; Archambault, M.; Caswell, J.L. Naturally occurring *Mycoplasma bovis*-associated pneumonia and polyarthritis in feedlot beef calves. *J. Vet. Diagn. Invest.* **2006**, *18*, 29–40. [CrossRef]
34. Ryan, M.J.; Wyand, D.S.; Hill, D.L.; Tourtellotte, M.E.; Yang, T.J. Morphologic changes following intraarticular inoculation of *Mycoplasma bovis* in calves. *Vet. Pathol.* **1983**, *20*, 472–487. [CrossRef]
35. Foster, A.P.; Naylor, R.D.; Howie, N.M.; Nicholas, R.A.; Ayling, R.D. *Mycoplasma bovis* and otitis in dairy calves in the United Kingdom. *Vet. J.* **2009**, *179*, 455–457. [CrossRef] [PubMed]
36. Ayling, R.; Nicholas, R.; Hogg, R.; Wessels, J.; Scholes, S.; Byrne, W.; Hill, M.; Moriarty, J.; O'Brien, T. *Mycoplasma bovis* isolated from brain tissue of calves. *Vet. Rec.* **2005**, *156*, 391–392. [CrossRef] [PubMed]
37. Kanci, A.; Wawegama, N.K.; Marenda, M.S.; Mansell, P.D.; Browning, G.F.; Markham, P.F. Reproduction of respiratory mycoplasmosis in calves by exposure to an aerosolised culture of *Mycoplasma bovis*. *Vet. Microbiol.* **2017**, *210*, 167–173. [CrossRef] [PubMed]
38. Jasper, D.E.; Al-Aubaidi, J.M.; Fabricant, J. Epidemiologic observations on mycoplasma mastitis. *Cornell Vet.* **1974**, *64*, 407–415.
39. Maunsell, F.P.; Woolums, A.R.; Francoz, D.; Rosenbush, R.F.; Step, D.L.; Wilson, D.J.; Janzen, E.D. *Mycoplasma bovis* infections in cattle. ACVIM Consensus Statement. *J. Vet. Intern. Med.* **2011**, *25*, 772–783. [CrossRef]
40. Lysnyansky, I.; Freed, M.; Rosales, R.S.; Mikula, I.; Khateb, N.; Gerchman, I.; van Straten, M.; Levisohn, S. An overview of *Mycoplasma bovis* mastitis in Israel (2004–2014). *Vet. J.* **2016**, *207*, 180–183. [CrossRef]
41. Hermeyer, K.; Peters, M.; Brügmann, M.; Jacobsen, B.; Hewicker-Trautwein, M. Demonstration of *Mycoplasma bovis* by immunohistochemistry and in situ hybridization in an aborted bovine fetus and neonatal calf. *J. Vet. Diagn. Invest.* **2012**, *24*, 364–369. [CrossRef]
42. Pfützner, H.; Sachse, K. *Mycoplasma bovis* as an agent of mastitis, pneumonia, arthritis and genital disorders in cattle. *Rev. Sci. Tech. Off. Int. Epiz.* **1996**, *15*, 1477–1494. [CrossRef]
43. Poumarat, F.; Longchambon, D.; Martel, J.L. Application of dot immunobinding on membrane filtration (MF dot) to the study of relationships within "M. mycoides cluster" and within "glucose and arginine-negative cluster" of ruminant mycoplasmas. *Vet. Microbiol.* **1992**, *32*, 375–390. [CrossRef]
44. Nicholas, R.A.J.; Baker, S.E. Recovery of mycoplasmas from animals. In *Mycoplasma Protocols*; Miles, R.J., Nicholas, R.A.J., Eds.; Humana Press: Totowa, NJ, USA, 1998; pp. 37–44.
45. Behera, S.; Rana, R.; Gupta, P.K.; Kumar, D.; Sonal; Rekha, V.; Arun, T.R.; Jena, D. Development of real-time PCR assay for the detection of *Mycoplasma bovis*. *Trop. Anim. Health Prod.* **2018**, *50*, 875–882. [CrossRef]
46. Andrés-Lasheras, S.; Zaheer, R.; Ha, R.; Lee, C.; Jelinski, M.; McAllister, T.A. A direct qPCR screening approach to improve the efficiency of *Mycoplasma bovis* isolation in the frame of a broad surveillance study. *J. Microbiol. Methods* **2020**, *169*, 105805. [CrossRef] [PubMed]
47. Appelt, S.; Aly, S.S.; Tonooka, K.; Glenn, K.; Xue, Z.; Lehenbauer, T.W.; Marco, M.L. Development and comparison of loop-mediated isothermal amplification and quantitative polymerase chain reaction assays for the detection of *Mycoplasma bovis* in milk. *J. Dairy Sci.* **2019**, *102*, 1985–1996. [CrossRef] [PubMed]
48. Parker, A.M.; House, J.K.; Hazelton, M.S.; Bosward, K.L.; Sheehy, P.A. Comparison of culture and a multiplex probe PCR for identifying *Mycoplasma* species in bovine milk, semen and swab samples. *PLoS ONE* **2017**, *12*, e0173422. [CrossRef] [PubMed]
49. Pansri, P.; Katholm, J.; Krogh, K.M.; Aagaard, A.K.; Schmidt, L.M.B.; Kudirkiene, E.; Larsen, L.E.; Olsen, J.E. Evaluation of novel multiplex qPCR assays for diagnosis of pathogens associated with the bovine respiratory disease complex. *Vet. J.* **2020**, *256*, 105425. [CrossRef] [PubMed]
50. Conrad, C.C.; Daher, R.K.; Stanford, K.; Amoako, K.K.; Boissinot, M.; Bergeron, M.G.; Alexander, T.; Cook, S.; Ralston, B.; Zaheer, R.; et al. A Sensitive and Accurate Recombinase Polymerase Amplification Assay for Detection of the Primary Bacterial Pathogens Causing Bovine Respiratory Disease. *Front. Vet. Sci.* **2020**, *7*, 208. [CrossRef] [PubMed]
51. Ashraf, A.; Imran, M.; Yaqub, T.; Tayyab, M.; Shehzad, W.; Mingala, C.N.; Chang, Y.-F. Development and validation of a loop-mediated isothermal amplification assay for the detection of *Mycoplasma bovis* in mastitic milk. *Folia Microb.* **2018**, *63*, 373–380. [CrossRef]
52. Itoh, M.; Hirano, Y.; Yamakawa, K.; Yasutomi, I.; Kuramoto, K.; Furuok, M.; Yamada, K. Combination of procedure for ultra rapid extraction (PURE) and loop-mediated isothermal amplification (LAMP) for rapid detection of *Mycoplasma bovis* in milk. *J. Vet. Med. Sci.* **2020**, 19–0695. [CrossRef]

53. Zhao, G.; Hou, P.; Huan, Y.; He, C.; Wang, H.; He, H. Development of a recombinase polymerase amplification combined with a lateral flow dipstick assay for rapid detection of the *Mycoplasma bovis*. *BMC Vet. Res.* **2018**, *14*, 412. [CrossRef]
54. Bokma, J.; Van Driessche, L.; Deprez, P.; Haesebrouck, F.; Vahl, M.; Weesendorp, E.; Deurenberg, R.H.; Pardon, P.; Boyen, P. Rapid identification of 1 *Mycoplasma bovis* from bovine bronchoalveolar lavage fluid with MALDI-TOF MS after enrichment procedure. *J. Clin. Microbiol.* **2020**, *58*, e00004-20. [CrossRef]
55. Thurmond, M.C.; Tyler, J.W.; Luiz, D.M.; Holmberg, C.A.; Picanso, J.P. The effect of pre-enrichment on recovery of *Streptococcus agalactiae*, *Staphylococcus aureus* and mycoplasma from bovine milk. *Epidemiol. Infect.* **1989**, *103*, 465–474. [CrossRef]
56. Punyapornwithaya, V.; Fox, L.K.; Gay, G.M.; Hancock, D.D.; Alldredge, J.R. Short communication: The effect of centrifugation and resuspension on the recovery of *Mycoplasma species* from milk. *J. Dairy Sci.* **2009**, *92*, 4444–4447. [CrossRef] [PubMed]
57. Li, Y.; Fan, P.; Zhou, S.; Zhang, L. Loop-mediated isothermal amplification (LAMP): A novel rapid detection platform for pathogens. *Microb. Pathog.* **2017**, *107*, 54–61. [CrossRef] [PubMed]
58. Nunoya, T.; Omori, T.; Tomioka, H.; Umeda, F.; Suzuki, T.; Uetsuka, K. Intracellular Localization of Mycoplasma bovis in the Bronchiolar Epithelium of Experimentally Infected Calves. *J. Comp. Path.* **2020**, *176*, 14–18. [CrossRef] [PubMed]
59. Kleinschmidt, S.; Spergser, J.; Rosengarten, R.; Hewicker-Trautwein, M. Long-term survival of *Mycoplasma bovis* in necrotic lesions and in phagocytic cells as demonstrated by transmission and immunogold electron microscopy in lung tissue from experimentally infected calves. *Vet. Microbiol.* **2013**, *162*, 949–953. [CrossRef] [PubMed]
60. Bell-Rogers, P.; Parker, L.; Cai, H.Y. Multi-locus sequence types of *Mycoplasma bovis* isolated from Ontario, Canada in the past three decades have a temporal distribution. *J. Vet. Diagn. Invest.* **2018**, *30*, 130–135. [CrossRef]
61. Register, K.B.; Lysnyansky, I.; Jelinski, M.D.; Boatwright, W.D.; Waldner, M.; Bayles, D.O.; Pilo, P.; Alt, D.P. Comparison of two multilocus sequence typing schemes for *Mycoplasma bovis* and revision of the PubMLST reference method. *J. Clin. Microbiol.* **2020**, *58*, e00283-20. [CrossRef]
62. Yair, Y.; Borovok, I.; Mikula, I.; Falk, R.; Fox, L.K.; Gophna, U.; Lysnyansky, I. Genomics-based epidemiology of bovine *Mycoplasma bovis* strains in Israel. *BMC Genom.* **2020**, *21*, 70. [CrossRef]
63. Parker, A.M.; Shukla, A.; House, J.K.; Hazelton, M.S.; Bosward, K.L.; Kokotovic, B.; Sheehy, P.A. Genetic characterization of Australian *Mycoplasma bovis* isolates through whole genome sequencing analysis. *Vet. Microbiol.* **2016**, *196I*, 118–125. [CrossRef]
64. Rasheed, M.A.; Qi, J.; Zhu, X.; Chenfei, H.; Menghwar, H.; Khan, F.A.; Guo, A. Comparative genomics of *Mycoplasma bovis* strains reveals that decreased virulence with increasing passages might correlate with potential virulence-related factors. *Front. Cell. Infect. Microbiol.* **2017**, *7*, 177. [CrossRef]
65. Sachse, K.; Pfützner, H.; Hötzel, H.; Demuth, B.; Heller, M.; Berthold, E. Comparison of various diagnostic methods for the detection of *Mycoplasma bovis*. *Rev. Sci. Tech.-Off. Int. Epiz.* **1993**, *12*, 571–580. [CrossRef]
66. Nielsen, P.K.; Petersen, M.B.; Nielsen, L.R.; Halasa, T.; Toft, N. Latent class analysis of bulk tank milk PCR and ELISA testing for herd level diagnosis of *Mycoplasma bovis*. *Prev. Vet. Med.* **2015**, *121*, 338–342. [CrossRef] [PubMed]
67. Gille, L.; Callens, J.; Supré, K.; Boyen, F.; Haesebrouck, F.; Van Driessche, L.; van Leenen, K.; Deprez, P.; Pardon, B. Use of breeding bull and absence of a calving pen as a risk factors for the presence of *Mycoplasma bovis* in dairy herds. *J. Dairy Sci.* **2018**, *101*, 8284–8290. [CrossRef] [PubMed]
68. Andersson, A.-M.; Aspán, A.; Wisselink, H.J.; Smid, B.; Ridley, A.; Pelkonen, S.; Autio, T.; Lauritsen, K.T.; Kensø, J.; Gaurivaud, P.; et al. A European inter-laboratory trial to evaluate the performance of three serological methods for diagnosis of *Mycoplasma bovis* infection in cattle using latent class analysis. *BMC Vet. Res.* **2019**, *15*, 369. [CrossRef] [PubMed]
69. Wawegama, N.K.; Browning, G.F.; Kanci, A.; Marenda, M.S.; Markham, F.F. Development of a Recombinant Protein-Based Enzyme-Linked Immunosorbent Assay for Diagnosis of *Mycoplasma bovis* Infection in Cattle. *Clin. Vaccine Immunol.* **2014**, *21*, 196–202. [CrossRef] [PubMed]
70. Petersen, M.B.; Wawegama, N.K.; Denwood, M.; Markham, P.F.; Browning, G.F.; Nielsen, L.R. *Mycoplasma bovis* antibody dynamics in naturally exposed dairy calves according to two diagnostic tests. *BMC Vet. Res.* **2018**, *14*, 258. [CrossRef] [PubMed]

71. Wisselink, H.J.; Smid, B.; Plater, J.; Ridley, A.; Andersson, A.-M.; Aspán, A.; Pohjanvirta, T.; Vähänikkilä, N.; Larsen, H.; Høgberg, J.; et al. A European interlaboratory trial to evaluate the performance of different PCR methods for *Mycoplasma bovis* diagnosis. *BMC Vet. Res.* **2019**, *15*, 86. [CrossRef]
72. Chazel, M.; Tardy, F.; Le Grand, D.; Calavas, D.; Poumarat, F. Mycoplasmoses of ruminants in France: Recent data from the national surveillance network. *BMC Vet. Res.* **2010**, *6*, 32. [CrossRef]
73. Mackie, D.P.; Finley, D.; Brice, N.; Ball, H.J. Mixed mycoplasma mastitis outbreak in a dairy herd. *Vet. Rec.* **2000**, *147*, 335–336. [CrossRef]
74. Jasper, D.E. Prevalence of mycoplasmal mastitis in the western states. *Calif. Vet.* **1980**, *43*, 24–26.
75. McAuliffe, L.; Ellis, R.J.; Lawes, J.R.; Ayling, R.D.; Nicholas, R.A.J. 16S rDNA PCR and denaturing gradient gel electrophoresis; a single generic test for detecting and differentiating *Mycoplasma* species. *J. Med. Microbiol.* **2005**, *54*, 731–739. [CrossRef]
76. Loy, J.D.; Leger, L.; Workman, A.M.; Clawson, M.L.; Bulut, E.; Wang, B. Development of a multiplex real-time PCR assay using two thermocycling platforms for detection of major bacterial pathogens associated with bovine respiratory disease complex from clinical samples. *J. Vet. Diagn. Invest.* **2018**, *30*, 837–847. [CrossRef] [PubMed]
77. Pereyre, S.; Tardy, F.; Renaudin, H.; Cauvin, E.; Del Prá Netto Machado, L.; Tricot, A.; Benoit, F.; Treilles, M.; Bébéar, C. Identification and Subtyping of Clinically Relevant Human and Ruminant Mycoplasmas by Use of Matrix-Assisted Laser Desorption Ionization–Time of Flight Mass Spectrometry *J. Clin. Microbiol.* **2013**, *51*, 3314–3323. [CrossRef] [PubMed]
78. O'Farrell, K.; Dillon, P.; Mee, j.; Crosse, S.; Nnolan, M.; Byrne, N.; Reidy, M.; Flynn, F.; Condon, T. Strategy for restocking Moorepark after depopulation following BSE. *Ir. Vet. J.* **2001**, *54*, 70–75.
79. Lysnyansky, I.; Mikula, I.; Ozeri, R.; Bellaiche, M.; Nicholas, R.A.J.; van Straten, M. Mycoplasma bovis Seroprevalence in Israeli Dairy Herds, Feedlots and Imported Cattle. *Isr. J. Vet. Med.* **2017**, *72*, 13–16.
80. Stabel, J.R.; Hurd, S.; Calvente, L.; Rosenbusch, R.F. Destruction of *Mycobacterium paratuberculosis*, *Salmonella* spp., and *Mycoplasma* spp. in raw milk by a commercial on-farm high-temperature, short-time pasteurizer. *J. Dairy Sci.* **2004**, *87*, 2177–2183. [CrossRef]
81. Gelsinger, S.L.; Heinrichs, A.J. Comparison of immune responses in calves fed heat-treated or unheated colostrum. *J. Dairy Sci.* **2017**, *100*, 4090–4101. [CrossRef] [PubMed]
82. Higuchi, H.; Gondaira, S.; Iwano, H.; Hirose, K.; Nakajima, K.; Kawai, K.; Hagiwara, K.; Tamura, Y.; Nagahata, H. *Mycoplasma* species isolated from intramammary infection of Japanese dairy cows. *Vet. Rec.* **2013**, *172*, 557. [CrossRef]
83. Kauf, A.C.; Rosenbusch, R.F.; Paape, M.J.; Bannerman, D.D. Innate immune response to intramammary *Mycoplasma bovis* infection. *J. Dairy Sci.* **2007**, *90*, 3336–3348. [CrossRef]
84. Punyapornwithaya, V.; Fox, L.K.; Hancock, D.D.; Gay, J.M.; Wenz, J.R.; Alldredge, J.R. Incidence and transmission of *Mycoplasma bovis* mastitis in Holstein dairy cows in a hospital pen: A case study. *Prev. Vet. Med.* **2011**, *98*, 74–78. [CrossRef]
85. Murai, K.; Lehenbauer, T.W.; Champagne, J.D.; Glenn, K.; Aly, S.S. Cost-effectiveness of diagnostic strategies using quantitative real-time PCR and bacterial culture to identify contagious mastitis cases in large dairy herds. *Prev. Vet. Med.* **2014**, *113*, 522–535. [CrossRef]
86. Mahdizadeh, S.; Sawford, K.; van Andel, M.; Browning, G.F. Efficacy of citric acid and sodium hypochlorite as disinfectants against *Mycoplasma bovis*. *Vet. Microbiol.* **2020**, *243*, 108630. [CrossRef] [PubMed]
87. Boddie, R.L.; Owens, W.E.; Ray, C.H.; Nickerson, S.C.; Boddie, N.T. Germicidal activities of representatives of five different teat dip classes against three bovine mycoplasma species using a modified excised teat model. *J. Dairy Sci.* **2002**, *85*, 1909–1912. [CrossRef]

15

Atypical Porcine Pestivirus Circulation and Molecular Evolution within an Affected Swine Herd

Alba Folgueiras-González [1,2], Robin van den Braak [1], Bartjan Simmelink [1], Martin Deijs [2], Lia van der Hoek [2] and Ad de Groof [1,*]

[1] Department Discovery & Technology, MSD Animal Health, Wim de Körverstraat 35, P.O. Box 31, 5830AA Boxmeer, The Netherlands; alba.folgueiras.gonzalez@merck.com (A.F.-G.); robin.braak.van.den@merck.com (R.v.d.B.); bartjan.simmelink@merck.com (B.S.)

[2] Laboratory of Experimental Virology, Department of Medical Microbiology, Amsterdam UMC Location AMC, University of Amsterdam, Meibergdreef 9, 1105AZ Amsterdam, The Netherlands; m.deijs@amsterdamumc.nl (M.D.); c.m.vanderhoek@amsterdamumc.nl (L.v.d.H.)

* Correspondence: ad.de.groof@merck.com

Abstract: Atypical porcine pestivirus (APPV) is a single-stranded RNA virus from the family Flaviviridae, which is linked to congenital tremor (CT) type A-II in newborn piglets. Here, we retrospectively investigated the molecular evolution of APPV on an affected herd between 2013 and 2019. Monitoring was done at regular intervals, and the same genotype of APPV was found during the entire study period, suggesting no introductions from outside the farm. The nucleotide substitutions over time did not show substantial amino acid variation in the structural glycoproteins. Furthermore, the evolution of the virus showed mainly purifying selection, and no positive selection. The limited pressure on the virus to change at immune-dominant regions suggested that the immune pressure at the farm might be low. In conclusion, farms can have circulation of APPV for years, and massive testing and removal of infected animals are not sufficient to clear the virus from affected farms.

Keywords: pestivirus; atypical porcine pestivirus (APPV); viral persistence; congenital tremor; swine; asymptomatic; genomic sequence; phylogenetic analysis; purifying selection

---

1. Introduction

The genus Pestivirus, belonging to the Flaviviridae family, includes single-stranded, positive-sense RNA viruses of veterinary importance, causing economically relevant diseases in livestock animals, but also affecting wildlife species [1]. While for decades the International Committee on Taxonomy of Viruses (ICTV) only recognized the four so-called classical pestiviruses, namely bovine viral diarrhea virus types 1 and 2 (BVDV-1 and BVDV-2), classical swine fever virus (CSFV) and border disease virus (BDV), the discovery of seven novel atypical pestiviruses in the last few years led to the proposal of a new species-independent classification from Pestivirus A to Pestivirus K. Thus, atypical porcine pestivirus (APPV) is now classified as Pestivirus K [2]. Moreover, new pestivirus genomes in bats [3] and piglets (LINDA virus [4]) have been discovered lately, but not yet classified.

Congenital tremor (CT) in newborn piglets, also known as myoclonia congenita, "shaker pigs" or "dancing pigs", was first reported in 1922 [5]. Its characteristic clinical signs involve tremors of the head and limbs which worsen on stress situations, but are almost gone during sleep. Even though most piglets are clinically healthy at weaning time, the earlier shivering hinders their ability to feed normally from their mother, thus increasing the risk for inadequate colostrum intake, growth retardation or even death by starvation [6]. CT is divided based on its pathology into type A, which displays morphological lesions on the central nervous system, and type B, which does not show any visible morphological lesion [7].

Regarding the distinct causes of disease, type A was further differentiated into five subtypes. Type A-I is associated with one of the classical pestiviruses, CSFV, and characterized by cerebellar hypoplasia in affected pigs [8]. Types A-III and A-IV are both related to different genetic defects only present in the Landrace breed and Saddleback breed, respectively [9,10]. Type-V, also defined by cerebellar hypoplasia, is caused by food poisoning by trichlorfon in pregnant sows [11]. Meanwhile, during the decades, the causing agent of CT type A-II remained unknown, although an infectious agent was suspected [12].

APPV was first characterized in 2015 by Hause et al. [13] through metagenomic sequencing performed on a sample positive for porcine reproductive and respiratory syndrome virus (PRRSV). After its discovery, two independent studies proved APPV's link to congenital tremor in newborn piglets via the inoculation of pregnant sows with infectious animal material [14,15]. However, Koch's postulates have not been fulfilled yet due to the difficulties in establishing an appropriate substrate for in vitro culture and retrieval of pure virus stocks [16]. In 2017, Lamb et al. [4] reported a novel pestivirus, named LINDA virus (lateral-shaking inducing neurodegenerative agent), in an Austrian cohort of CT piglets. Although the clinical manifestations and pathology were similar to the ones of APPV, further phylogenetic analysis showed its proximity to Bungowannah virus, a pestivirus never detected outside Australia.

A research study by Postel et al. [17] analyzed 1460 samples of apparently healthy pigs from different countries. They showed that the prevalence of APPV genotypes was around 10% and up to 60% of the tested animals were seropositive. Kaufmann et al. [18] showed that APPV has been circulating in Switzerland at least since 1986, which was the earliest detection point worldwide. To date, APPV has been reported on four continents and fourteen different countries [19]. Mortality is high in CT-affected litters, from around 10% to as high as 30% in some affected farms [14–16].

APPV is a highly variable enveloped virus which contains a linear, non-segmented, positive-sense RNA strand of around 11–12 kb. A single open-reading frame (ORF) encodes a single polyprotein of 3635 amino acids on average, which is assumed to be cleaved co- and post-translationally into four structural (the core protein C and the envelope glycoproteins Erns, E1 and E2) and eight non-structural proteins (Npro, p7, NS2, NS3, NS4A, NS4B, NS5A and NS5B) [13]. Several novel APPV sequences have been described since the first report in 2015, further dividing the phylogenetic tree and proposing distinct divisions into three, four or five different genotypes and into numerous particular subclades [20]. To date, 58 unique full-genome sequences are available in NCBI GenBank (access date: 1 April 2020). The APPV full-genome sequences have 80–99% identity, showing high variability even within the same country, with difficulty to infer the origin, dissemination and common ancestor of several strains of the virus [19,21].

High variability in RNA viruses, caused by the lack of proofreading repair mechanisms in RNA polymerases, provides them with a selective advantage, promoting rapid adaptation to novel hosts and environments [22]. On the other hand, excessive error rates can also lead to lethal mutagenesis and threaten the viability of the viral populations [23]. Therefore, hypervariable regions that are thought to contribute to immune escape and adaptation, as well as hyperconserved elements that are fundamental for virus replication and maintenance in the population are main research topics for molecular evolution studies [24].

In the current study, we retrospectively investigated the molecular evolution and functional implication of nucleotide and amino acid substitutions in the APPV genome in a farm in the North Brabant province of The Netherlands over a period of seven years. Sampling was done consistently over time in the controlled environment of a closed-herd farm, where the full farming process is carried out within the farm, and the breeding stock is replaced by gilts from the farm itself. Therefore, by eliminating the input of animals from outside, the risk of novel viral introductions is minimized. In 2013, a first CT outbreak with positive cases of APPV was reported in the farm. Two years later, in 2015, a second APPV outbreak occurred in the same farm with clinically affected, trembling piglets that tested positive. Since then, serum samples were taken from CT piglets at the time of the outbreaks, as well as from apparently healthy pigs as part of regular farm monitoring for APPV and other porcine viruses. Pigs that tested positive were removed from the breeding population to stop the spread of the virus via persistently infected animals. However, several re-emerging peaks of viremic animals were been detected in the farm during the monitoring period, suggesting the continued circulation of APPV in clinically healthy animals.

To assess the possible biological significance of the selective pressures that shape the evolution of APPV within the farm, we looked for evidence of purifying and diversifying selection in the APPV genome. Although viral surface glycoproteins like E2 are well-known targets of positive selection, and variations in these regions can help in immune escape, we also took a full-genome study approach to get a more general, helicopter view and investigate other regions that might have been underestimated until now. The correlation of clinical CT outbreaks with fixation events of non-synonymous, but also synonymous, substitutions can reveal the link to pathogenicity and infectivity of the virus. Here, we reported, to our knowledge, the first longitudinal study on the evolution of the full-length APPV genome within a controlled farm environment. We compared molecular evolution and variability in the genome sequences found on the farm with full-genome sequences from different locations around the world.

2. Materials and Methods

2.1. Sample Collection

In 2013, the farm under study increased the population of breeding sows from 280 to 570 sows and relocated to new facilities. Piglets stayed in the farrowing unit after weaning (i.e., litters were not mixed). Piglets were vaccinated with a porcine reproductive and respiratory syndrome virus (PRRSV) live vaccine at 2 weeks of age, and with a combined porcine circovirus type 2 (PCV2) and *Mycoplasma hyopneumoniae* (*M. hyo*) vaccine at 3 weeks of age. PRRSV was regularly diagnosed in the farm and therefore a vaccination strategy in sows and piglets was set up. There were no other pathogens diagnosed in regular screenings.

Serum and fecal samples were obtained from gilts and congenitally trembling piglets during the CT outbreaks in 2013 and 2015. Between January 2016 and April 2016, serum was collected from all gilts selected for breeding (196 animals) at the age of first insemination for APPV monitoring and removal of positive animals.

To monitor the presence of APPV in serum over time, five litters with CT born from gilts during the 2015/2016 outbreak were repeatedly sampled until the age of 18 weeks. Moreover, 6 gilts (4 APPV-positive at 5 and 18 weeks of age, and 2 negative) and 2 boars (1 APPV-positive at 5 and 18 weeks of age, and 1 negative), were followed for APPV presence in serum and fecal shed until the age of 10 months. Two APPV-positive gilts were co-housed with one negative gilt, and the boars were housed next to each other with direct contact.

From April 2016 to 2019, clinically healthy 10-week-old gilts in the sow breeding line maintained on the farm were regularly monitored for the presence of APPV in serum. Samples from animals with congenital tremor symptoms were also taken for analysis. In total, 1498 samples were taken during this period.

Blood was collected using the Vacuette 5/8 mL Sep Clot Activator (Greiner-Bio One, Kremsmünster, Austria) and serum was obtained by centrifugation for 10 min at 3200× *g* at 4 °C. Fecal samples were collected using Sigma Virocult swabs and vials (MWE, Corsham, UK), vortexed, transferred to 1.5 mL Eppendorf tubes and centrifuged for 10 min at 10,000× *g* at 4 °C.

RNA was extracted from 200 μL samples by the automated MagNA Pure 96 system (Roche Applied Science, Manheim, Germany) using the protocol 'Viral NA plasma external lysis SV3.1'.

2.2. *Quantitative Reverse Transcription*

A universal, quantitative, reverse transcription PCR (qRT-PCR) was used to quantitatively detect APPV in samples using primers in the 5′-untranslated region (UTR) of the genome (APPV-PAN2-F3-B: CGYGCCCAAAGAGAAATCGG and APPV-PAN2-R3-B: CCGGCACTCTATCAAGCAGT) [14]. One-step qPCR reactions were performed in a final volume of 50 μL containing 1 μL SuperScript III RT/Platinum Taq Mix (Thermo Fisher Scientific, Waltham, MA, USA), 25 μL 2× SYBR Green Reaction Mix (Thermo Fisher Scientific, Waltham, MA, USA), 17 μL water, 1 μL forward primer (10 μM), 1 μL reverse primer (10 μM) and 5 μL of the RNA isolate. Thermocycling was performed in the CFX96 Touch real-time PCR detection system (Bio-Rad Laboratories, Hercules, CA, USA) starting with an RT reaction for 3 min at 55 °C, a pre-denaturation step for 5 min at 95 °C and 40 cycles of 15 s at 95 °C (denaturation) and 30 s at 60 °C (annealing and elongation). The specificity of SYBR Green qPCR was validated by melting curve analysis between 65 °C and 95 °C with an increasing gradient of 0.5 °C per 5 s. Results were analyzed with the CFX Manager software (Bio-Rad Laboratories, Hercules, CA, USA).

To obtain a standard curve for the quantitative analysis, a recombinant bacterial plasmid containing the 5′-UTR PCR target was made (GenScript, Piscataway, NJ, USA). The copy number of the recombinant plasmid was calculated, and eight dilution series (10^8–10^1 copies/μL) were included in duplicate in RT-qPCR to calculate the number of virus copies per μL.

2.3. *Viral Genome Amplification and Sanger Sequencing*

A starting sequence of 1073 bp obtained from a previous study using Illumina Sequencing (Amsterdam UMC, Amsterdam, The Netherlands) was used as reference [14]. This short read was mapped to the 58 full-genome sequences available in NCBI GenBank (access date: 1 April 2020). The three most similar full-genome sequences (GenBank accession numbers: KY624591.1, MH885413.1 and KX778724.1) were aligned by CLUSTALW using Geneious Prime v2019.0.4 (http://www.geneious.com) (Geneious, Auckland, New Zealand), and the consensus sequence was extracted for primer design.

The cDNA from the extracted RNA of the clinical samples (Section 2.1) was synthesized using the QuantiTect reverse transcription kit (Qiagen, Hilden, Germany) following the manufacturer's manual. The entire viral genome from the 2013 sample was amplified using an initial series of twelve overlapping PCRs. Gaps and faulty PCRs were solved following a genome walking strategy (amplification and sequencing primers available in Supplementary Table S1). PCR reactions were performed in a final volume of 25 μL containing 12.5 μL 2× Phusion High-Fidelity PCR Master Mix with HF Buffer (New England BioLabs, Ipswich, MA, USA), 0.75 μL DMSO 100%, 6.75 μL water, 1.25 μL FW 10 μM primer, 1.25 μL REV 10 μM primer and 2.5 μL of template cDNA. Thermocycling was performed in the CFX96 Touch real-time PCR detection system (Bio-Rad Laboratories, Hercules, CA, USA) using an initial denaturation step at 98 °C for 5 min, 40 cycles of 30 s at 98 °C (denaturation), 30 s at the annealing temperature optimal for the primer set and 1 min and 30 s at 72 °C (elongation), followed by 7 min at 72 °C. The PCR products were stored at 4 °C until further analysis. Five microliters of the PCR products were analyzed by agarose gel electrophoresis (1.4% *w*/*v* agarose) to check the fragment size and the specificity of the amplification. PCR products were purified using the QiaQuick PCR purification kit (Qiagen, Hilden, Germany) following the manufacturer's manual.

Sequencing PCR reactions were performed using the BigDye Terminator v3.1 cycle sequencing kit (Applied Biosystems, Carlsbad, CA, USA) in a final volume of 20 μL containing 4 μL BigDye Terminator ready reaction mix, 3 μL 2× Phusion High-Fidelity PCR Master Mix with HF Buffer (New England BioLabs, Ipswich, MA, USA), 0.5 μL DMSO 100%, 2.5 μL WFI, 2.5 μL FW or REV 10 μM primer and 7.5 μL of the purified PCR product. Thermocycling was performed in 30 cycles of 10 s at 95 °C (denaturation), 10 s at the annealing temperature optimal for the primer set and 2 min at 60 °C (elongation). The PCR products were stored at 4 °C for further analysis. The cycle sequencing products were purified using the DyeEx 2.0 Spin kit (Qiagen, Hilden, Germany) following the manufacturer's manual. Capillary electrophoresis was performed using the 3500 Genetic Analyzer (Applied Biosystems,

Carlsbad, CA, USA) and data were analyzed using the Sequencher 5.4.6 (Gene Codes, Ann Arbor, MI, USA) and Geneious Prime v2019.0.4 (Biomatters Ltd., Auckland, New Zealand) software.

Based on the obtained sequence, Sanger sequencing was performed following the same methodology on the other five samples (years 2015, 2016, 2017, 2018 and 2019) by GenScript (Piscataway, NJ, USA).

2.4. Determination of E2 Sequences

The amplification of E2-coding sequences was performed using a two-step RT-PCR protocol as described in Section 2.3. The amplification and sequencing PCR reactions of 857 bp and 953 bp fragments were performed using two primer pairs flanking the E2-coding region (E2-F1: 5′-TGGTGCCTATTGTTGTCAGG-3′, E2-R1: 5′-AGTTCTTCCTTGACGGCTAG-3′, E2-F2: 5′-GCCCTGGTGAACATAGTCAC-3′ and E2-R2: 5′-TCCTTGACGGCTAGCATTATG-3′). Capillary electrophoresis was performed using the 3500 Genetic Analyzer (Applied Biosystems, Carlsbad, CA, USA) and trimmed sequences (702 bp) were analyzed using Geneious Prime v2019.0.4 (Biomatters Ltd., Auckland, New Zealand).

2.5. Submission of Sequences

The sequences of the APPV genomes were deposited in GenBank under the accession numbers MT512531–MT512537. The partial E2-coding sequences were deposited in GenBank under the accession numbers MW011356–MW011406.

2.6. Nucleotide and Amino Acid Analysis of Variants

The obtained partial E2-coding sequences were aligned using the CLUSTALW translation alignment in Geneious Prime v2019.0.4 (Biomatters Ltd., Auckland, New Zealand) with BLOSUM cost matrix, a gap open cost of 5 and a gap extended cost of 4.

The fifty-eight full-genome APPV sequences from NCBI GenBank database (access date: 1 April 2020) were aligned along with the sequences obtained in the current study [25]. Multiple sequence alignment was performed using the CLUSTALW translation alignment in Geneious Prime v2019.0.4 (Biomatters Ltd., Auckland, New Zealand) with BLOSUM cost matrix, a gap open cost of 10 and a gap extended cost of 6.66. For the farm dataset, we called single nucleotide substitutions on the aligned genomes using Geneious Prime v2019.0.4 and differentiated them into synonymous and non-synonymous. Ambiguous nucleotide and amino acid calls, which are considered by the software as variants, were treated as missing data.

The prediction of *O*-glycosylation and *N*-glycosylation motifs in the Erns, E1 and E2 glycoproteins were performed with DictyOGlyc1.1, NetOGlyc4.0 and NetNGlyc1.0 prediction algorithms via the webserver from the Technical University of Denmark Department of Bio and Health Informatics (DTU Bioinformatics, http://www.cbs.dtu.dk/services/) [26,27].

2.7. Phylogenetic Analysis and Estimation of Evolutionary Rates within the Farm

The Recombination Detection Program version 4 (RDP4) was used to screen for recombination events on the multiple sequence alignment of the six APPV genomes found in the farm, using RDP, GENECONV, BootScan, Maxchi, Chimaera, Siscan and 3Seq methods. Recombination was considered when p-value was <0.0001 and the recombinant score was >0.6 [28].

The full-genome APPV sequences available in NCBI and the six APPV in-farm sequences obtained in this study were aligned using the CLUSTALW translation alignment in Geneious Prime v2019.0.4 (Biomatters Ltd., Auckland, New Zealand) with BLOSUM cost matrix, a gap open cost of 10 and a gap extended cost of 6.66. The phylogenetic tree was created with the MEGA X software using the neighbor-joining method with the Kimura two-parameter substitution model [29,30]. Complete deletion was done in case of gaps or missing data. The analysis was performed for 500 bootstrap replicates.

An estimation of the evolutionary rates was calculated for the obtained E2-coding sequences, as well as for the six full-genome sequences using the TempEst v1.5.3 software [31].

2.8. Selection Pressure Analysis

Selection pressure analyses were done for the multiple sequence alignment of the six farm sequences as well as for the multiple sequence alignment including the NCBI full-genome APPV sequences. Selection pressure analyses were performed on the full ORF, using mixed-effects model of evolution (MEME) and fixed-effects likelihood (FEL). All these algorithms were implemented on the HyPhy (Hypothesis Testing using Phylogenies) open-source software package and can be accessed through the Datamonkey webserver (https://www.datamonkey.org/) [32].

MEME uses a mixed-effect maximum likelihood approach. The algorithm estimates a synonymous α parameter (d_S) and a two-category mixture of non-synonymous (d_N) β parameters for each site. MEME infers two ω (d_N/d_S) classes and uses a likelihood ratio test to compare between the models and check for episodic diversifying selection. A significance threshold of $p < 0.1$ was used on the analysis [33].

The fixed-effects likelihood (FEL) algorithm was used in order to detect negatively selected sites on the alignment. FEL uses a maximum likelihood approach to infer non-synonymous (d_N) and synonymous (d_S) substitution rates, also assuming a constant selection pressure for each site on the alignment. All branches were tested for selection. A model with synonymous rate variation, where the d_S parameter in the codon model is allowed to vary across sites, was used for the analysis. A significance threshold of $p < 0.1$ was used on the analysis [24].

3. Results

3.1. 2013–2016: Congenital Tremor Outbreaks, Follow Up Studies and Eradication Strategy Design

In 2013, the farm increased the internal population of breeding sows, aimed to breed gilts for the replacement of production sows (sows breeding line) from 280 to 570 sows and, at the same time, relocated to new facilities with state-of-the-art climate control and housing conditions. Piglets stayed in the farrowing unit after weaning, thus litters were not mixed. In the same year, a first large-scale CT outbreak was reported on the farm and a second large-scale outbreak occurred at the end of 2015/early 2016. Both outbreaks were related with positive cases of APPV and various other clinical observations (e.g., reduced vitality and mortality of the piglets, and increased return to estrus percentage). In the time between 2013 and 2015, no major abnormalities were observed, although incidentally few piglets with tremors were seen, but with no impact on production.

During the 2015–2016 outbreak, CT prevalence varied from 5% in litters from fourth parity sows, up to 55% in litters from first and second parity sows. In the latter case, the mortality in the farrowing unit ranged from 25% in litters from second parity sows to 69% in the ones from first parity sows. The related effects on the production data are shown in Supplementary Table S2.

After the second large-scale outbreak, it was decided to monitor all gilts selected for breeding for the presence of APPV, both purebred line gilts and production gilts. Serum of those animals was analyzed at the age of first insemination with the aim to remove positive gilts from the breeding population. A universal, quantitative, reverse transcription PCR (qRT-PCR) was used to quantitatively detect APPV on pig serum samples. This strategy was applied between January and April 2016, during which time 196 gilts were tested and 15% of them tested positive for APPV (Supplementary Table S3).

During parallel monitoring of pigs born with CT and positive for APPV in serum, we observed that a significant percentage of pigs turned PCR-negative for APPV in serum around the age of 18 weeks. The piglets born with CT were considered as persistent carriers of the virus and, at the time of weaning, the virus was still present in the piglets that still showed recognizable, but less severe, tremors. A follow-up of these piglets showed that the percentage of APPV-positive PCR scores in serum was reduced to 45% at 18 weeks of age, with viral copy numbers in serum also being greatly reduced (Supplementary Table S4).

To gain further insight into the dynamics of APPV viremia, 6 gilts (4 APPV-positive at 5 and 18 weeks of age, and 2 negative), and 2 boars (1 APPV-positive at 5 and 18 weeks of age, and 1 negative), were followed for APPV presence in serum until the age of 10 months. Two APPV-positive gilts were co-housed with one negative gilt, in separate cages, and the boars were housed next to each other with direct contact. No APPV was detected in any of the 8 animals at the age of 24 weeks and at any time point thereafter, with the exception of 1 boar testing PCR-positive at the age of 32 weeks (Supplementary Table S5). Fecal shed from the same animals was also monitored until the age of 10 months via qPCR. Results showed, in the age range between 24 and 44 weeks, intermittent shedding in the feces of the persistently infected (PI) gilts and temporary presence in the feces of horizontally infected gilts (Supplementary Table S6).

3.2. 2016–2019: Re-Emergence of Congenital Tremor and Monthly Quantitative Detection of APPV

Since April 2016, when regular sampling from clinically healthy 10-week-old gilts in the sow breeding line maintained on the farm started, serum samples were received monthly for APPV monitoring purposes. Until December 2019, a total of 1505 serum samples from 10–16-week-old pigs were analyzed.

Figure 1 shows the percentage of APPV-positive animals among the tested set for each month since the screening started in April 2016 until the last analyzed data from December 2019. In this period, two peaks of CT symptoms in newborn piglets were detected in the farm in April 2016 and May 2017 (blue columns in Figure 1). In order to diminish horizontal transmission of the virus in the sow breeding population, infected APPV pigs detected during the monitoring were removed from the population as these were likely persistently infected.

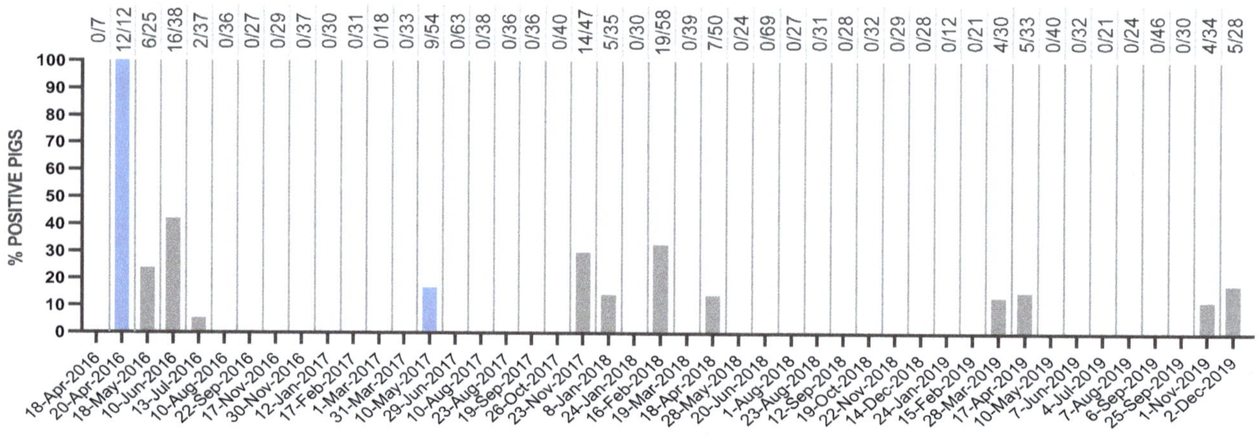

Figure 1. Percentage of atypical porcine pestivirus (APPV)-positive pigs detected during monthly screening in the farm by RT-qPCR analysis. The x-axis shows the sampling date from April 2016 to December 2019. The percentage of positive samples is shown in the y-axis. Blue-colored columns show that positive PCR results were accompanied by clinical CT symptoms on those specific months—i.e., April 2016 and May 2017. The number of PCR-positive animals in relation to the total number tested each specific month is shown above the columns.

3.3. Characterization of APPV Sequences

Forty-eight E2-coding sequences were determined from the APPV-positive samples collected during monthly monitoring in the farm at different time points between 2016 and 2019, along with three sequences obtained previously in 2013 and 2015 during the large-scale CT outbreaks (Supplementary Table S7). The E2-coding sequences showed a maximum pairwise genetic distance of only 0.71%. The low genetic diversity observed within the farm supported the hypothesis that only one viral strain was circulating in the herd with no viral introductions from the outside.

The amino acid sequences were also compared according to the collection date (Supplementary Figure S1). Samples obtained from different animals at the same time point showed a completely identical genome, with the exception of the highly mutated codon D752, varying to either Gly, Ser or Asn residues (Section 3.5). Besides, a more thorough approach was taken for the samples obtained from affected animals at the time of the CT outbreaks, with 8 out of 12 sequences obtained in April 2016 and 8 out of 9 in May 2017. No characteristic differences were seen at those time points that could lead to an explanation of the distinct symptoms in relation to the nucleotide or amino acid sequences.

3.4. Phylogenetic Analysis and Estimation of Evolutionary Rates of APPV within the Farm

A phylogenetic analysis of the full-length APPV sequences available worldwide and obtained from the NCBI database and six APPV sequences obtained in the present study (Section 3.5) confirmed the division of APPV into three different clades, two of them containing only sequences from China (Figure 2). APPV sequences from the current study clustered in one subtree together with two German sequences (NC_030653 and KU041639, from 2015), one Austrian sequence (KX778724, from 2016), two Chinese sequences (MH885413, from 2018, and KY624591, from 2016) and one South Korean sequence (MF979135, from 2016). The other full-APPV genome from The Netherlands available in NCBI was clustered within the same clade, but into a different subtree, together with eight sequences from Switzerland and two from the US (Figure 2).

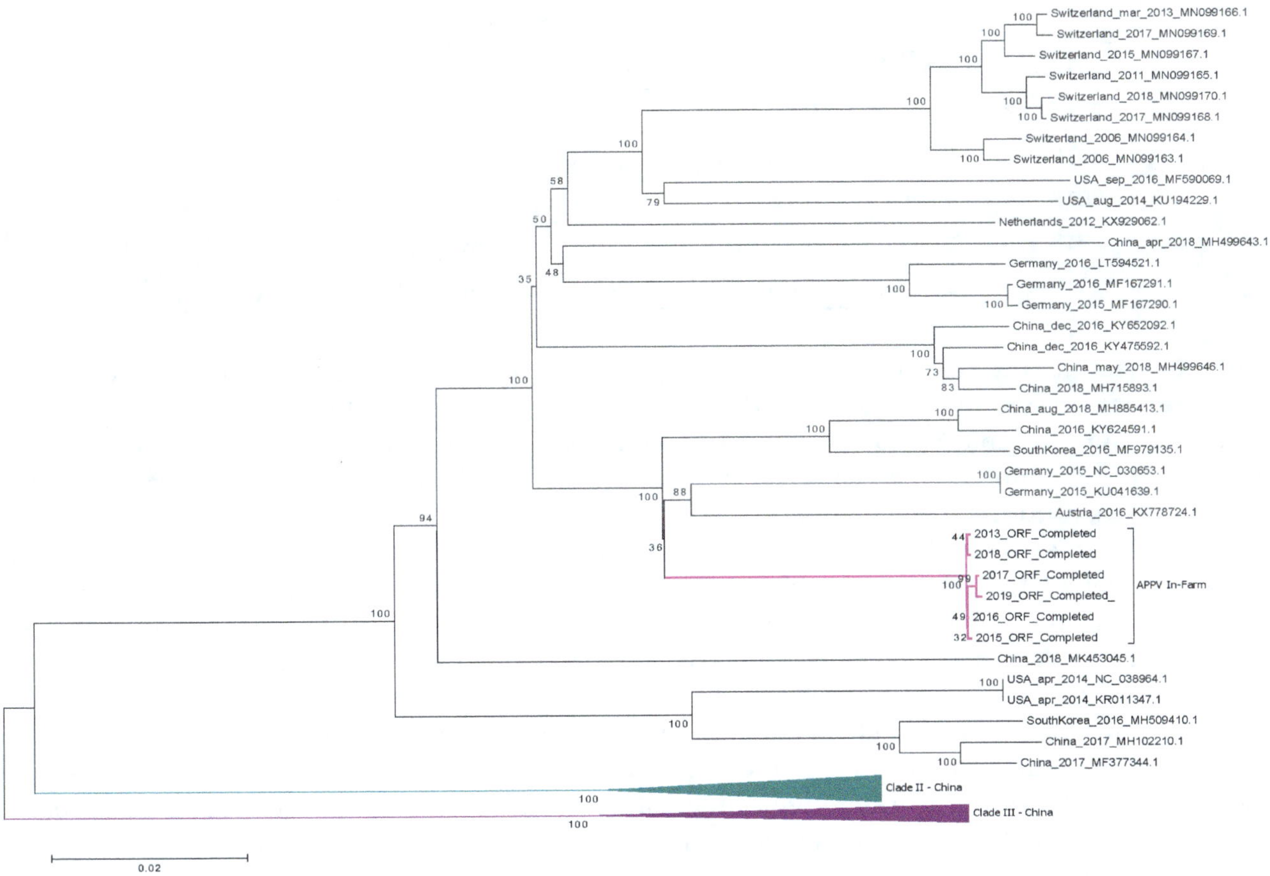

Figure 2. Phylogenetic analysis of the complete coding region alignment of atypical porcine pestivirus (APPV) sequences worldwide obtained from NCBI database and six APPV sequences retrieved in the present longitudinal study on the Dutch swine farm between 2013 and 2019. The neighbor-joining method with the Kimura two-parameter substitution model was used. Gaps and missing data were

subjected to complete deletion. Bootstrap values are provided at the root of the clusters. The scale bar is a measure of the proportion of divergence. Run for 500 bootstrap replicates. Clade I shown as expanded tree. Clades II and III, containing only sequences from China, are collapsed and shown in green and purple in the lower part of the tree. APPV branches obtained in the current study are shown in pink.

3.5. *Genome and Protein Variations of APPV within the Farm*

The samples with the highest numbers of APPV genome copies were selected from each of the years, and six full-length APPV genomic sequences from samples collected in the farm on 2013 and each year between 2015 and 2019, were determined. The 2013 and 2015 APPV genome sequences were obtained from serum samples from CT-affected piglets at the time of the large-scale outbreaks. The length of the complete APPV in-farm coding sequence (excluding the 5′-UTR region) was 10,908 nt, in line with the previously reported length of the coding region [14]. Multiple sequence alignment was performed on these six sequences using the CLUSTALW translation alignment in Geneious Prime v2019.0.4. The sequences from the different years showed a high similarity at the nucleotide level, between 99.74% and 99.90%. The number of nucleotide differences ranged from only 10 nucleotide substitutions between 2017 and 2019 genomes to 26 nucleotide substitutions between 2013 and 2017 genomes. On the amino acid level, the differences ranged from only 1 amino acid substitution between 2017 and 2019 to 7 amino acid substitutions between 2013 and 2017 and between 2016 and 2017 (Table 1).

Table 1. Distance matrix from the multiple sequence alignment of six in-farm APPV sequences.

	2013	2015	2016	2017	2018	2019
2013		3 aa	7 aa	6 aa	3 aa	5 aa
2015	18 nt		4 aa	3 aa	2 aa	3 aa
2016	17 nt	15 nt		7 aa	6 aa	6 aa
2017	26 nt	18 nt	23 nt		4 aa	1 aa
2018	16 nt	13 nt	15 nt	19 nt		5 aa
2019	25 nt	21 nt	21 nt	10 nt	20 nt	

The nucleotide substitutions found in the alignment were classified regarding their protein location and differentiating synonymous substitutions and non-synonymous substitutions. All substitutions are shown in Supplementary Table S8. Forty-five nucleotide substitutions were found along the APPV genome during the monitoring years in the farm from which thirty-four positions corresponded to synonymous substitutions. Eleven non-synonymous substitutions occurred on the APPV genome in the farm between 2013 and 2019. Among those, one amino acid change, V563A, was in the structural glycoprotein gene E1, while two amino acid changes, I726V and D752G, were in the E2 structural glycoprotein encoding region. The other eight non-synonymous substitutions occurred in the genes of non-structural proteins: two in Npro (S48P and H152L), one in NS2 (R1122K), three in NS5A (K2437R, G2550E and A2824T) and two in NS5B (D2979N and N3166T) (Supplementary Table S8).

Some amino acid changes in the strains have not been described before. The E1 non-synonymous substitution V563A only occurred within the farm, while the genotype of this site worldwide was always conserved as a Val residue. The synonymous substitution found on the same coding gene, V567, was also exclusive, when compared with other sequences in Clade I. Interestingly, site T608 in the in-farm sequences possessed a unique genotype compared with the consensus I608, and the V608 variant present as well in Clades II and III. Moreover, site I790 also showed a unique genotype, found only in one sequence from Switzerland from 2011 (accession number MN099165), while a Val residue is encoded on that position in the sequences worldwide. The glycosylation status of the pestivirus glycoproteins plays an important role in virulence. In this line, the substitution on E2 glycoprotein D752 to a Gly, Ser or Asn residue (Supplementary Table S8, Supplementary Figure S1) modified the 752NDT754 N-glycosylation motif predicted by NetNGlyc1.0 server (http://www.cbs.dtu.dk/services/). In the non-structural proteins, a unique motif was found in the N-terminal protease. The site 126KPAPASR132 was unique within the APPV sequences retrieved from the current farm study, including up to four modifications on its amino acid chain, in comparison with other geographically distinct APPV full genome sequences.

An estimation of the evolutionary rates within the farm was calculated for the full ORF of the APPV genome, as well as for the E2 glycoprotein-the coding sequence using TempEst v1.5.3 software [31]. An evolutionary rate of 3.224×10^{-4} substitutions/site/year (correlation coefficient = 0.9009; $R^2 = 0.8117$) was estimated for the full ORF of APPV over a period of six years of evolution, from 2013 to 2019, within the studied farm. The envelope glycoprotein E2, considered in all pestiviruses as the main antigen eliciting immune response, had an estimated evolutionary rate of 9.347×10^{-4} substitutions/site/year (correlation coefficient = 0.7706; $R^2 = 0.5938$). Both evolutionary rates were in line with the ones reported in other pestivirus species. The evolution of the CSFV E2 gene was estimated between 1.73×10^{-3} and 5.76×10^{-4} substitutions/site/year [34,35], while the full genome estimation was 1.03×10^{-4} substitutions/site/year [36]. For BVDV, evolutionary rates of 1.40×10^{-4} substitutions/site/year for the full genome and 1.26×10^{-3} substitutions/site/year for the E1-E2 coding region were reported [37]. A recombination analysis was done using the RDP4 software in order to find breakpoints within the multiple sequence alignment that might have undergone recombination, and to screen them for evidence of phylogenetic incongruence previous to phylogenetic tree building [28]. No recombination events were found at the farm level.

3.6. *Selection Patterns within a Farm: Six-Year Evolution Study on an APPV in-Farm Variant*

Negative, also called purifying, selection consists of the evolutionary pressure hindering the fixation of non-beneficial or deleterious protein variations in the population. On the other hand, positive or diversifying selection is the evolutionary pressure that promotes the fixation of beneficial protein variations in the population. This last one can be considered pervasive, when it is constant through time, or episodic, when it is sporadic and affecting only some lineages. Using the algorithms implemented in the HyPhy software packages via the Datamonkey webserver [32], we were able to identify a number of codons potentially subjected to selection pressures on our APPV genome between 2013 and 2019.

No positively selected codons, neither episodic nor pervasive, were found by any of the methods. Thus, positive selection cannot be considered as an evolution pattern within the farm during the six years of the study. On the other hand, FEL (fixed-effects likelihood) found evidence of pervasive negative/purifying selection at 9 sites among the 3635 codons, with a p-value threshold of 0.1. The nine codons subjected to purifying selection were found to be in the N-terminal protease (codon 132), the Erns glycoprotein (codon 418), the NS2 protein (codons 1054 and 1198), the NS3 protein (codon 1814), the NS5A protein (codons 2676 and 2848) and the NS5B protein (codons 2905 and 3243). FEL algorithm indicated, under the global MG94xREV model, a total non-synonymous/synonymous rate ratio for the in-farm alignment equal to 0.172, indicating the prevalence of negative selection within the APPV genome sequence.

4. Discussion

In 2013, a first large-scale CT outbreak was reported in a farm in The Netherlands, with a second large-scale outbreak at the end of 2015/early 2016, both related to APPV infections. After the second outbreak, all gilts selected for breeding were monitored by serum PCR screening at the age of first insemination for the presence of APPV with the aim of removing infected animals from the breeding population. However, there were some practical limitations to this approach: (1) The removal of a high percentage of the selected gilts at the age of first insemination severely disrupted the normal farm sow replacement strategy. (2) Serological tests were not available at the time and thus, the difference between persistent carriers and gilts with horizontal infections could not be established. (3) Parallel monitoring of persistently infected pigs from the second outbreak revealed that, in contrast to what it may have been expected based on experience with other pestiviruses, APPV disappeared from the serum in adult pigs. The data published by Schwartz et al. [16] showed stable presence of APPV in serum until 14 weeks of age, but our observations on a larger number of animals showed that a significant percentage of pigs turned PCR-negative for APPV around the age of 18 weeks.

Fecal shed was also monitored to potentially identify persistently APPV-infected pigs. In the age range between 24 and 44 weeks, monitoring APPV infection is difficult due to the absence of the virus in serum and intermittent shedding in the feces of PI gilts. Horizontally infected gilts show temporary presence in feces and serum. Therefore, a gilt-monitoring strategy was technically complicated and could lead to false-negative test results and consequently, the maintenance of persistently infected animals in the breeding population. It is of note that APPV-positive fecal shed has not proven to be infectious.

Based on these considerations, we reasoned that the early removal of PI animals in the purebred gilt breeding population, by performing qPCR analysis on serum samples before the age of 16 weeks, was the best strategy to control APPV at the farm level. Hence, a monthly monitoring program for APPV infections in 10-week-old selected breeding gilts of the sow breeding line was set up in the "closed" CT-affected farm with the purpose of reducing the risk of horizontal APPV infections to pregnant gilts and subsequent vertical infection of newborn piglets. It was assumed that these persistent carriers of APPV, often born without showing clinical symptoms after vertical transmission of the virus and with subsequent use in the farm sow replacement breeding program, contributed significantly to the risk of infections of pregnant gilts and low-parity sows in group housing. The results of our analysis showed that even with stringent removal of APPV PCR-positive, assumed persistently infected replacement gilts, the virus cannot be completely eliminated from the farm. The genotype remained unchanged throughout the years, as demonstrated by the low genetic diversity observed in the partial E2-coding sequences from the samples obtained during monthly monitoring, making it unlikely that new introductions via sperm were involved in the continuing APPV infections in the farm. Re-emerging peaks of viremic animals, often without symptoms of the disease but incidentally with the birth of CT piglets during these six years within this closed-herd farm, even with infected breeding animals removed from the population, showed that the virus was difficult to control let alone eliminate. Besides, the E2-coding sequences obtained from the majority of affected animals at the time of the CT outbreaks did not show any characteristic difference at the nucleotide nor amino acid level when compared to the asymptomatic carriers that could lead to an explanation for the clinical manifestation.

The hypervariable regions, which contribute to virus escape from the immune system, as well as the conserved elements involved in crucial virus replication processes and maintenance of the viral population, are obvious targets for drug and vaccine design [24]. Moreover, it can be hypothesized that certain substitutions in the viral coding sequence may be involved in the cyclic peaks of viremia and/or correlate with the pathogenicity of the virus. In the present study, forty-five nucleotide substitutions were found along the APPV genome during the monitoring years in the farm, eleven of them causing an amino acid change. Among those, two occurred on the E2 protein-coding gene, usually recognized as the main antigen able to elicit neutralizing antibodies in infected animals [38,39]. Recent studies on subunit E2 vaccines from APPV have shown strong immune responses in mice [40]. Moreover, E1–E2 heterodimers have been considered in other pestivirus species as key for viral infectivity [38]. Although the results obtained after the analysis of the APPV sequences on the followed farm did not point at any positively selected sites, two of the non-synonymous substitutions found on the heterodimer-coding genes were almost unique to the farm under study. More interestingly, the substitution D752G in E2 glycoprotein, which showed high variability throughout the fifty-one partial E2 sequences analyzed, modified the predicted 752NDT754 *N*-glycosylation motif. Generally, E2 glycosylation sites are highly conserved due to their primary role in viral entry and infection and their removal has shown viral attenuation in other pestivirus species [41]. Further research needs to be done to decipher the functionality of this highly variable motif.

The unique motif 126KPAPASR132 was found in the N-terminal protease in all APPV sequences retrieved from the farm. This motif included up to four modifications on its amino acid chain, in comparison with other geographically distinct APPV full-genome sequences. Although the exact functionality of this site is not known, Npro plays an important role in viral evasion of the innate immune response in other pestivirus species. Npro activity decreases the levels of the interferon regulatory factor 3 (IRF3) via proteasomal degradation, inhibiting its downstream signaling and thus suppressing type-I interferon responses in infected animals [42]. Previous research studies have related the functionality of this protein with the enhancement of co-infections with bovine respiratory syncytial virus (BRSV) in cattle [43]. APPV in persistently infected animals is commonly found together with other viruses and, it may therefore intensify those secondary infections. More importantly, experimental Erns and Npro mutations in the BVDV genome have failed to induce persistent infections in cattle [44].

The other 34 substitutions found along the APPV genome during the six years evolution in the farm, but not leading to amino acid changes, are not less important as the codon usage bias has been related to virus translation efficiency [45], RNA structures critical for replication and packing [46] and enhanced virulence [47]. Future studies on the codon usage and effects on RNA structure using reverse genetics may therefore shed light on the actual effect of synonymous substitutions. We are aware of the fact that, with only six full-genome sequences included in the current study, our results were based on a limited amount of sequence data. However, given the dynamics of the virus at the farm, we had maximized our analysis possibilities. Pigs with high APPV loads in serum, which are needed for a successful sequencing strategy, were only occasionally observed and, in addition, pigs from the same litter were expected to have the same viral genotype, as demonstrated by the partial E2 sequences obtained from a large number of samples, and further sequence analysis would not add meaningful data. Moreover, the limited genome variation shown within the farm suggested that more sequences obtained during the same years would not radically change the observations and conclusions drawn in the present study. Nonetheless, we acknowledge that an increase in the number of APPV full-length sequences available, especially within longitudinal studies, will be key for the scientific community to further understand the evolutionary dynamics and genomic features of this pestivirus.

With regard to the evolutionary pressures of APPV, the present study showed a general genome-wide purifying pressure, especially strong on the non-structural proteins. These results indicated the importance for the virus to maintain the functionality of the non-structural viral proteins, avoiding the fixation of detrimental amino acid substitutions that might hinder the virus ability to evade the host immune system and cause persistent infections. In Flaviviridae, non-structural proteins have been determined as key players in viral escape from the host immune system. Hepatitis C virus (HCV) NS3 protein inhibits tumor necrosis factor alpha (TFN-α) stimulated NF-κB activation to evade the host innate immunity [48]; NS4A proteins of dengue virus 1 (DENV-1) inhibit the interferon- β (IFN-β) signaling pathway mediated by the retinoic acid-inducible gene I (RIG-I) and TANK-binding kinase-1 (TBK1) proteins [49]; and NS5 protein of several flaviviruses is also involved in the inhibition of IFN signaling by degrading the signal transducer and activator of transcription 1 (STAT1) or STAT2 [50,51]. Even though the signaling pathways and target sites of the majority of the non-structural proteins remain unknown for several virus species, these examples acknowledge their potential function in the host innate immune evasion. The strong purifying selection we found could be explained by a lack of pressure from the host immune system, as the persistently infected animals may potentially be immunotolerant, although experimental evidence is needed to ultimately confirm this hypothesis. Regular use of ELISA systems, to monitor whether immunity is raised to the virus, would bring light to this issue [39].

Monitoring studies in APPV-infected farms during the last years showed that APPV caused persistent infections in piglets when they were infected in-utero, occasionally developing congenital tremors, while horizontal infections within the herd were transient and without visible clinical signs [39]. As aforementioned, this is similar to BVDV infections in cattle, which only causes persistent infections in the calves when the virus is transmitted in-utero before 120 days of gestation. While some persistently infected calves are born with congenital malformations, others are clinically healthy with BVDV infections going unnoticed until the onset of clinical signs in the new parities [52]. A widely accepted hypothesis, supported by several research studies, is that non-cytopathic BVDV strains fail to induce type-I interferon responses in the infected fetus developing persistent infections and immunotolerant calves [52,53]. These persistently infected animals shed the virus continuously during their lifetimes, provoking transient horizontal infections within the herds, but more importantly infecting pregnant cows leading to the birth of persistently infected calves [54].

Our study results of APPV circulation on the affected sow farm showed similarities with the ways that BVDV persists within the cattle populations. Persistently APPV-infected animals remained undetected in a population that was not continuously monitored by PCR because they did not always show congenital tremors. Although our control strategy did not result in full elimination of the virus, at least it resulted in no further large-scale outbreaks since early 2016. Our approach was based on the hypothesis that persistently infected gilts are the main contributors to the spread of the virus and thus, removing those indirectly leads to the prevention of infections of pregnant sows. Nevertheless, the combination with a direct approach based on the elimination of infected pregnant animals could further improve the eradication strategy, as experimental studies have shown that virus infection during early stages of gestation leads to viremia and transplacental transfer.

Research on APPV vaccines is still limited. High strain heterogenicity and persistent infections have been a major bottleneck in the case of BVDV vaccination [55], and for APPV the same problems will be encountered when vaccines are designed and tested. Importantly, effective controlling strategies in closed farm situations should start with intensive testing of all the animals in the herd, followed by removal of positive carriers from the population. Testing should not only be done via RT-qPCR in serum, but also in fecal swabs, as it has been observed that the virus disappears from blood while it can still (intermittently) be present in feces [14]. The strategy presented in this study was not adequate to fully eliminate the virus; APPV kept circulating in the sow population after removal of persistent carriers in the sow breeding herd, suggesting that all gilts should be monitored. In addition, serological data could reveal if the virus is still circulating within the herd via horizontal infections. Vaccination of seronegative gilts and sows is an option that can be considered if removal of carriers alone does not sufficiently control APPV infections.

Supplementary Materials:
Table S1: List of amplification and sequencing primers used in the study; Table S2: Details on the production data of the studied farm during the 2015–2016 CT outbreak; Table S3: Serum APPV monitoring of gilts selected for breeding at the age of first insemination between January and April in 2016; Table S4: Follow-up of five litters with CT born from gilts for the presence of APPV in serum over time (2015/2016 outbreak); Table S5: Follow-up of boars and gilts until the age of 10 months for the presence of APPV in serum (2015/2016 outbreak); Table S6: Follow-up of boars and gilts until the age of 10 months for the presence of APPV in fecal shed (2015/2016 outbreak); Table S7: APPV E2 sequencing sample list and corresponding APPV viral loads; Table S8: Nucleotide substitutions in the APPV in-farm multiple sequence alignment; Figure S1: Multiple sequence alignment of the partial APPV E2 amino acid sequences chronologically ordered.

Author Contributions: Conceptualization, A.F.-G., A.d.G. and L.v.d.H.; methodology, A.F.-G., L.v.d.H., M.D., R.v.d.B. and B.S.; software, A.F.-G., R.v.d.B. and B.S.; data analysis, A.F.-G.; writing—original draft preparation, A.F.-G.; writing—review and editing, A.d.G., L.v.d.H. and R.v.d.B.; supervision, A.d.G. and L.v.d.H. All authors have read and agreed to the published version of the manuscript.

Acknowledgments: The authors wish to acknowledge the input of the veterinarian Jolanda Rooijendijk, from DAC de Peelhorst, and the farmers who sent in samples of diseased animals. We thank Ignacio Postigo-Hidalgo for useful discussions on bioinformatics.

References

1. Blome, S.; Beer, M.; Wernike, K. New Leaves in the Growing Tree of Pestiviruses. *Adv. Virus Res.* **2017**, *99*, 139–160. [CrossRef] [PubMed]
2. Smith, D.B.; Meyers, G.; Bukh, J.; Gould, E.A.; Monath, T.; Scott Muerhoff, A.; Pletnev, A.; Rico-Hesse, R.; Stapleton, J.T.; Simmonds, P.; et al. Proposed revision to the taxonomy of the genus Pestivirus, family Flaviviridae. *J. Gen. Virol.* **2017**, *98*, 2106–2112. [CrossRef] [PubMed]
3. Wu, Z.; Liu, B.; Du, J.; Zhang, J.; Lu, L.; Zhu, G.; Han, Y.; Su, H.; Yang, L.; Zhang, S.; et al. Discovery of Diverse Rodent and Bat Pestiviruses With Distinct Genomic and Phylogenetic Characteristics in Several Chinese Provinces. *Front. Microbiol.* **2018**, *9*, 2562. [CrossRef]
4. Lamp, B.; Schwarz, L.; Hogler, S.; Riedel, C.; Sinn, L.; Rebel-Bauder, B.; Weissenbock, H.; Ladinig, A.; Rumenapf, T. Novel Pestivirus Species in Pigs, Austria, 2015. *Emerg. Infect. Dis.* **2017**, *23*, 1176–1179. [CrossRef]
5. Kinsley, A.T. Dancing pigs. *Vet. Med.* **1922**, *17*, 123.
6. Done, J.T.; Woolley, J.; Upcott, D.H.; Hebert, C.N. Porcine congenital tremor type AII: Spinal cord morphometry. *Br. Vet. J.* **1986**, *142*, 145–150. [CrossRef]
7. Done, J.T. Congenital Nervous Diseaseas of Pigs: A Review. *Lab. Anim.* **1968**, *2*, 207–217. [CrossRef]
8. Bradley, R.; Done, J.T.; Hebert, C.N.; Overby, E.; Askaa, J.; Basse, A.; Bloch, B. Congenital tremor type AI: Light and electron microscopical observations on the spinal cords of affected piglets. *J. Comp. Pathol.* **1983**, *93*, 43–59. [CrossRef]
9. Blakemore, W.F.; Harding, J.D.; Done, J.T. Ultrastructural observations on the spinal cord of a Landrace pig with congenital tremor type AIII. *Res. Vet. Sci.* **1974**, *17*, 174–178. [CrossRef]
10. Patterson, D.S.; Sweasey, D.; Brush, P.J.; Harding, J.D. Neurochemistry of the spinal cord in British Saddleback piglets affected with congenital tremor, type A-IV, a second form of hereditary cerebrospinal hypomyelinogenesis. *J. Neurochem.* **1973**, *21*, 397–406. [CrossRef]
11. Knox, B.; Askaa, J.; Basse, A.; Bitsch, V.; Eskildsen, M.; Mandrup, M.; Ottosen, H.E.; Overby, E.; Pedersen, K.B.; Rasmussen, F. Congenital ataxia and tremor with cerebellar hypoplasia in piglets borne by sows treated with Neguvon vet. (metrifonate, trichlorfon) during pregnancy. *Nord. Vet. Med.* **1978**, *30*, 538–545. [PubMed]
12. Patterson, D.S.; Done, J.T.; Foulkes, J.A.; Sweasey, D. Neurochemistry of the spinal cord in congenital tremor of piglets (type AII), a spinal dysmyelimogenesis of infectious origin. *J. Neurochem.* **1976**, *26*, 481–485. [CrossRef] [PubMed]
13. Hause, B.M.; Collin, E.A.; Peddireddi, L.; Yuan, F.; Chen, Z.; Hesse, R.A.; Gauger, P.C.; Clement, T.; Fang, Y.; Anderson, G. Discovery of a novel putative atypical porcine pestivirus in pigs in the USA. *J. Gen. Virol.* **2015**, *96*, 2994–2998. [CrossRef] [PubMed]
14. de Groof, A.; Deijs, M.; Guelen, L.; van Grinsven, L.; van Os-Galdos, L.; Vogels, W.; Derks, C.; Cruijsen, T.; Geurts, V.; Vrijenhoek, M.; et al. Atypical Porcine Pestivirus: A Possible Cause of Congenital Tremor Type A-II in Newborn Piglets. *Viruses* **2016**, *8*, 271. [CrossRef]
15. Arruda, B.L.; Arruda, P.H.; Magstadt, D.R.; Schwartz, K.J.; Dohlman, T.; Schleining, J.A.; Patterson, A.R.; Visek, C.A.; Victoria, J.G. Identification of a Divergent Lineage Porcine Pestivirus in Nursing Piglets with Congenital Tremors and Reproduction of Disease following Experimental Inoculation. *PLoS ONE* **2016**, *11*, e0150104. [CrossRef]
16. Schwarz, L.; Riedel, C.; Hogler, S.; Sinn, L.J.; Voglmayr, T.; Wochtl, B.; Dinhopl, N.; Rebel-Bauder, B.; Weissenbock, H.; Ladinig, A.; et al. Congenital infection with atypical porcine pestivirus (APPV) is associated with disease and viral persistence. *Vet. Res.* **2017**, *48*, 1–14. [CrossRef]
17. Postel, A.; Meyer, D.; Cagatay, G.N.; Feliziani, F.; De Mia, G.M.; Fischer, N.; Grundhoff, A.; Milicevic, V.; Deng, M.C.; Chang, C.Y.; et al. High Abundance and Genetic Variability of Atypical Porcine Pestivirus in Pigs from Europe and Asia. *Emerg. Infect. Dis.* **2017**, *23*, 2104–2107. [CrossRef]
18. Kaufmann, C.; Stalder, H.; Sidler, X.; Renzullo, S.; Gurtner, C.; Grahofer, A.; Schweizer, M. Long-Term Circulation of Atypical Porcine Pestivirus (APPV) within Switzerland. *Viruses* **2019**, *11*, 653. [CrossRef]

19. Yan, X.L.; Li, Y.Y.; He, L.L.; Wu, J.L.; Tang, X.Y.; Chen, G.H.; Mai, K.J.; Wu, R.T.; Li, Q.N.; Chen, Y.H.; et al. 12 novel atypical porcine pestivirus genomes from neonatal piglets with congenital tremors: A newly emerging branch and high prevalence in China. *Virology* **2019**, *533*, 50–58. [CrossRef]
20. Xie, Y.; Wang, X.; Su, D.; Feng, J.; Wei, L.; Cai, W.; Li, J.; Lin, S.; Yan, H.; He, D. Detection and Genetic Characterization of Atypical Porcine Pestivirus in Piglets With Congenital Tremors in Southern China. *Front. Microbiol.* **2019**, *10*, 1406. [CrossRef]
21. Beer, M.; Wernike, K.; Drager, C.; Hoper, D.; Pohlmann, A.; Bergermann, C.; Schroder, C.; Klinkhammer, S.; Blome, S.; Hoffmann, B. High Prevalence of Highly Variable Atypical Porcine Pestiviruses Found in Germany. *Transbound. Emerg. Dis.* **2017**, *64*, e22–e26. [CrossRef] [PubMed]
22. Steinhauer, D.A.; Domingo, E.; Holland, J.J. Lack of evidence for proofreading mechanisms associated with an RNA virus polymerase. *Gene* **1992**, *122*, 281–288. [CrossRef]
23. Bull, J.J.; Sanjuan, R.; Wilke, C.O. Theory of lethal mutagenesis for viruses. *J. Virol.* **2007**, *81*, 2930–2939. [CrossRef] [PubMed]
24. Kosakovsky Pond, S.L.; Frost, S.D. Not so different after all: A comparison of methods for detecting amino acid sites under selection. *Mol. Biol. Evol.* **2005**, *22*, 1208–1222. [CrossRef] [PubMed]
25. Sayers, E.W.; Cavanaugh, M.; Clark, K.; Ostell, J.; Pruitt, K.D.; Karsch-Mizrachi, I. GenBank. *Nucleic Acids Res.* **2019**, *47*, D94–D99. [CrossRef] [PubMed]
26. Gupta, R.; Jung, E.; Gooley, A.A.; Williams, K.L.; Brunak, S.; Hansen, J. Scanning the available Dictyostelium discoideum proteome for O-linked GlcNAc glycosylation sites using neural networks. *Glycobiology* **1999**, *9*, 1009–1022. [CrossRef]
27. Steentoft, C.; Vakhrushev, S.Y.; Joshi, H.J.; Kong, Y.; Vester-Christensen, M.B.; Schjoldager, K.T.; Lavrsen, K.; Dabelsteen, S.; Pedersen, N.B.; Marcos-Silva, L.; et al. Precision mapping of the human O-GalNAc glycoproteome through SimpleCell technology. *EMBO J.* **2013**, *32*, 1478–1488. [CrossRef]
28. Martin, D.P.; Murrell, B.; Golden, M.; Khoosal, A.; Muhire, B. RDP4: Detection and analysis of recombination patterns in virus genomes. *Virus Evol.* **2015**, *1*, vev003. [CrossRef]
29. Kimura, M. A simple method for estimating evolutionary rates of base substitutions through comparative studies of nucleotide sequences. *J. Mol. Evol.* **1980**, *16*, 111–120. [CrossRef]
30. Kumar, S.; Stecher, G.; Li, M.; Knyaz, C.; Tamura, K. MEGA X: Molecular Evolutionary Genetics Analysis across Computing Platforms. *Mol. Biol. Evol.* **2018**, *35*, 1547–1549. [CrossRef]
31. Rambaut, A.; Lam, T.T.; Max Carvalho, L.; Pybus, O.G. Exploring the temporal structure of heterochronous sequences using TempEst (formerly Path-O-Gen). *Virus Evol.* **2016**, *2*, vew007. [CrossRef] [PubMed]
32. Delport, W.; Poon, A.F.; Frost, S.D.; Kosakovsky Pond, S.L. Datamonkey 2010: A suite of phylogenetic analysis tools for evolutionary biology. *Bioinformatics* **2010**, *26*, 2455–2457. [CrossRef] [PubMed]
33. Murrell, B.; Wertheim, J.O.; Moola, S.; Weighill, T.; Scheffler, K.; Kosakovsky Pond, S.L. Detecting individual sites subject to episodic diversifying selection. *PLoS Genet.* **2012**, *8*, e1002764. [CrossRef] [PubMed]
34. Choe, S.; Le, V.P.; Shin, J.; Kim, J.H.; Kim, K.S.; Song, S.; Cha, R.M.; Park, G.N.; Nguyen, T.L.; Hyun, B.H.; et al. Pathogenicity and Genetic Characterization of Vietnamese Classical Swine Fever Virus: 2014–2018. *Pathogens* **2020**, *9*, 169. [CrossRef]
35. Yoo, S.J.; Kwon, T.; Kang, K.; Kim, H.; Kang, S.C.; Richt, J.A.; Lyoo, Y.S. Genetic evolution of classical swine fever virus under immune environments conditioned by genotype 1-based modified live virus vaccine. *Transbound. Emerg. Dis.* **2018**, *65*, 735–745. [CrossRef] [PubMed]
36. Kwon, T.; Yoon, S.H.; Kim, K.W.; Caetano-Anolles, K.; Cho, S.; Kim, H. Time-calibrated phylogenomics of the classical swine fever viruses: Genome-wide bayesian coalescent approach. *PLoS ONE* **2015**, *10*, e0121578. [CrossRef]
37. Chernick, A.; van der Meer, F. Evolution of Bovine viral diarrhea virus in Canada from 1997 to 2013. *Virology* **2017**, *509*, 232–238. [CrossRef]
38. Ronecker, S.; Zimmer, G.; Herrler, G.; Greiser-Wilke, I.; Grummer, B. Formation of bovine viral diarrhea virus E1-E2 heterodimers is essential for virus entry and depends on charged residues in the transmembrane domains. *J. Gen. Virol.* **2008**, *89*, 2114–2121. [CrossRef]
39. Cagatay, G.N.; Meyer, D.; Wendt, M.; Becher, P.; Postel, A. Characterization of the Humoral Immune Response Induced after Infection with Atypical Porcine Pestivirus (APPV). *Viruses* **2019**, *11*, 880. [CrossRef]
40. Zhang, H.; Wen, W.; Hao, G.; Chen, H.; Qian, P.; Li, X. A Subunit Vaccine Based on E2 Protein of Atypical Porcine Pestivirus Induces Th2-type Immune Response in Mice. *Viruses* **2018**, *10*, 673. [CrossRef]

41. Risatti, G.R.; Holinka, L.G.; Fernandez Sainz, I.; Carrillo, C.; Lu, Z.; Borca, M.V. N-linked glycosylation status of classical swine fever virus strain Brescia E2 glycoprotein influences virulence in swine. *J. Virol.* **2007**, *81*, 924–933. [CrossRef] [PubMed]
42. Hilton, L.; Moganeradj, K.; Zhang, G.; Chen, Y.H.; Randall, R.E.; McCauley, J.W.; Goodbourn, S. The NPro product of bovine viral diarrhea virus inhibits DNA binding by interferon regulatory factor 3 and targets it for proteasomal degradation. *J. Virol.* **2006**, *80*, 11723–11732. [CrossRef] [PubMed]
43. Alkheraif, A.A.; Topliff, C.L.; Reddy, J.; Massilamany, C.; Donis, R.O.; Meyers, G.; Eskridge, K.M.; Kelling, C.L. Type 2 BVDV N(pro) suppresses IFN-1 pathway signaling in bovine cells and augments BRSV replication. *Virology* **2017**, *507*, 123–134. [CrossRef] [PubMed]
44. Meyers, G.; Ege, A.; Fetzer, C.; von Freyburg, M.; Elbers, K.; Carr, V.; Prentice, H.; Charleston, B.; Schurmann, E.M. Bovine viral diarrhea virus: Prevention of persistent fetal infection by a combination of two mutations affecting Erns RNase and Npro protease. *J. Virol.* **2007**, *81*, 3327–3338. [CrossRef]
45. Coleman, J.R.; Papamichail, D.; Skiena, S.; Futcher, B.; Wimmer, E.; Mueller, S. Virus attenuation by genome-scale changes in codon pair bias. *Science* **2008**, *320*, 1784–1787. [CrossRef]
46. Simmonds, P.; Smith, D.B. Structural constraints on RNA virus evolution. *J. Virol.* **1999**, *73*, 5787–5794. [CrossRef]
47. Lauring, A.S.; Acevedo, A.; Cooper, S.B.; Andino, R. Codon usage determines the mutational robustness, evolutionary capacity, and virulence of an RNA virus. *Cell Host Microbe* **2012**, *12*, 623–632. [CrossRef]
48. Chen, Y.; He, L.; Peng, Y.; Shi, X.; Chen, J.; Zhong, J.; Chen, X.; Cheng, G.; Deng, H. The hepatitis C virus protein NS3 suppresses TNF-alpha-stimulated activation of NF-kappaB by targeting LUBAC. *Sci. Signal.* **2015**, *8*, ra118. [CrossRef]
49. Dalrymple, N.; Cimica, V.; Mackow, E. Dengue Virus NS Proteins Inhibit RIG-I/MAVS Signaling by Blocking TBK1/IRF3 Phosphorylation: Dengue Virus Serotype 1 NS4A Is a Unique Interferon-Regulating Virulence Determinant. *mBio* **2015**, *6*, e00553-15. [CrossRef]
50. Kumthip, K.; Chusri, P.; Jilg, N.; Zhao, L.; Fusco, D.N.; Zhao, H.; Goto, K.; Cheng, D.; Schaefer, E.A.; Zhang, L.; et al. Hepatitis C virus NS5A disrupts STAT1 phosphorylation and suppresses type I interferon signaling. *J. Virol.* **2012**, *86*, 8581–8591. [CrossRef]
51. Grant, A.; Ponia, S.S.; Tripathi, S.; Balasubramaniam, V.; Miorin, L.; Sourisseau, M.; Schwarz, M.C.; Sanchez-Seco, M.P.; Evans, M.J.; Best, S.M.; et al. Zika Virus Targets Human STAT2 to Inhibit Type I Interferon Signaling. *Cell Host Microbe* **2016**, *19*, 882–890. [CrossRef] [PubMed]
52. Charleston, B.; Fray, M.D.; Baigent, S.; Carr, B.V.; Morrison, W.I. Establishment of persistent infection with non-cytopathic bovine viral diarrhoea virus in cattle is associated with a failure to induce type I interferon. *J. Gen. Virol.* **2001**, *82*, 1893–1897. [CrossRef] [PubMed]
53. Peterhans, E.; Jungi, T.W.; Schweizer, M. BVDV and innate immunity. *Biologicals* **2003**, *31*, 107–112. [CrossRef]
54. Brock, K.V. The persistence of bovine viral diarrhea virus. *Biologicals* **2003**, *31*, 133–135. [CrossRef]
55. Griebel, P.J. BVDV vaccination in North America: Risks versus benefits. *Anim. Health Res. Rev.* **2015**, *16*, 27–32. [CrossRef]

16

An Assessment of Secondary Clinical Disease, Milk Production and Quality and the Impact on Reproduction in Holstein Heifers and Cows from a Single Large Commercial Herd Persistently Infected with Bovine Viral Diarrhea Virus Type 2

Natália Sobreira Basqueira [1], Jean Silva Ramos [1], Fabricio Dias Torres [1], Liria Hiromi Okuda [2], David John Hurley [3], Christopher C. L. Chase [4], Anny Raissa Carolini Gomes [5] and Viviani Gomes [1,*]

1 Department of Internal Medicine, College of Veterinary Medicine and Animal Science, University of São Paulo, São Paulo 05508-270, Brazil; na_sobreira@usp.br (N.S.B.); ramos.jan@outlook.com (J.S.R.); torres@axysanalises.com.br (F.D.T.)
2 Biological Institute, 1252 Conselheiro Rodrigues Alves Ave, Vila Mariana, São Paulo 04014-900, Brazil; okuda@biologico.sp.gov.br
3 Food Animal Health and Management Program, College of Veterinary Medicine, University of Georgia, Athens, GA 30602, USA; djhurley@uga.edu
4 Department of Veterinary and Biomedical Sciences, South Dakota State University, Brookings, SD 57007, USA; christopher.Chase@SDSTATE.EDU
5 Department of Veterinary Medicine, Federal University of Paraná, Curitiba 80040-380, Brazil; anny.gomes7@gmail.com
* Correspondence: viviani.gomes@usp.br.

Abstract: The aim of this study was to evaluate secondary clinical disease, milk production efficiency and reproductive performance of heifers and cows persistently infected (PI) with bovine viral diarrhea virus type 2 (BVDV type 2). PI animals (n = 25) were identified using an antigen capture ELISA of ear notch samples. They were distributed into three age groups: ≤ 12 (n = 8), 13 to 24 (n = 6) and 25 to 34 (n = 11) months old. A control group of BVDV antigen ELISA negative female cattle that were age matched to the PI animals was utilized from the same herd. The PI group had a 1.29 higher odds ratio for diarrhea than controls (p = 0.001, IC95% = 1.032–1.623) and 1.615 greater chance of developing bovine respiratory disease (BRD) (p = 0.012, IC95% = 1.155–2.259). The age at first insemination (p = 0.012) and number of insemination attempts required to establish the first pregnancy (p = 0.016) were both higher for PI than controls. Milk production was higher for control cows than PI cows during most of the sampling periods. Somatic cell counts (SCC) were higher in PI cows than the controls at all sampling points across lactation ($p \leq 0.042$). PI cattle had a higher incidence of disease, produced less milk, a higher SCC, and poorer reproductive performance than control cattle in this study.

Keywords: diarrhea; bovine respiratory disease; milk production; somatic cells count (SCC); reproductive performance; BVDV persistent infection

---

1. Introduction

Bovine viral diarrhea virus (BVDV) is a ubiquitous infectious agent that affects the productivity and reproduction efficiency of both dairy and beef cattle. BVDV is responsible for significant monetary losses to producers that have been estimated to range between $0.50 to $687.80 US dollars per infected animal per year [1]. Losses have been reported to be associated with morbidity, mortality, premature voluntary culling, reduced slaughter value, stillbirths, abortion and other reproductive losses, the cost of veterinary services and treatments, the cost of replacement stock, the costs of additional labor and reduction in milk production [1–3].

The documented clinical impacts of BVDV infection provide the rationale for continual BVDV testing in the herd [4]. The clinical disease associated with BVDV infected cattle can present as a myriad of effects. These range from mild and unapparent infection to severe disease, leading to rapid death. The disease observed depends on the properties of the infecting strain, and the immune and physiological state of the host. Host factors such as gestational age at the time of exposure, general immunocompetence, immunotolerance to BVDV viral antigens due to prior exposure or vaccination, and the level of physical, social and environmental stress impact the severity and outcome of the disease [5].

The typical clinical signs and symptoms associated with BVDV infection have been reported in both acutely infected and persistently infected (PI) cattle [6,7]. These signs and symptom can routinely be induced during experimental challenge with any of several commonly used strains [8–10]. However, challenge with BVDV under experimental conditions often does not reproduce the full variety of manifestations of the disease seen in the field. Specifically, there is a lack of authoritative information about the typical clinical findings throughout the lifespan of PI cattle [11]. This is, in part, due to the short lifespan of PI cattle, which is often less than one year [12].

We have observed that there are few studies that have been published detailing the associated clinical picture of BVDV-associated secondary diseases in PI cattle. The diseases most frequently detected in PI cattle infected with the major BVDV 1 subtypes (a, b, c) were diarrhea (41%), bronchopneumonia (20%), and their combination (9%). In addition, neurological signs were observed at necropsy in 10% of the BVDV infected PI cattle. Further, abortion, laminitis and other diseases of the hoof, weakness, and anemia were only occasionally observed in PI animals [13].

Kane et al. (2015) described an outbreak of BVDV type 2a that results in abortion and PI births, despite neonatal deaths. Many of the PI cattle died as yearlings. Seventeen of 36 died with lesions consistent with mucosal disease, whereas six died without gross lesions, and two were euthanized because of chronic ill thrift. The 11 PI animals appeared healthy and were sold for slaughter. The virus population of BVDV type 2a in PI animals from this outbreak differs in size and diversity, and it could be used as a quantifiable phenotype correlated with clinical presentation of BVDV such as growth rate, congenital defects, viral shed and cytokine expression [14].

BVDV PI animals are often difficult to breed successfully. Further, herds with PI cattle can have reproductive problems. BVDV has been identified in the ovaries and uterus of PI animals [15]. The virus appears to inhibit conception through physiological alterations that induce morphologic changes in the ovaries leading to an increased interval between calving. In addition, BVDV inhibits normal embryo cleavage and reduces the number of viable embryos produced during in vitro fertilization [15–17]. BVDV can also induce congenital defects during fetal development, abortions (in 6% to 10% of fetuses), and stillbirth at any point in gestation [18]. Thus, PI cattle may have a significant role in poor reproductive function in herds.

A dairy herd containing PI infected animals generally has a higher incidence of mastitis (both subclinical and clinical), and frequently has a higher somatic cell count (SCC) than comparably managed BVDV free herds [19–22]. The effects of BVDV on milk production include: an average loss of 368 kg of milk, 9.35 kg of protein and 10.2 kg of fat per cow per lactation [23].

The majority of studies estimating the losses caused by BVDV infection have been reported for animals with acute infection. There is little reliable information about the impact of PI cattle with respect to secondary clinical disease, efficacy of reproduction, or its impact on milk production and quality. Thus, the aim of this study was to collect data about associated secondary clinical diseases, document reproductive efficacy, and document milk production and quality for Holstein PI heifers and cows that had naturally acquired infection with BVDV type 2 viruses.

Here, we present data collected from one large commercial herd with a well-documented history of BVDV infections over a long period. Prior to the PI screening in this herd, BVDV-associated diseases and production losses were inferred from farm records. Historically, this farm had a high incidence and recurrence of bronchopneumonia in young calves, characterized by an interstitial bronchopneumonia or fibrinosuppurative bronchopneumonia. In August 2013, the etiological cause of bovine respiratory disease (BRD) was investigated for ten young heifers. Two of these animals were positive in transtracheal wash for BVDV as detected by RT-PCR [24]. Between 2013 and 2015, BVDV was confirmed for some cases of fetal infection by the detection of serum BVDV antibody in calves before colostrum intake. In addition, neonate calves were found to be BVDV positive by RT-PCR [25,26]. In this herd, our team investigated the evidence of specific antibodies against the BVDV p80 protein in heifers from 1 to 390 days of age (n = 585). We detected low levels of p80 antibody in serum over the first 120 days in 10–20% of the calves. There was an abrupt rise in the number of p80 positive to 70% of the calves being serum positive after 120 days of age. This was associated with a higher mortality of calves in the post-weaning period due to anaplasmosis and babesiosis [27]. In 2015, mucosal disease was observed in a heifer during the post-weaning period. This herd also had a decline in reproductive performance. The associated reduction in the production of calves was not initially associated with BVDV infection. However, evidence linking BVDV to calf disease lead to a global screening for PI cattle in the herd in 2016.

Based on this history, the study presented here was conducted to determine the impact of naturally occurring BVDV PI animals on production parameters.

2. Materials and Methods

2.1. Herd Management

This study was performed on the largest commercial dairy farm in Brazil. It is located in São Paulo State (22°21′25″ S and 47°23′03″ W). The research was approved by the Committee for Ethics in Animal Use of the School of Veterinary Medicine and Animal Science from University of São Paulo in 1 May 2017 (Protocol number 5131190216). Written informed consent was obtained from the farm responsible.

This dairy herd was composed of approximately 3700 Holstein cattle. There were 1750 cows in lactation, with an average daily milk production of 38.5 L per cow. Calves were housed in individual suspended cages (1.0 × 0.9 m) from birth until they were abruptly weaned at about day 75 of age. They were transferred to group housing of 9, 18 or 36 heifers as they got older. The pens contained a sand bed, common drinking water trough, and a bunker with free choice calf starter diet (Guabi, São Paulo, Brazil). The calves had free access to grass (Tifton) pasture inside the pen.

Beginning at 10 months of age, heifers were kept in a confinement pasture with about 100 animals per unit. These heifers were enrolled into the standard reproductive protocols for the farm at about 13 months of age when they reached about 1.20 m tall at the withers. The majority of the heifers had entered the reproductive protocol by 13 to 14 months of age and their average weight was 380 kg. In the reproduction protocol, each heifer received a dose of prostaglandin (MSD Animal Health, Montes Claros, Minas Gerais) weekly. The heifers were inseminated when they demonstrated they were in heat. Pregnancy diagnosis using ultrasound (Mindray, Shenzhen, China) was performed every 21 days, and heifers previously inseminated, but not pregnant at this time were submitted to the fixed-time artificial insemination protocol, or fixed-time embryo transfer. A majority of the heifers (92–93%) were pregnant by 17 months of age. They were kept in a confinement pasture with about 100 animals per pasture with free choice TMR ration formulated and produced in the farm, water and access to grass pasture until the seventh month of gestation.

In the eighth month of pregnancy, heifers were moved to the maternity pen. This pen had a cross-ventilation system and held 200 heifers or dry cows. After calving, lactating cows were housed in a force cross-ventilated barn, divided into six pens, with about 290 animals in each pen.

During early calfhood, passive BVDV control was assumed to be provided by the transfer of maternal BVDV antibody in colostrum (see BVDV vaccine protocol below). Calves were fed a total volume of 5 L of fresh maternal colostrum (containing ≥50 g/L of IgG, documented using a colostrometer (MS Schippers, Campinas, Brazil), divided into two feedings. Both feedings were delivered within the first 18 h after birth.

2.2. Herd Vaccination History

The young heifers were vaccinated against BVDV (using a killed commercial vaccine—Cattle Master® GOLD FP 5/L5, Zoetis, Parsippany-Troy Hills, NJ, USA), beginning at 60 days of age with a priming dose. This was followed by a booster dose of the same vaccine 30 days after the first vaccination. From this point forward, all animals in this herd (heifers ≥2 months of age and cows) were vaccinated biannually with the same vaccine in April and October. This herd previously used a commercial vaccine without BVDV type 2 for several decades until 2012 (Cattle Master 4 + L5®, Zoetis). Subsequent vaccination utilized an inactivated BVDV 1 (5960) and BVDV 2 (53637) containing vaccine with the addition of a thermosensitive BoHV-1 (Cooper) and BPIV-3 (RLB 103), a modified-live BRSV (375), and five species of killed *Leptospira* spp. This vaccine was diluted in an immune stimulating complexes (ISCOM) adjuvant (Cattle Master® GOLD FP 5/L5, Zoetis).

2.3. PI Screening and Choice of Experimental Groups

Ear skin samples (ear notches measuring 1 cm × 0.5 cm), were obtained from the dorsal pinna margin of each young heifer or calf (n = 2247) using a stainless-steel ear notching clamp (type V pig, Walmur, Porto Alegre, Rio Grande do Sul). The sample obtained was stored in a sterile microtube (Eppendorf, São Paulo, Brazil), then frozen at −20 °C until it was processed. Each sample was assessed individually for BVDV using an antigen capture, Erns antigen specific ELISA test (IDEXX BVDV Ag/Serum Plus Test, IDEXX, Westbrook, ME, USA). After 30 days, animals positive at initial screening were retested using the same protocol with new biopsy samples. This was followed by testing of all live dams and grandams of the animals identified as PI among the heifers and calves. After the removal of all PI animals identified in this herd, all newborn calves were tested monthly by ear notch sampling. The duration of PI screening lasted about 13 months from September of 2015 until October of 2016.

A total of 26 PI cattle, including 19 calves and heifers, 4 dams and 3 neonates (born after removal of PI animals from the investigated herd) were found. Twenty-five of the 26 heifers and cows were included in this study. Animals were distributed by age: ≤12 months (n = 8), 13 to 24 months (n = 6) and 25 to 36 months (n = 11). The control group was composed of animals free of persistent BVDV (n = 25). They were selected as aged matched pairs for the PI cows and heifers.

2.4. Virus Characterization

Blood samples were collected via jugular venipuncture using an 18 gauge × 2.5 cm single sample needles into two 8 L glass tubes (Vacutainer ACD Solution A REF 364606, BD Diagnostics, San Jose, CA, USA) from all animals in the study. The blood collected in ACD solution A were processed for buffy coat isolation as previously described by Harpin et al. [28] and stored at −80 °C.

For BVDV characterization, the RNA was extracted from the buffy coat using TRIZOL LS reagent (Invitrogen, Thermo Fisher Scientific Inc., Waltham, MA, USA), according to manufacturer's instructions and stored at −80 °C until molecular testing was performed. For RT-PCR, a one-step RT-PCR kit (Access Quick RT-PCR System, Promega Corporation, Madison, WI, USA) was utilized and a set of primers from the 5′ UTR region (5′ TAG CCA GCT CCT TAG TAG GAC 3′ and 5′ ACT CCA TGT GCC ATG TAC AGC 3′) were selected. This allowed the detection of all BVDV strains (types I, II and Hobi-like) [23]. Using a total volume of 25 μL, the reaction was performed using 12.5 μL AcessQuick Master mix 1× (Tris-HCl, KCl, dNTP, $MgCl_2$ and Taq Polymerase), 1.25 μL of sense primer and 1.25 μL of anti-sense primer (1 mol/μL), 0.5 μL of reverse transcriptase enzyme AMV, 4.5 μL of nuclease-free water and 5 μL of isolated RNA. The amplification cycle was 45 °C for 45 min for disassociation and reverse transcriptase activation at 94 °C for 5 min. This was followed by 40 cycles of 94 °C for 30 s, 57 °C for 30 s and 72 °C for 30 s. An incubation at 72 °C for 5 min allowed the final extension. The assay was held at 4 °C following amplification. Amplicons were visualized on 1.5% agarose gels by horizontal electrophoresis. The gels were stained with Gel Red at a dilution of 1:150 (Biotium, Fremont, CA, USA). The products were visualized and measured using a transilluminator under ultraviolet light (302 nm). The samples were considered positive, as compared to the BVDV positive control, if the product was 29 bp. The standard 100 bp ladder (Thermo Fisher Scientific Inc. Waltham, MA, USA) was used to establish the product size.

From 19 BVDV positive samples by RT-PCR, five were submitted to sequencing to verify which type was involved in this herd. Three PIs aged from 1 to 12 months of age, 1 PI from 14 to 24 months of age, and 1 PI from 25 to 32 months of age were selected so that there was at least one PI representative of each age group. The PCR products were purified using the Wizard DNA and PCR Clean-up kit (Promega™, Madison, WI, USA) following manufacturer's instructions. The reaction consisted of the BigDye 3.1 Xterminator kit® (Applied Biosystems™, Foster City, CA, USA) and universal BVDV primers (3.2 pmol/μL) from the 5′ UTR region. The total reaction volume was 10 μL. The sequencing cycle consisted of 1 cycle of 95 °C for 1 min, 35 cycles of 95 °C for 30 s, 50 °C for 15 s and 60 °C for 4 min. This amplification was followed by holding the product at 4 °C to preserve the DNA. The sequencing reaction plate was precipitated using the BigDye Xterminator purification kit according to manufacturer's instructions. Finally, the plate was applied to a 350 L Sequencer (Applied Biosystems™). The quality of sequences generated was analyzed using Sequence Analyzer software (Applied Biosystems™). The BVDV sequence data was edited using the BioEdit program, and after obtaining a consensus sequence fit, it was assessed using Blast and aligned with published BVDV sequences using the ClustalW program. The criteria utilized for building the phylogeny tree were based on a better than 98% identity with the core BVDV sequence. The MEGA 7.0 program was used to determine which algorithm method [29] could be applied to these samples for relatedness analysis, and a bootstrap of 1000 replicates was used to build a relational tree.

2.5. *Data from the Farm Record*

The farm records were utilized to document the reproductive performance, milk production and milk quality. Retrospective data correspond to the longevity of PI animals, since they were diagnosed as persistently infected at different ages and were immediately slaughtered after diagnosis. The digital record of each animal from the Dairy Comp Program® (Valley Agricultural Software, Tulare, CA, USA) was used to generate the milk production records.

The reproduction records were collected from the farm register. The parameters collected were: age at first insemination, number of artificial insemination (AI) attempts required to achieve conception, the frequency of abortion, and the age of each heifer at the first calving. Fourteen of 16 PI heifers (12 to 36 months of age) were presented for artificial insemination. The success in reproduction (based on the parameters collected), was compared to control heifers paired for age and size (n = 14).

Eight PI heifers calved. These PI heifers were assessed relative to their BVDV negative pair heifer (n = 8). Data were also collected comparatively for the quantity and quality of the milk produced from the monthly milk report of the farm based on program records. All data collected were assessed relative to windows for days in milk: M1 = 15–39 days; M2 = 44–73 days; M3 = 74–104 days; M4 = 107–132 days; M5 = 139–166 days and M6 = 167–195 days. Not all data was recorded for each cow at each interval, because all PI cows were slaughtered immediately after being confirmed positive for BVDV by antigen ELISA results, removing them from the study in different phrases of lactation.

We were able to collect data for immediate post-partum diseases in eight PI and eleven paired cows with respect to the treatment given. The data for the treatment of cows for metritis, mammary edema, retained placenta, ketosis, clinical mastitis and bovine respiratory disease were collected.

2.6. Clinical Scores

Clinical scores were collected for the heifers (both PI and paired controls) at the initiation of the study. Over the course of the study, all pairs remaining at each assessment point were collected for health status. The health status of each heifer (or cow) was evaluated using a scoring system developed at the University of Wisconsin (https://www.vetmed.wisc.edu/fapm/svm-dairy-apps/calf-health-scorer-chs/). At each assessment point, a clinical examination was performed for each pair of heifers or cows, beginning on the day of the second BVD ear notch collection. The fecal score was recorded as 0 (normal consistency), 1 (pasty, semi-formed), 2 (pasty with large amount of water), or 3 (watery, fluid feces with fecal content in the perineum and on tail). The BRD Score was compiled from the rectal temperature, evidence of cough, character of nasal secretion, presence of ocular secretion, observation of abnormal head and ear positioning. These were classified on a scale from 0 to 3 for each observation, representing the intensity of each clinical manifestation. Animals having a fecal score of 2 or 3, or a summed BRD score of ≥4.0 were considered to have clinical disease.

2.7. Statistical Analysis

Statistical analysis was performed using the Statistical Package for the Social Science (SPSS) version 19.0 (IBM Corporation, Armonk, NY, USA).

The association between experimental groups (PI and paired control) for the prevalence of diarrhea, BRD, post-partum disease and the rate of successful calving was evaluated using either Chi-square or Fisher's exact test. Fisher's exact test was chosen when the groups had less than 5 pairs represented. Binary logistic regression was performed to estimate the odds ratios and confidence intervals of 95% between outcomes in the paired heifers (cows).

The normality of continuous variables was tested using the Shapiro–Wilk test. If the data were not normally distributed, the variables were transformed using one of the following: quadratic root, log10 or inverse transformation. Student's t-test for normally distributed independent samples, and the Mann–Whitney U test for samples that were not normally distributed were performed to compare between groups for parametric and non-parametric analysis, respectively. The time-series analyses of milk production and milk composition were evaluated by using a one-way ANOVA for repeated measures coupled with a Bonferroni post-hoc test to compare data across time within each experimental group.

3. Results

3.1. Identification of PI Animals and the Outcomes for PI Heifers and Cows

PI screening was conducted on samples from 2247 heifers and calves from young animals born prior to the start of the testing program, and on the cows in the herd that had male or stillborn calves. Thirty-four of 2247 (1.5%) were BVDV infected. BVDV positive animals included: 19 aged 1 to 12; seven aged 13 to 24, and eight aged 25 to 36 months.

Results of the second round of testing indicated that 19 of the remaining 30 animals (four animals died or were euthanized before retesting) were confirmed as PI. Following this round of testing, all live dams (n = 11) and grandams (n = 4) of the PI heifers and calves were tested. Four dams (25 to 36 months of age) were found to be PI. After the removal of the PI cows from the herd, all newborn calves were tested on a monthly basis as they were born. Three additional PI calves (of 103 new calves) born over the next two months were identified with no additional PI calves identified during the next nine months on this farm.

3.2. Virus Characterization

Nineteen of 25 (76%) buffy coat samples from confirmed PI cows tested were positive for BVDV. All positive samples in the RT-PCR appeared to be closely related BVDV type 2 viruses. Five of these positive samples were subjected to sequencing to confirm the genetic relatedness based on their having suitable quality for sequencing and representing the diversity of the age groups established in the study. The BVDV virus 5′ UTR sequences were analyzed and grouped in a maximum likelihood tree. The phylogenetic tree is shown in Figure 1, and it was observed that the five samples were all identified as BVDV II strains with 98% of confidence. This was based on published BVDV II strain sequences. No BVDV virus was recovered from any of the control animals using the RT-PCR test.

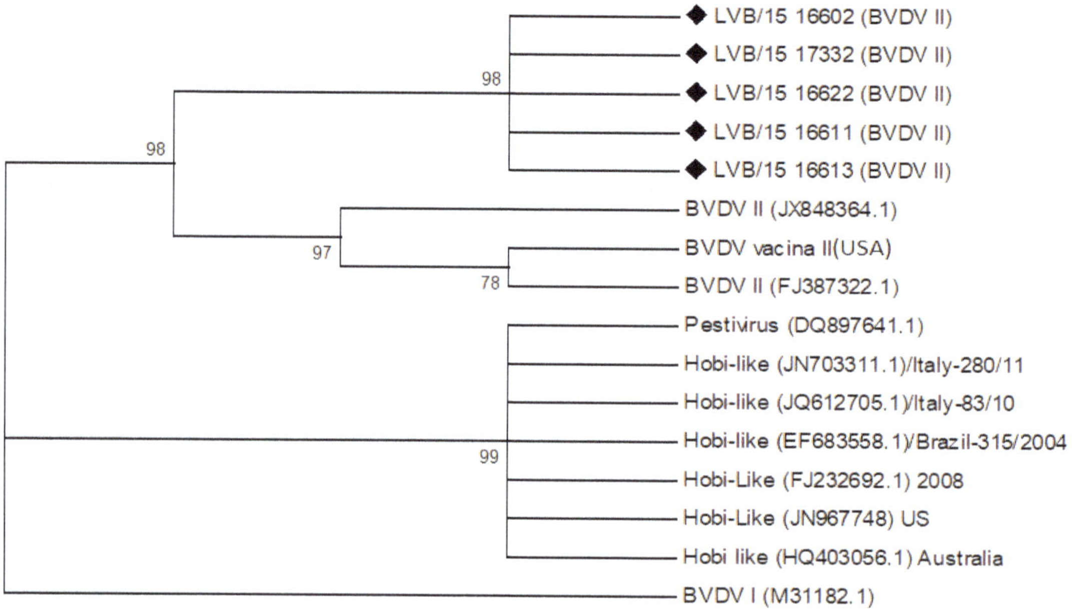

Figure 1. Phylogram displaying the relationships of the nucleotide sequences obtained in the current study as aligned against bovine viral diarrhea virus (BVDV) and other pestivirus sequences reported in GenBank. The phylogenetic tree was constructed using a maximum likelihood algorithm under the Kimura 2 evolutionary model with 1000 bootstrap replicates testing.

3.3. Impact of Being PI on Reproductive Performance

Reproductive performance was evaluated in sexually mature females (13 to 36 months of age). Artificial insemination of control pair heifers was initiated earlier (14.3 ± 1.19 months) than for PI heifers (15.58 ± 1.42 months) ($p = 0.012$). In addition, the number of artificial insemination attempts required to achieve the first successful pregnancy was greater for the PI heifers (mean of 4.0) than the paired control heifers (mean of 1.0) ($p = 0.016$). Only half of the 16 PI heifers calved during this study. All 16 paired control heifers produced a calf during the course of the study. There was an association observed between successful calving if a heifer was PI in the study ($p = 0.003$).

Only eight PI within a total of 14 heifers calved following artificial insemination. Failure to calf by PI heifers was generally due to abortion of her calf or being sent to slaughter before she could calve. In contrast, all paired control heifers ($n = 14$) calved following the first insemination. Control heifers were 1.75 more times more likely to deliver a calf than PI heifers (IC 95%, 1.112–2.755).

3.4. The Quantity of Milk Produced and Quality and Composition of Milk

A summary of the quantity of milk produced and of milk quality measurements are shown in Table 1. The difference between groups means (PI vs. control) for quantity of milk produced were: 4.71, 10.46, 11.38, 12.98, 21.23 and 16.63 L, respectively for the periods designated M1 to M6. Higher quantities of milk production were observed in control cows relative to PI cows during the sampling periods M2 ($p = 0.019$), M4 ($p = 0.013$), M5 ($p = 0.002$) and M6 ($p = 0.004$).

Table 1. Mean and standard deviation (±SD) of the quantity of milk produced and the composition of the milk produced by PI and paired control cows (NI) over the course of lactation. SCC: somatic cell count.

Variables	Groups	M1 (15–39 DIM)		M2 (44–73 DIM)		M3 (74–104 DIM)		M4 (107–132 DIM)		M5 (139–166 DIM)		M6 (167–195 DIM)		*p*-Value
		Mean ± SD	*N*	Mean ± SD	*N*	Mean ± SD	*N*	Mean ± SD	*N*	Mean ± SD	*N*	Mean ± SD	*N*	
Yield (Liters)	PI	26.29 ± 11.77	7	24.29 ± 10.61	7	27.5 ± 5.28	6	28.4 ± 4.56	5	23.4 ± 12.82	5	26 ± 2.16	4	0.217
	NI	31 ± 13.06	7	34.75 ± 14.71	8	38.88 ± 15.42	8	41.38 ± 8.57	8	44.63 ± 7.29	8	42.63 ± 7.82	8	0.948
	p-value	0.492	-	0.143	-	0.112	-	0.010	-	0.003	-	0.002	-	-
SCC ($\times 10^5$)	PI	203.43 ± 246.21	7	308.86 ± 380.88	7	530 ± 476.28	6	1046.2 ± 970.37	5	919.2 ± 979.85	5	1045.25 ± 1156.22	4	0.555
	NI	50.57 ± 50.21	7	23.88 ± 16.99	8	41.38 ± 72.17	8	372.38 ± 978.72	8	21.75 ± 18.61	8	24 ± 14.4	8	0.445
	p-value	0.042	-	0.001	-	0.001	-	0.004	-	0.001	-	0.006	-	-
Lactose (%)	PI	4.66 ± 0.53	7	4.86 ± 0.3	7	4.75 ± 0.48	6	4.6 ± 0.49	5	4.72 ± 0.37	5	4.7 ± 0.44	4	0.954
	NI	4.63 ± 0.51	7	4.84 ± 0.16	8	4.79 ± 0.22	8	4.85 ± 0.18	8	4.79 ± 0.2	8	4.84 ± 0.2	8	0.941
	p-value	0.920	-	0.438	-	0.734	-	0.380	-	0.904	-	0.901	-	-
Fat (%)	PI	3.4 ± 0.81	7	3.77 ± 0.8	7	3.3 ± 0.36	6	3.34 ± 0.63	5	3.86 ± 0.46	5	3.38 ± 0.69	4	0.673
	NI	3.11 ± 0.38	7	3.45 ± 0.46	8	3.49 ± 0.57	8	3.18 ± 0.52	8	3.38 ± 0.27	8	3.23 ± 0.49	8	0.574
	p-value	0.475	-	0.712	-	0.512	-	0.710	-	0.054	-	0.961	-	-
Protein (%)	PI	2.91 ± 0.21a	7	3.07 ± 0.18ab	7	3.13 ± 0.16ab	6	3.22 ± 0.13ab	5	3.24 ± 0.05ab	5	3.35 ± 0.13b	4	0.001
	Control	2.83 ± 0.26a	7	2.88 ± 0.21a	8	2.96 ± 0.18ab	8	3.06 ± 0.16ab	8	3.16 ± 0.16b	8	3.26 ± 0.21b	8	0.003
	p-value	0.586	-	0.082	-	0.094	-	0.078	-	0.403	-	0.175	-	-

N = sample size. Difference between group means was assessed using Student's *t* test, and changes over time using a one-way ANOVA. *p*-value was considered significant if $p < 0.05$, and tendency declared when $p > 0.05$–1.00.

The SCC was higher in PI than paired control cows at each timepoint analyzed during the course of lactation. The differential in the quantity of milk produced between the PI and paired control cows increased over the course of lactation ($p \leq 0.001$). In general, PI milk was more concentrated than milk from the paired controls. PI had higher fat content (in %) at the M5 sampling ($p = 0.054$), and showed a tendency for a higher percent of protein at the samplings M2 ($p = 0.082$), M3 ($p = 0.094$) and M4 ($p = 0.078$). The level of lactose was not different between the PI and paired control cows at any sampling point. No differences were observed within either of the experimental groups over the course of the experiment (M1–M6).

3.5. The Assessment of Clinical Signs and Disease

There was an association between the prevalence of diarrhea and the incidence of BRD that was different between the PI and control groups (Table 2). An analysis of the dataset, without respect to age, demonstrated an association between a higher diarrhea score ($p = 0.012$) and higher BRD score ($p = 0.001$) linked to the PI group of animals. When age was added as a factor in analysis, a tendency was detected ($p = 0.074$) toward a higher frequency of diarrhea in PI (33%) than control (0%) cattle of 25 to 36 months of age. There was no difference observed in diarrhea frequency among calves <12 months of age ($p = 0.500$), or heifers 12 to 24 months of age ($p = 0.455$) between groups. The PI heifers had a 1.29 greater odds ratio for development of diarrhea (fecal score $\geq$ 2.0) than the control heifers ($p = 0.001$, IC 95% = 1.032–1.623). This was assessed using binary logistic regression of the global PI population, without respect to age.

Table 2. The percentage (number of cases/number of subjects *100) of diarrhea and bovine respiratory disease (BRD) in persistently infected (PI) and control Holstein heifers and cows.

Clinical Scores	Groups	Results	Global Population	Age (Months)		
				<12	13–24	25–36
Diarrhea (Score ≥2.0)	PI	Positive	22.7 (5/22)	12.5 (1/8)	20.0 (1/5)	33.3 (3/9)
		Negative	77.3 (17/22)	87.5 (7/8)	80.0 (4/5)	66.7 (6/9)
	Control	Positive	0 (0/25)	0	0	0
		Negative	100 (25/25)	100 (8/8)	100 (6/6)	100 (11/11)
	p-value		0.012	0.500	0.455	0.074
BRD (Sum of Score ≥4.0)	PI	Positive	38.1 (8/21)	37.5 (3/8)	20.0 (1/5)	50 (4/8)
		Negative	61.9 (13/21)	62.5 (5/8)	80.0 (4/5)	50 (4/8)
	Control	Positive	0 (0/25)	0 (0/8)	0 (0/6)	0 (0/11)
		Negative	100 (25/25)	100 (8/8)	100 (6/6)	100 (11/11)
	p-value		0.001	0.055	0.251	0.008

Global population means all PI and non-infected BVDV, without respect to age. Difference between groups was considered significant if $p \leq 0.05$, and a tendency declared if $p > 0.05 \leq 0.10$, using the Chi-square or Fisher exact test as necessary.

The frequency of animals with BRD (sum of scores $\geq$ 4) was higher for PI heifers (38.5%) than the paired control heifers (0%) based on analysis of the global data ($p = 0.001$). Similar results were observed for cows 25 to 36 months of age and young heifers (<12 month). For these cows, PI animals had a higher frequency of BRD (50.0%) than control cows (0%). No difference in BRD was observed for heifers 12 to 24 months of age ($p = 0.251$) between experimental groups in this study. The PI heifers had a 1.615 greater chance of developing BRD (sum of scores > 4.0) than the control heifers ($p = 0.012$, IC 95% = 1.155–2.259) when assessed using binary logistic regression analysis applied to the global population.

The relative occurrence of mammary edema ($p = 0.322$), retained placenta ($p = 0.183$), ketosis ($p = 0.421$), clinical mastitis ($p = 0.297$) and BRD ($p = 0.297$) in PI cows was determined by assessing values from eight lactating PI cows and 11 control cows (originally paired with PI heifers). We observe a higher frequency of the occurrence of metritis in PI (37.5%, 3/8) than the control cows (0%, 0/11) ($p = 0.058$). The PI cows had a 1.6 greater chance of developing metritis than the control cows (IC 95% = 0.935–2.737).

When all types of post-partum disease were combined, the total occurrence was higher in the PI cows (100%, 8/8) than in control cows (36.4%, 4/11) ($p = 0.007$). The PI heifers had a three-times greater chance of developing post-partum disease than paired control heifers (IC 95% = 1.348–6.678).

4. Discussion

This research was focused on understanding the impact of persistent infection with BVDV type 2 on secondary clinical disease, the quantity of milk produced and its quality, and on factors affecting reproductive efficacy in Holstein heifers and cows. The study comprehensively tested the herd and discovered a significant number of PI heifers, calves and even established cows (25–36 months of age). To our knowledge, this paper represents the first study to examine the impacts of BVDV type 2 persistent infection relevant to dairy cattle production and reproduction in a large dairy herd. Previously, Kane et al. (2015) reported information about clinical presentation in PI caused by a single strain of BVDV2, however it was in a Angus and Angus-cross beef herd.

This study collected all of the data from PI cattle with naturally acquired infections. Previous papers in the literature have almost exclusively presented the effects of induced, or naturally acquired, acute infection, or induced PI resulting from BVDV challenge. The experimental challenge cannot induce disease that has identical complexity as naturally acquired infections. It is likely that challenge models do not fully replicate the interaction between virus, host and the environment that occur in a true production setting.

The investigated herd was not closed. Animals from southern Brazil were added to the herd continually. To accelerate the genetic improvement in the herd, heifers and cows from the farm were sent to an embryo harvesting center in Paraná state in the south of Brazil. The embryos resulting from their utilization of this reproductive technology were implanted in cows from the farm of origin. The embryo transfer facility also had cows and heifers from other farms that did not utilize formal BVDV control programs. BVDV testing and vaccination for these animals from other farms was not implemented until the cows and heifers arrived at the embryo facility. After delivery of the calves, half of the new heifers resulting from this program were returned to the farm where the cows originated. Among the PI cows in this study, at least one animal infected with BVDV type 2 came from this embryo harvesting facility.

During the last two decades (1998–2018), over 300 bovine pestiviruses have been partially or fully sequenced in Brazil. These include viruses identified in a number of geographical regions, representing different backgrounds of the cattle, and from cattle presenting with diverse clinical pictures. Phylogenetic analysis of these viruses demonstrated a predominance of BVDV 1 (54.4%) in Brazil. The BVDV type 1 subgenotypes identified were: 1a (33.9%) and 1b (16.3%) most frequently, and subgenotypes-1d, -1e, and -1i at very low frequencies. The overall BVDV type 2 frequency was 25.7%, but it varied considerably by the region of the country. It reached as high as 48% of the BVDV identified in one state. HobiPeV accounted for 19.9% of the viruses identified. HobiPeV had the highest frequency in northeast Brazil [30].

Understanding regional genetic diversity of ruminant pestiviruses is important for establishing appropriate vaccine protocols. It makes sense that vaccines should include viral genotypes that are present in each region [31]. In Brazil, most commercial vaccines against BVDV contain only BVDV type 1 strains. This is in the face of epidemiological evidence of a broad distribution of the BVDV type 2 viruses among several Brazilian states. The farm where this research was conducted utilized a vaccine containing BVDV type 1a for several decades prior to our study. The vaccine protocol was changed in 2012. This was due to the introduction of the first commercial BVDV vaccine containing both BVDV type 1 and type 2 genotypes of virus.

The detection of 17 persistently infected cattle of 13 to 36 months of age was a surprise. Taylor et al. reported that only 4/51 PI animals survived longer than one year in a beef herd that was studied.

Noncytopathic (NCP) BVDV establish lifelong PI in fetal calves following infection between 40 and 120 days of gestation, prior to functional immune system development. Cytopathic BVDV strains arise from NCP strain via mutation in the NS23 gene. Superinfection of PI animals with a closely related CP virus will generate mucosal disease [32]. Darweesh et al. reported a mortality rate of 23/41 (56%) in PI cattle also infected with BVDV type 2a that subsequently developed mucosal disease. The adult PI reported in this research did not develop fatal mucosal disease [33].

The prevalence of diarrhea disease and BRD in PI cattle infected with BVDV type 2 was established by scoring fecal and respiratory signs into disease scores in this study. PI cattle had a higher prevalence of both diarrhea (22.7%) and BRD (38.1%) than the paired control animals (0%). This finding was most clear in adult animals (25–36 months of age). It is our contention that while these animals did not develop mucosal disease they did develop subacute chronic intestinal and/or pulmonary inflammatory problems that resulted in the development of secondary disease.

Bachofen et al. published a retrospective and prospective study that analyzed 86 clinical reports of PI animals (median: 12 months of age) between January 1995 to 2005. The animals were under the care of the ruminant clinic at the Department of Farm Animals, University of Zurich. Within this population, 26% (about 30 cattle) were 24 months of age, and four animals were more than three years old. Most of the cases had a history of recurrent, or untreated, diarrhea (41%), pneumonia (20%) or both together (9%). These finding are similar to the findings reported from our study.

Unfortunately, the short time between the completion of the second PI testing cycle and the PI slaughter by the farm did not allow us to conduct a complete physical examination of all PI animals. Therefore, our clinical findings were limited to an examination of the intestinal and respiratory tract in the slaughtered cattle. However, our physical examination of lactating cows allowed us to detect enlarged lymph nodes and enlarged hemolymphatic nodules throughout the body under the skin. We were also able to observe any asymmetry of the mammary gland (quarters), and identify vulvovaginitis, periodontitis and circular alopecia lesions around the eyeball. Further, all lactating PI cows had at least one post-partum disease. These included hypocalcemia, mammary edema, mastitis, retained placenta, metritis, ketosis or BRD. It is our position that this is the first report of the spectrum of post-partum disease that occurs within PI cows.

BRD is frequently reported in cattle when acutely or persistently infected with BVDV. The nasopharynx and respiratory tract are the main routes of entry for BVDV virus. BVDV antigen has routinely been detected in both the upper and lower respiratory tract of animals with BRD [34,35]. Moreover, the genetic material of BVDV has been previously detected using trans-tracheal lavage from both slaughterhouse and necropsied animals, some showing no symptoms [36,37].

This assessment of reproductive records indicated that PI heifers were older than their paired controls at their first artificial insemination attempt. This was due to a delay in the development of sexual maturity in the PI heifers. The earliest inseminations were done at 12 to 13 months of age. The heifers weighed about 350 kg and were about 1.20 m tall at the withers. Heifers should have attained at least 40% to 50% of their adult body weight (~300 kg) by the time of the first service. Stokstad and Loken reported that the PI calves born to heifers that were challenged with an experimental infection during pregnancy were found to be smaller, less active and to grow more slowly than calves from uninfected heifer dams [38].

The number of inseminations required to achieve the first pregnancy was greater for PI heifers than the paired control heifers. BVDV has been localized in ovarian tissue for prolong periods of the following acute infection with cytophatic and noncytophatic strains [18,39]. Altamiranda et al. identified NCP BVDV throughout the ovarian tissue of PI cattle. This virus appeared to be associated with alterations in the structure of the follicular regions of the ovaries. These alterations are believed to directly impact embryo development, leading to reduced rates of ovum cleavage and impaired embryo development.

Grooms, Ward and Brock evaluated the morphological differences in ovaries of six PI cows, compared to six cows with no documented BVDV, using classical histological methods. PI cows appeared to have ovarian hypoplasia and significant morphological changes in the number of tertiary, graafian, atretic, corpus luteum hemorrhagic and albicans body follicles.

Fray et al. suggested that BVDV compromises ovarian function through three mechanisms: (1) BVDV may affect the gonadotrophic function of the pituitary; (2) BVDV suppresses the plasma estrogen level affecting ovulation and estrus; (3) BVDV induces generalized leukopenia, affecting the leukocyte population of the ovaries and impairing follicular dynamics [40].

The reproductive impact in PI cows continues after calving. PI cows have reduced milk production volume and produce more concentrated milk. It is important to note that the decrease in milk production and the increase in SCC are gradual processes that persist throughout the entire lactation period. We found no previously published data about individual PI cows with respect to milk production or quality. However, the reduced milk production, high SCC, and higher occurrence of subclinical and clinical mastitis have been reported in herds with very high BVDV antibody titers. This was observed both before and immediately after the institution of significant BVDV eradication and control programs in Europe [19–23].

To summarize, in a single large dairy herd, we identified 25 PI cattle infected with BVDV type 2. The impact of the virus on production measures (both reproduction and milk production) appears to be significant and consistent. It appears that PI heifers are only half as successful in achieving a first calf as paired controls, and that milk production and quality are significantly poorer in PI cows. Further, PI cattle had diarrhea disease at a higher frequency and in older cows than the paired controls, and PI cattle had a greater frequency of BRD.

5. Conclusions

PI cattle suffered more diarrhea and BRD than their paired controls. The PI heifers had a delayed initial breeding success, and only half of PI heifers delivered a calf following their initial series of AI service. In addition, the PI cows had reduced milk production and poorer milk quality, with an increased SCC throughout lactation.

Author Contributions: V.G., N.S.B., F.D.T., D.J.H. and C.C.L.C. designed the experiments. V.G., N.S.B., L.H.O. and F.D.T. performed the experiments. V.G., J.S.R., N.S.B. and A.R.C.G. analyzed the data. V.G., N.S.B., D.J.H., A.R.C.G. and C.C.L.C. wrote the manuscript. V.G., D.J.H., A.R.C.G. and C.C.L.C. reviewed the manuscript. All authors have read and agreed to the published version of the manuscript.

References

1. Richter, V.; Lebl, K.; Baumgartner, W.; Obritzhauser, W.; Käsbohrer, A.; Pinior, B.A. Systematic Worldwide Review of the Direct Monetary Losses in Cattle due to Bovine Viral Diarrhoea Virus Infection. *Vet. J.* **2017**, *220*, 80–87. [CrossRef] [PubMed]
2. Chi, J.; Weersink, A.; VanLeeuwen, J.A.; Keefe, G.P. The Economics of Controlling Infectious Diseases on Dairy Farms. *Can. J. Agric. Econ.* **2002**, *50*, 237–256. [CrossRef]
3. Yarnall, M.J.; Thrusfield, M.V. Engaging Veterinarians and Farmers in Eradicating Bovine Viral Diarrhoea: A Systematic Review of Economic Impact. *Vet. Rec.* **2017**, *181*, 347. [CrossRef] [PubMed]
4. Grooms, D.L.; Givens, M.D.; Sanderson, M.W.; White, B.J.; Grotelueschen, D.M.; Smith, D.R. Integrated BVD control plans for beef operations. *Bov. Pract.* **2009**, *43*, 106–116.
5. Baker, J.C. The Clinical Manifestations of Bovine Viral Diarrhea Infection. *Vet. Clin. N. Am. Food. Anim. Pr.* **1995**, *11*, 425–445. [CrossRef]
6. Givens, M.D.; Marley, M.S.D. Infectious Causes of Embryonic and Fetal Mortality. *Theriogenology* **2008**, *70*, 270–285. [CrossRef]
7. Walz, P.H.; Grooms, D.L.; Passler, T.; Ridpath, J.F.; Tremblay, R.; Step, D.L.; Callan, R.J.; Givens, M.D. Control of Bovine Viral Diarrhea Virus in Ruminants. *J. Vet. Intern. Med.* **2010**, *24*, 476–486. [CrossRef]
8. Zimmerman, A.D.; Buterbaugh, R.E.; Schnackel, J.A.; Chase, C.C. Efficacy of a Modified-live Virus Vaccine Administered to Calves with Maternal Antibodies and Challenged Seven Months Later with a Virulent Bovine Viral Diarrhea type 2 virus. *Bov. Pract.* **2009**, *43*, 35–43.

9. Zimmerman, A.D.; Klein, A.L.; Buterbaugh, R.E.; Hartman, B.; Rinehart, C.L.; Chase, C.C. Vaccination with a Multivalent Modified-live Virus Vaccine Administered One Year Prior to Challenge with Bovine Viral Diarrhea Virus Type 1b and 2a in Pregnant Heifers. *Bov. Pract.* **2013**, *47*, 22–33.
10. Falkenberg, S.M.; Dassanayake, R.P.; Neill, J.D.; Ridpath, J.F. Evaluation of Bovine Viral Diarrhea Virus Transmission Potential to Naïve Calves by Direct and Indirect Exposure Routes. *Vet. Microbiol.* **2018**, *217*, 144–148. [CrossRef]
11. Kane, S.E.; Holler, L.D.; Braun, L.J.; Neill, J.D.; Young, D.B.; Ridpath, J.F.; Chase, C.C.L. Bovine viral diarrhea virus outbreak in a beef cow herd in South Dakota. *J. Am. Vet. Med. Assoc.* **2015**, *246*, 1358–1362. [CrossRef] [PubMed]
12. Smirnova, N.P.; Bielefeldt-Ohmann, H.; Van Campen, H.; Austin, K.J.; Han, H.; Montgomery, D.L.; Shoemaker, M.L.; van Olphen, A.L.; Hansen, T.R. Acute non-cytopathic bovine viral diarrhea virus infection induces pronounced type I Interferon Response in Pregnant Cows and Fetuses. *Virus Res.* **2008**, *132*, 49–58. [CrossRef] [PubMed]
13. Bachofen, C.; Braun, U.; Hilbe, M.; Ehrensperger, F.; Stalder, H.; Peterhans, E. Clinical Appearance and Pathology of Cattle Persistently Infected with Bovine Viral Diarrhoea Virus of Different Genetic Subgroups. *Vet. Microbiol.* **2010**, *141*, 258–267. [CrossRef]
14. Ridpath, J.F.; Bayles, D.O.; Neill, J.D.; Falkenberg, S.M.; Bauermann, F.V.; Holler, L.; Braun, L.J.; Young, D.B.; Kane, S.E.; Chase, C.C.L. Comparison of the breadth and complexity of bovine viral diarrhea (BVDV) populations circulating in 34 persistently infected cattle generated in one outbreak. *Virology* **2015**, *485*, 297–304. [CrossRef] [PubMed]
15. Grooms, D.L.; Ward, L.A.; Brook, K.V. Morphologic Changes and Immunohistochemical Detection of Viral Antigen in Ovaries from Cattle Persistently Infected with Bovine Viral Diarrhea Virus. *Am. J. Vet. Res.* **1996**, *57*, 830–833. [PubMed]
16. Pinto, V.D.S.C.; Alves, M.F.; Martins, M.D.S.N.; Basso, A.C.; Tannura, J.H.; Pontes, J.H.F.; Romaldini, A.H.C.N. Effects of Oocytes Exposure to Bovine Diarrhea Viruses BVDV-1, BVDV-2 and Hobi-like Virus on In Vitro Produced Bovine Embryo Development and Viral Infection. *Theriogenology* **2017**, *97*, 67–72. [CrossRef]
17. Altamiranda, E.A.G.; Kaiser, G.G.; Mucci, N.C.; Verna, A.E.; Campero, C.M.; Odeón, A.C. Effect of Bovine Viral Diarrhea Virus on the Ovarian Functionality and in Vitro Reproductive Performance of Persistently Infected Heifers. *Vet. Microbiol.* **2013**, *165*, 326–332. [CrossRef] [PubMed]
18. Grooms, D.L. Reproductive Consequences of Infection with Bovine Viral Diarrhea Virus. *Vet. Clin. North. Am. Food. Anim. Pract.* **2004**, *20*, 5–19. [CrossRef]
19. Waage, S. Influence of New Infection with Bovine Virus Diarrhoea Virus on Udder Health in Norwegian Dairy Cows. *Prev. Vet. Med.* **2000**, *43*, 123–135. [CrossRef]
20. Berends, I.M.G.A.; Swart, W.A.J.M.; Frankena, K.; Muskens, J.; Lam, T.J.G.M.; Van Schaik, G. The Effect of Becoming BVDV-free on Fertility and Udder Health in Dutch Dairy Herds. *Prev. Vet. Med.* **2008**, *84*, 48–60. [CrossRef]
21. Laureyns, J.; Piepers, S.; Ribbens, S.; Sarrazin, S.; De Vliegher, S.; Van Crombrugge, J.M.; Dewulf, J. Association Vetween Herd Exposure to BVDV-Infection and Bulk Milk Somatic Cell Count of Flemish Dairy Farms. *Prev. Vet. Med.* **2013**, *109*, 148–151. [CrossRef] [PubMed]
22. Tschopp, A.; Deiss, R.; Rotzer, M.; Wanda, S.; Thomann, B.; Schüpbach-Regula, G.; Meylan, M. A Matched Case-control Study Comparing Udder Health, Production and Fertility Parameters in Dairy Farms Before and After the Eradication of Bovine Virus Diarrhoea in Switzerland. *Prev. Vet. Med.* **2017**, *144*, 29–39. [CrossRef] [PubMed]
23. Tiwari, A.; Vanleeuwen, J.A.; Dohoo, I.R.; Keefe, G.P.; Haddad, J.P.; Tremblay, R.; Scott, H.M.; Whiting, T. Production Effects of Pathogens Causing Bovine Leukosis, Bovine Viral Diarrhea, Paratuberculosis, and Neosporosis. *J. Dairy Sci.* **2007**, *90*, 659–669. [CrossRef]
24. Basqueira, N.S.; Martin, C.C.; França, J.; Okuda, L.H.; Pituco, M.E.; Batista, C.F.; Maria, A.; Paiva, M.; Gomes, V. Bovine Respiratory Disease (BRD) Complex as a Signal for Bovine Viral Diarrhea Virus (BVDV) Presence in the Herd. *Acta Sci. Vet.* **2017**, *55*, 1–6. [CrossRef]
25. Silva, B.T.; Baccili, C.C.; Henklein, A.; Oliveira, P.L.; Oliveira, S.M.F.N.; Sobreira, N.M.; Gomes, V. Transferência de Imunidade Passiva (TIP) e Dinâmica de Anticorpos Específicos em Bezerros Naturalmente Expostos para as Viroses Respiratórias. *Arq. Bras. Med. Vet. Zootec.* **2018**, *70*, 1414–1422. [CrossRef]

26. Martin, C.C.; Baccili, C.C.; Silva, B.T.; Novo, S.M.F.; Sobreira, N.M.; Pituco, E.M.; Gomes, V. Detection of Bovine Viral Diarrhea Virus Infection in Newborn Calves Before Colostrum Intake. *Semina Ciências Agrárias* **2016**, *37*, 1379–1388. [CrossRef]
27. Baccili, C.C.; Sobreira, N.M.; Silva, B.T.; Pituco, E.M.; Gomes, V. Interface Between Maternal Antibodies and Natural Challenge for Bovine Viral Diarrhea Virus (BVDV) in Holstein Heifers. *Acta Sci. Vet.* **2016**, *44*, 1–6. [CrossRef]
28. Harpin, S.; Hurley, D.J.; Mbikay, M.; Talbot, B.; Elazhary, Y. Vaccination of Cattle with a DNA Plasmid Encoding the Bovine Viral Diarrhoea Virus Major Glycoprotein E2. *J. Gen. Virol.* **1999**, *80*, 3137–3144. [CrossRef] [PubMed]
29. Kumar, S.; Hedges, S.B. Advances in Time Estimation Methods for Molecular Data. *Mol. Biol. Evol.* **2016**, *33*, 863–869. [CrossRef]
30. Flores, E.F.; Cargnelutti, J.F.; Monteiro, F.L.; Bauermann, F.V.; Ridpath, J.F.; Weiblen, R. A genetic profile of bovine pestiviruses circulating in Brazil (1998–2018). *Anim. Health Res. Rev.* **2018**, *19*, 134–141. [CrossRef]
31. Mahony, T.J.; McCarthy, F.M.; Gravel, J.L.; Corney, B.; Young, P.L.; Vilcek, S. Genetic Analysis of Bovine viral Diarrhoea Viruses from Australia. *Vet. Microbiol.* **2005**, *106*, 1–6. [CrossRef]
32. Taylor, L.F.; Janzen, E.D.; Ellis, J.A.; Van Den Hurk, J.V.; Ward, P. Performance, Survival, Necropsy, and Virological Findings from Calves Persistently Infected with the Bovine Viral Diarrhea Virus Originating from a Single Saskatchewan Beef Herd. *Can. Vet. J.* **1997**, *38*, 29–37. [PubMed]
33. Darweesh, M.F.; Rajput, M.K.; Braun, L.J.; Ridpath, J.F.; Neill, J.D.; Chase, C.C. Characterization of the Cytopathic BVDV Strains Isolated from 13 Mucosal Disease Cases Arising in a Cattle Herd. *Virus Res.* **2015**, *195*, 141–147. [CrossRef] [PubMed]
34. Shin, T.; Acland, H. Tissue Distribution of Bovine Viral Diarrhea Virus Antigens in Persistently Infected Cattle. *J. Vet. Sci.* **2001**, *2*, 81–84. [CrossRef] [PubMed]
35. Liebler-Tenorio, E.M.; Ridpath, J.E.; Neill, J.D. Distribution of Viral Antigen and Tissue Lesions in Persistent and Acute Infection with the Homologous Strain of Noncytopathic Bovine Viral Diarrhea Virus. *J. Vet. Diagn. Investig.* **2004**, *16*, 388–396. [CrossRef]
36. Weinstock, D.; Bhudevi, B.; Anthony, E.C. Single-tube Single- enzyme Reverse Transcriptase PCR Assay for Detection of Bovine Viral Diarrhea Virus in Pooled Bovine Serum. *J. Clin. Microbiol.* **2001**, *39*, 343–346. [CrossRef]
37. Fulton, R.W.; Purdy, C.W.; Confer, A.W.; Saliki, J.T.; Loan, R.W.; Briggs, R.E.; Burge, L.J. Bovine Viral Diarrhea Viral Infections in Feeder Calves with Respiratory Disease: Interactions with Pasteurella spp., Parainfluenza-3 Virus, and Bovine Respiratory Syncytial Virus. *Can. J. Vet. Res.* **2000**, *64*, 151–159.
38. Stokstad, M.; Loken, T. Pestivirus in Cattle: Experimentally Induced Persistent Infection in Calves. *J. Vet. Med. B Infect. Dis. Vet. Public Health* **2002**, *49*, 494–501. [CrossRef]
39. Grooms, D.L.; Brock, K.V.; Pate, J.L.; Day, M.L. Changes in ovarian follicles following acute infection with bovine viral diarrhea virus. *Theriogenology* **1998**, *49*, 595–605. [CrossRef]
40. Fray, M.D.; Paton, D.; Alenius, S. The Effects of Bovine Viral Diarrhoea Virus on Cattle Reproduction in Relation to Disease Control. *Anim. Reprod. Sci.* **2000**, *60*, 615–627. [CrossRef]

17

Efficacy of Two Antibiotic-Extender Combinations on *Mycoplasma bovis* in Bovine Semen Production

Tarja Pohjanvirta [1,*], Nella Vähänikkilä [1], Henri Simonen [2], Sinikka Pelkonen [1] and Tiina Autio [1]

1 Finnish Food Authority, Laboratory and Research Division, Veterinary Bacteriology and Pathology Unit, Neulaniementie 4, 70210 Kuopio, Finland; nella.vahanikkila@foodauthority.fi (N.V.); sinikka.pelkonen@foodauthority.fi (S.P.); tiina.autio@foodauthority.fi (T.A.)

2 VikingGenetics, Korpikyläntie 77, 15870 Hollola, Finland; hesim@vikinggenetics.com

* Correspondence: tarja.pohjanvirta@foodauthority.fi;

Abstract: *Mycoplasma bovis* is an important bovine pathogen. Artificial insemination (AI) using contaminated semen can introduce the agent into a naïve herd. Antibiotics, most often gentamycin, tylosin, lincomycin, spectinomycin (GTLS) combination are added to semen extender to prevent transmission of pathogenic bacteria and mycoplasmas. In a commercial AI straw production system with industrial scale procedures, we analyzed the mycoplasmacidal efficacy of GTLS and ofloxacin on *M. bovis* ATCC and wild type strain isolated from commercial AI straws. The strains were spiked at two concentrations (10^6 and 10^3 CFU/mL) into semen. Viable *M. bovis* in frozen semen straws was detected by enrichment culture and real-time PCR. We also compared different protocols to extract *M. bovis* DNA from spiked semen. None of the antibiotic protocols had any effect on the viability of either of the *M. bovis* strains at high spiking concentration. At low concentration, the wild type was inhibited by all other protocols, except low GTLS, whereas the ATCC strain was inhibited only by high GTLS. The InstaGene™ matrix was the most effective method to extract *M. bovis* DNA from semen. When there is a low *M. bovis* contamination level in semen, GTLS used at high concentrations, in accordance with Certified Semen Services requirements, is more efficient than GTLS used at concentrations stated in the OIE Terrestrial Code.

Keywords: *Mycoplasma bovis*; bovine semen; antibiotics; prevention; DNA extraction

---

1. Introduction

Mycoplasma bovis is a major bovine pathogen causing substantial economic losses and has a debilitating effect on animal welfare. *M. bovis* causes a variety of diseases including mastitis, pneumonia, arthritis, otitis media, and genital infections [1]. Efforts to develop efficacious vaccines have not been successful [2]. Once established in a cattle farm, *M. bovis* can be difficult to eradicate [3]. Consequently, it is of paramount importance to prevent the introduction of the agent into naïve herds.

One *M. bovis* transmission route into a herd is artificial insemination (AI) [4]. Recently, we reported on how contaminated semen used in AI, introduced *M. bovis* infection into closed naïve dairy herds [5]. In a previous study, heifers inseminated with semen containing *M. bovis* became repeat breeders, and only half of them finally conceived [6]. *M. bovis* could be isolated from cervico-vaginal mucus of some of the heifers, 8–32 weeks after insemination. Kissi et al. [7] showed that insemination with frozen *Mycoplasma sp.* containing semen often resulted in prolonged diestrus, suggesting that mycoplasma could initiate a pathological process in the uterus. However, very little is known about the concentration of *M. bovis* in naturally infected bull semen and the infectious dose needed to initiate an infection in the female genital system.

There are several viral and bacterial pathogens that can be transmitted via semen [8]. Semen used for AI should be free of infectious agents. Several types of antibiotics have been added to seminal extenders before freezing to control bacterial contamination, including mycoplasmas. The World Organization for Animal Health OIE lists, in the OIE Terrestrial Code [9], the following three different antibiotic combinations to be used in international trade of bovine semen: gentamicin (250 μg), tylosin (50 μg), lincomycin-spectinomycin (150/300 μg) (GTLS) in each mL of frozen semen; penicillin (500 IU), streptomycin (500 μg), lincomycin-spectinomycin (150/300 μg) (PSLS); or amikacin (75 μg), divekacin (25 μg). The European Union directive 88/407/1993 includes the use of the above mentioned PSLS, or an alternative combination of antibiotics with an equivalent effect against campylobacters, leptospires, and mycoplasmas. Shin et al. [10], in 1988, developed a method where GTLS concentration was doubled as compared with the concentration stated in OIE Code, and GTLS was first added into raw semen before extending with GTLS containing extender. Nowadays, GTLS is widely used in bovine semen production, and Certified Semen Services (CSS) in USA has a special protocol in place for GTLS use [11]. However, Visser et al. conducted two studies, in 1995 and 1999 [12,13], in which they questioned the ability of even the high GTLS concentration to control *M. bovis* in AI. Since the studies of Shin et al. [10] and Visser et al. [12,13], animal protein sources in commercial extenders have often been replaced with plant protein sources such as soybean lecithin to avoid disease transmission through the use of animal source protein [14]. Most commercially available soy-lecithin-based extenders contain GTLS as standard antibiotics. However, recent *M. bovis* isolates have shown a marked increase in MIC90 values for tylosin, lincomycin, and spectinomycin, but resistance against fluoroquinolones is still quite rare [15–17]. Recently a fluoroquinolone antibiotic, ofloxacin, was shown to be non-toxic to spermatozoa and effective in protecting semen from bacteria, although the authors did not analyze its effect on mycoplasmas [18].

Introductions of *M. bovis* into countries free of the organism have recently been reported (Finland 2012 [19], New Zealand 2017, (https://www.mpi.govt.nz/protection-and-response/mycoplasma-bovis/). Although these introductions have not been directly linked to semen, *M. bovis* risk, due to global semen trade, continues to be a concern, especially in New Zealand where eradication of *M. bovis* has been attempted. In this study, we evaluated the efficacy of the low OIE Code and the high CSS guideline GTLS concentrations and two ofloxacin concentrations on the viability of two different *M. bovis* strains in spiked frozen semen. We used an ATCC strain, as well as a wild type strain recently isolated from commercial AI semen straws [5]. Unlike in previous GTLS efficacy studies [10,12,13], we used a commercial animal protein free extender. We wanted to study if it was possible to achieve mycoplasmacidal effect, in other words, no detection of *M. bovis* in AI semen straws after semen was enriched in mycoplasma broth, and an aliquot of the broth culture was directly analyzed using *M. bovis* real-time polymerase chain reaction (PCR).

Mycoplasmas are fastidious organisms needing special culture media and expertise in isolation. Instead of mycoplasma culture, PCR could be an option in AI centers to ensure *M. bovis*-free semen lots. There are only a few studies about PCR detection of *M. bovis* in bovine semen. Therefore, we also evaluated sensitivity of different DNA extraction methods to detect *M. bovis* in semen.

Experiments to produce *M. bovis* contaminated AI straws were conducted, in a commercial AI straw producing laboratory, using industrial scale procedures. This was possible because semen production ceased in this center after these experiments.

2. Results

Raw pooled semen showed no growth in mycoplasma culture. *M. bovis* or Friis broth did not have any detrimental effect on quality parameters of semen (Table 1).

After storage of the AI straws for five weeks in liquid nitrogen, at high spiking concentrations (10^6 CFU/mL), viable *M. bovis* bacteria were detected in processed semen regardless of the processing protocol. When low *M. bovis* concentrations were inoculated, differences among processing protocols were seen (Table 2). At a low spiking concentration, the ATCC strain was more resistant than the wild type strain to different antibiotics. The only protocol inhibiting the growth of the ATCC strain was the high GTLS 500/100/300/600 μg/mL (final concentration in extended semen) supplement added in the semen lab to the extender. All protocols, except EU GTLS 250/50/150/300 µg/mL (final concentration in extended semen) and extender without antibiotics, inhibited the growth of the wild type at a low spiking concentration.

Table 1. Semen quality parameters of raw and spiked semen.

Semen	Strain (CFU/mL)	Motility %	Viability %	Sperm Concentration (10^6/mL)
Raw semen		75.0	82.5	1850
Processed semen	ATCC 10^3	55 ± 2.9	53 ± 3.0	65 ± 2.9
	ATCC 10^6	56 ± 6.1	53 ± 2.5	67 ± 2.3
	wild type 10^3	52 ± 5.5	52 ± 2.1	67 ± 2.1
	wild type 10^6	57 ± 5.5	52 ± 4.6	67 ± 2.3
	unspiked	53 ± 5.1	54 ± 2.3	61 ± 1.3

Table 2. Detection of *M. bovis* wild type and ATCC 27368 by culture (+/-) from three parallel pooled samples (e.g., + + +) from different antibiotic/extender protocols after five-week storage of the straws in liquid nitrogen. Concentration used in spiking and culture dilution are shown in the table.

	10^3 CFU/mL			10^6 CFU/mL		
Culture dilution	−2	−3	−4	−2	−3	−4
Wild type strain						
GTLS 500/100/300/600 [a]	- - -	- - -	- - -	- - -	+ + +	+ + +
CSS GTLS [b]	- - -	- - -	- - -	- - -	- - -	+ + +
EU GTLS [c]	- - -	- - +	- - -	- - -	+ + +	+ + +
OF 400 µg [d]	- - -	- - -	- - -	- - -	+ + +	+ + +
OF 100 µg	- - -	- - -	- - -	- - -	+ + +	+ + +
no antibiotic	+ + +	+ - +	+ - -	+ + +	+ + +	+ + +
ATCC strain						
GTLS 500/100/300/600	- - -	- - -	- - -	+ - -	- - -	+ + +
CSS GTLS	- - -	- - -	- + -	+ + +	- + -	+ + +
EU GTLS	- - -	+ + +	+ - -	- - -	+ + +	+ + +
OF 400 µg	- - -	- - +	+ - +	+ - +	+ + +	+ + +
OF 100 µg	- - -	+ + +	- + +	+ - -	+ + +	+ + +
no antibiotic	+ + +	+ + +	+ + -	+ + +	+ + +	+ + +

[a] gentamycin (500 µg/mL), tylosin (100 µg/mL), lincomycin (300 µg/mL), spectinomycin (600 µg/mL); [b] Certified Semen Services gentamycin (500 µg/mL), tylosin (100 µg/mL), lincomycin (300 µg/mL), spectinomycin (600 µg/mL) protocol; [c] gentamycin (250 µg/mL), tylosin (50 µg/mL), lincomycin (150 µg/mL), spectinomycin (300 µg/mL); [d] ofloxacin.

Antimicrobials present in extended semen affect the mycoplasma culture, and thus several dilutions were made. In samples with high concentration of antimicrobials, viable *M. bovis* could be detected only in the highest culture dilution (Table 2).

We compared three different DNA extraction methods for spiked semen samples. At a high spiking concentration (10^6 CFU/mL), all pools were positive in PCR regardless of the DNA extraction method. Ct values varied between 24.7 and 28.5, and no significant differences in Ct values among extraction methods were seen (data not shown).

At a low spiking concentration, the method using InstaGene™ (method three) was the most effective. Using this method, we detected *M. bovis* in 94% (17/18) of pools spiked with 10^3 CFU/mL of ATCC strain, and in 72% (13/18) spiked with 10^3 CFU/mL of wild type strain. With method one, 67% (12/18) and with method two, 56% (10/18) of pools spiked with ATCC strain were positive in PCR, respectively. For the wild type strain, respective figures were for method one 61% (11/18) and 33% (6/18) for method two (Table 3). The Ct values varied between 34.3 and 36.7, and no significant differences in Ct values among extraction methods were seen (data not shown).

Table 3. Comparison of three different DNA extraction methods for detection of *M. bovis* in semen using *oppD* real-time PCR. Results (+/-) from three parallel pools (e.g., + + +) from each antibiotic protocol are shown.

	10^3 CFU/mL						10^6 CFU/mL					
	ATCC			Wild Type			ATCC			Wild Type		
	Method 1 [a]	Method 2 [b]	Method 3 [c]	Method 1	Method 2	Method 3	Method 1	Method 2	Method 3	Method 1	Method 2	Method 3
GTLS 500/100/300/600	- + +	+ + -	+ + +	+ - -	+ - +	+ - -	+ + +	+ + +	+ + +	+ + +	+ + +	+ + +
CSS GTLS	+ - -	- + +	+ + +	- + +	- - -	+ + +	+ + +	+ + +	+ + +	+ + +	+ + +	+ + +
EU GTLS	+ + +	+ + -	+ + +	+ + +	+ - +	- + +	+ + +	+ + +	+ + +	+ + +	+ + +	+ + +
OF 400 µg	+ + +	+ - +	+ + +	+ - +	- - -	+ + -	+ + +	+ + +	+ + +	+ + +	+ + +	+ + +
OF 100 µg	- + -	- - +	+ - +	- + -	- - -	+ + +	+ + +	+ + +	+ + +	+ + +	+ + +	+ + +
Control	- + +	- - +	+ + +	- + +	+ + -	+ - +	+ + +	+ + +	+ + +	+ + +	+ + +	+ + +

[a] QIAamp DNA mini kit (Qiagen, Hilden, Germany); [b] 2% Triton-X 100 and QIAamp DNA mini kit (Parker et al. 2017); [c] InstaGene™ matrix (Bio-Rad, Helsinki, Finland).

Minimum inhibitory concentration values of the strains used in spiking are shown in Table 4.

Table 4. MIC values (μg/mL) of ATCC 27368 and wild type strains (dilution range of antibiotic tested).

Antibiotic	**Dilution Range Tested μg/mL**	**ATCC 27368**	**Wild Type**
Tylosin	0.5–32	≤0.5	16
Lincomycin	0.25–32	2	1
Spectinomycin	2–128	4	≤2
Enrofloxacin	0.03–2	0.25	0.25
Danofloxacin	0.03–2	0.25	0.25

3. Discussion

Our study showed that it is challenging to rely on the use of antibiotics in bovine semen production to control *M. bovis*. None of the studied antibiotics had any effect on viability of *M. bovis* at 10^6 CFU/mL in extended semen, and the lower spiking concentration of 10^3 CFU/mL gave discrepant results. The high GTLS concentration reduced the number of viable *M. bovis* below the level of detection in all but one pool when 10^3 CFU/mL was spiked. In contrast, using the low concentration EU GTLS protocol, four out of six pools were positive in culture, suggesting that the GTLS concentration stated in the OIE Code is not high enough to eliminate even a low concentration of *M. bovis* in semen.

Our results on efficacy of GTLS are in line with previous studies by Shin et al. [10] and Visser et al. [12,13], although there are marked differences in experimental setup among the studies. In our study, an AI straw production system was performed in a commercial facility using industrial scale procedures, the wild type study strain had been recently isolated from AI straws, different extenders and treatments were used, and survival of *M. bovis* was measured using a different method. In the earlier studies [10,12,13], animal protein containing extenders were used, as well as a plate counting method was used to detect viable *M. bovis*. Shin et al. [10] found that a high GTLS concentration in 20% egg yolk citrate extender showed 85% reduction of viable *M. bovis*. GTLS in other extenders was less mycoplasmacidal, thus, extender composition seemed to affect the efficacy of GTLS on *M. bovis*. However, the opinion of Shin et al. [10] was that the reduction of *M. bovis* concentration was so notable that it made the semen safe to use, and Shin's GTLS protocol was implemented for use in the Unites States AI industry. Later, Visser et al. [12,13] studied the effect of high GTLS in egg yolk tris extender. They noticed a one to two decimal reduction in *M. bovis* numbers in some batches, and in some batches the number of viable *M. bovis* was even higher in the GTLS-treated semen as compared with non-treated semen. We did not attempt to analyze the number of colony-forming units after liquid nitrogen storage. Instead, we aimed to find any viable *M. bovis* cells by enrichment culture and using real-time PCR to detect *M. bovis* in broth cultures. Previously, we showed that the limit of detection of this method was 1.4×10^2 CFU/mL of *M. bovis* PG45 in fresh, non-frozen extended bull semen [20]. Animal protein-free extender used in this study did not seem to enhance the efficacy of antibiotics as compared with earlier studies. The inclusion of further field strains isolated from AI semen in this study would have been appropriate, but these were not readily available.

Macrolide and linco/spectinomycin resistance, in recent *M. bovis* isolates from Europe, has increased as compared with isolates before 2000 [15,17]. This may have an impact on the effect of GTLS in *M. bovis* in semen as the highest dilutions tested in recent European studies [16,21] were from 64 to 256 μg/mL, and several strains had MIC values higher than the highest tested concentration. Antimicrobial susceptibility studies [15–17,21,22] showed that contemporary *M. bovis* strains are susceptible to fluoroquinolones, except for a few strains that had MIC_{90} over 32 μg/mL. Gloria et al. [18] reported that ofloxacin, a fluoroquinolone antibiotic, had non-significant effects on sperm quality and controlled bacteria efficiently in semen doses, although they did not study the effect on mycoplasmas. This tempted us to examine the effect of two different ofloxacin concentrations on *M. bovis* in semen. To our knowledge, this is the first publication on efficacy of a fluoroquinolone on *M. bovis* in commercial semen production. Although the ATCC strain used for spiking had an MIC value of 0.25 μg/mL for enrofloxacin and danofloxacin, the 100 μg/mL ofloxacin concentration in extender had no effect on the viability of the ATCC strain, and two out of three tested pools of the high ofloxacin concentration were also culture positive. Antimicrobial resistance, in the strains we used in this study did not explain the results, as MIC values for tylosin, lincomycin, and spectinomycin, as well as for fluoroquinolones, were well below the concentrations of antibiotics in semen extenders. The biological conditions for antibiotics to act with *M. bovis* in MIC testing are remarkably different as compared with conditions in semen production.

Most antibiotics require ongoing cell activity or cell division to be able to destroy bacteria. Low temperature can keep bacteria in a stationary phase of growth, thus, making the antibiotics almost ineffective. This is considered in the EU directive 88/407/1993 which states that extended semen with antibiotics must be kept a minimum of 45 min at 5 °C, and in the CSS protocol that requires, first, adding antibiotics in raw semen, and then keeping extended semen at 5 °C for a minimum of two hours before freezing. In our study, extended semen with different antibiotics was kept for 3–3.5 h at temperatures (decreasing from 34 °C to 17 °C) that, in theory, allowed replication of mycoplasmas. Thus, the negative effect of low temperature on antimicrobial effect cannot explain our results.

A possible way to control the dissemination of *M. bovis* via AI could be testing of raw semen or multiple straws of extended semen using PCR. However, PCR inhibitors present in semen can pose problems for detecting *M. bovis*. Semen contains very high amounts of DNA and protein, potassium ions, citric acids, and fructose. Therefore, it is essential to have a highly sensitive method for DNA isolation from bull semen. We compared three different DNA extraction methods and found that InstaGene™ proved to be the most efficient and robust method to detect *M. bovis* DNA in extended bull semen. To our knowledge, Parker et al. [23] and McDonald [24] are the only studies on the sensitivity of real-time PCR detection of *M. bovis* in semen. Parker et al. [23] used the Triton-X extraction method which, in our study, had lower sensitivity than the InstaGene™ method. Together with the *uvrC* gene-based real-time PCR, their limit of detection was 1.3×10^5 CFU/mL, which was higher than for our method. McDonald [24] used a commercial DNA isolation kit on spiked semen and multiplex real-time PCR targeting *fusA* and *oppD/F* genes. These assays detected 3.1×10^3 *M. bovis* genomes per mL semen, which was a similar level of detection to our InstaGene™ method. Little is known about shedding of *M. bovis* into semen during different stages of infection. It is generally known that shedding of mycoplasmas into semen can be intermittent. Ball et al. [25] showed that at least three semen lots from a bull needed to be analyzed to find out if the bull was shedding mycoplasmas into semen. This has also been shown for the secretion of *M. bovis* to semen. A clinically healthy bull in the AI center was shown to shed *M. bovis* in semen for a very short period and intermittently [5]. Our culture and PCR results also highlight the problem that *M. bovis* seems to be unequally distributed in extended semen, a phenomenon we also saw when examining the straws from the naturally infected bull semen. Therefore, it is important to analyze several straws, even from the same lot, when trying to detect *M. bovis* in semen. We also found that, within the same lot, some straws were positive only in PCR, but unculturable [5]. This can lead to unnecessary disposing of semen lots that contain only dead bacteria.

AI using *M. bovis*-contaminated semen can introduce the agent into naïve dairy herds. We showed that even using modern commercial extender and industrial procedures, neither GTLS nor ofloxacin reached 100% bactericidal effect on *M. bovis*. Our results suggest that regarding *M. bovis* in semen, it is safer to use the high 500/100/300/600 μg/mL GTLS concentration. To be able to fully understand the risk of *M. bovis* contaminated semen in dairy herds and to know if it is even necessary to have zero tolerance for *M. bovis* in commercial semen, we need to know what is the *M. bovis* load that would initiate a pathological process in the female genital system.

Another option, although very laborious, is to test processed semen for the presence of *M. bovis*, considering the special features of *M. bovis* infection in bulls and occurrence in semen. However, the increasing antimicrobial resistance in contemporary *M. bovis* strains, the difficulties achieving 100% mycoplasmacidal effect using antibiotics in semen, and the pressure to reduce the amount of antibiotics used in semen industry calls for future attempts to allow only *M. bovis* negative bulls into semen production.

4. Materials and Methods

4.1. Semen Collection and Quality Assessment

All studies were done in a commercial AI straw producing AI center's laboratory using industrial scale procedures. This was possible because the semen production ceased in this center after these experiments. Semen from three bulls was collected into sterile collection tubes at the AI center of VikingGenetics, Hollola, Finland. The motility of each semen batch was evaluated microscopically at 200× magnification using prewarmed glass slides and coverslips. Viability and concentration of each batch was analyzed using flow cytometry (CyFlow, Partec, Germany). Pooled raw semen (0.3 mL) was cultured in Friis broth [26] to detect possible *Mycoplasma* contamination. The final sperm cell concentration was 12–13 million per straw. On the basis of the weight and concentration, the volume of extender was calculated.

4.2. Mycoplasma Bovis Strains

Two *M. bovis* strains were used in spiking, i.e., a wild type isolate from commercial AI straws (strain 198, [5]) and a reference strain ATCC 27368. Strains were cultured in Friis broth in closed tubes at 37 °C, for 70 ± 2 h. High (10^8 CFU/mL) and low (10^5 CFU/mL) concentration stock solutions were made from the cultures in Friis broth. To verify the *M. bovis* concentration of the stocks, ten-fold dilutions were made and plated on Friis plates. Plates were incubated at 37 °C, in 5% CO_2, for 7 days, and colony-forming units were counted.

4.3. Protocols Used for Processing Semen

Semen from the three bulls was pooled and divided into 30 aliquots which were kept at 32 °C. Commercial animal protein-free extender base containing 7% glycerol was used in all protocols. Six antibiotic protocols were compared as follows: (1) GTLS (500/100/300/600 µg/mL, respectively) fresh antibiotic supplemented extender; (2) raw semen was treated with GTLS fresh antibiotics for 3 min and further extended with GTLS (500/100/300/600 µg/mL, respectively) fresh antibiotic supplemented extender (according to Certified Semen Services (CSS) requirements), later called CSS GTLS; (3) GTLS (250/50/150/300 µg/mL, respectively), antibiotic supplemented extender (ready to use liquid concentrate containing antibiotics), according to the OIE Code, Article 4.7.7, later called EU GTLS; (4) ofloxacin 100 µg/mL (Sigma Aldrich 33703) antibiotic supplemented extender; or (5) ofloxacin 400 µg/mL antibiotic supplemented extender; and (6) extender without antibiotics, control. The final concentration of the *M. bovis* strains in extended semen was either 10^6 CFU/mL or 10^3 CFU/mL. Friis broth was used as a negative control in each different antibiotic/extender aliquot. The protocols are described in Table 5. All extenders, antibiotics, and Friis broth were kept at 32 °C before being added into the semen. All protocols, except number two (CSS GTLS), included diluting the semen in 1:1extender (with or without antibiotics) and Friis broth containing either 10^8 or 10^5 CFU *M. bovis* ATCC or wild type. In protocol two (CSS GTLS), GTLS was first diluted 1:4 in sterile water and 38 µL added into neat semen (380 µL), *M. bovis* culture (118 µL) yielding the same antibiotic concentration as if 20 µL GTLS mixture (500/100/300/600) would have been added directly to raw semen. After 3 min of incubation at 32 °C, the semen was further diluted 1:1 with extender containing GTLS. Then, all aliquots were incubated for one hour at 34 °C, after which they were diluted further with extender with or without antibiotics to give the final concentration of 56 million sperm cells/mL. Then, the temperature of the aliquots was allowed to stabilize to room temperature (approximately one hour) after which automatic semen straw filling and sealing machine (MPP Quattro, Minitube, Germany) was used. Semen was packed into 0.25 mL straws. After packing, the straws were cooled to 17 °C for one hour and further cooled quickly to 4 °C. The straws were kept at 4 °C overnight and they were deep-frozen with industrial semen straw freezer (Digitcool 5300, IMV, France) the next morning. Cryopreserved straws were stored in liquid nitrogen storage tank (−196 °C) until they were analyzed.

Table 5. Antibiotic/extender protocols used for processing semen.

GTLS (500/100/300/600)	CSS GTLS (500/100/300/600)	EU GTLS (250/50/150/300)	OF400	OF100	Control
0.38 mL semen	0.38 mL semen	0.38 mL semen	0.38 mL semen	0.38 mL semen	0.38 mL semen
+	+	+	+	+	+
0.38 mL GTLS extender	0.118 mL *M.bovis*	0.38 mL GTLS extender	0.38 mL OF extender	0.38 mL OF extender	0.38 mL extender no antibiotic
+	+	+	+	+	+
0.118 mL *M. bovis*	38 µL GTLS 1:4 3 min	0.118 mL *M. bovis*	0.118 mL *M. bovis*	0.118 mL *M. bovis*	0.118 mL *M. bovis*
+	+	+	+	+	+
	0.38 mL GTLS extender				
	+				
1 h 34 °C	1 h 34 °C	1 h 34 °C	1 h 34 °C	1 h 34 °C	1 h 34 °C
+	+	+	+	+	+
10.875 mL GTLS extender	10.875 mL GTLS extender	10.875 mL GTLS extender	10.875 mL OF extender	10.875 mL OF extender	10.875 mL extender no antibiotic
Room temperature 50–90 min and packing in straws (0.25 mL per straw)					
1 h + 17 °C					
21 h + 4 °C					
Storage in liquid nitrogen					

4.4. Semen Quality Parameters after Thawing

After 18 days storage in liquid nitrogen, two straws from each trial lot were thawed. The motility was assessed under phase contrast microscope. Flow cytometric analysis was used to evaluate viability and concentration of sperm cells.

4.5. Viability Testing of M. Bovis from Semen Straws Stored in Liquid Nitrogen

After storage of five weeks in liquid nitrogen, 18 straws from each of the 30 trial lots were randomly retrieved from the nitrogen tank. They were divided into three pools, each consisting of six straws. Straws were thawed and the content of the six straws was pooled. From each pool, 0.6 mL of semen was used in three different DNA extraction procedures described in Section 4.6., and 0.3 mL of semen was placed into 2.7 mL of Friis broth. Ten-fold dilutions, up to 10^{-5}, were made into Friis broth in tightly closed tubes. Broth cultures were incubated at 37 °C for 14 days. The growth and color change of the medium were monitored every other day, and broths suspected of mycoplasma growth were plated on Friis agar and tested for *M. bovis* using real-time PCR targeting *M. bovis oppD* gene [27]. From each trial lot, all broth culture dilutions from 10^{-2} to 10^{-4} were tested for *M. bovis*, as described above, at the latest, immediately after the 14-day incubation period.

4.6. DNA Extraction from Semen Straws after Storage in Liquid Nitrogen

Three different protocols to extract DNA from spiked semen were compared. In each method, 200 µL of semen was used as a starting material. Method one was automated DNA extraction using a QIAcube (Qiagen, Hilden, Germany) robot and blood and body fluids protocol with QIAamp DNA mini kit. The elution volume was 150 µL. In method two [25], 200 µL of semen was combined with 200 µL of 2% Triton-X 100 (Sigma Aldrich) in 10 mM Tris and 1 mM EDTA (pH 8) buffer. The sample was thoroughly vortexed and pelleted at 13,000× *g* for 5 min. DNA was extracted from the pellet using the QIAcube robot and bacterial pellet protocol with QIAamp DNA mini kit. The elution volume was 150 µL. Method three was modified from the OIE Terrestrial Manual method to isolate DNA from bovine semen for herpesvirus PCR (chapter 3.4.11, adopted May 2017). In method three, 200 µL of semen was centrifuged at 13,000× *g* for 10 min and supernatant was discarded. The pellet was mixed with 200 µL of InstaGene™ matrix (Bio-Rad, Helsinki, Finland), 5.8 µL proteinase K (20 mg/mL), and 7.5 µL DL-dithiothreitol (1 M). Samples were incubated at 56 °C, for 30 min, and then vortexed at high speed for 10 s. The tubes were boiled in water bath (100 °C) for 8 min, and then vortexed at high speed for 10 s. Then, the tubes were centrifuged at 10,000× *g* for 3 min. The supernatant was transferred into a new microtube and stored at −20 °C.

4.7. M. bovis Real-Time PCR

Broth cultures and DNA extracted from semen straw pools were examined by real-time PCR (CFX96 Touch Real-Time PCR Detection System, Bio-Rad, CA, USA) targeting *opp*D-gene of *M. bovis*, as described previously by Sachse et al [27]. Friis broth cultures were prepared for real-time PCR as follows: First, 200 µL of broth culture was incubated for 15 min at 95 °C and centrifuged at 10,000× *g* for 5 min. Two µL of culture supernatant or DNA was used as PCR template. Commercially available plasmid pUC19 was used as internal amplification control, according to Fricker et al. [28].

4.8. Determining Minimal Inhibitory Concentration (MIC) of Wild Type Strain and ATCC 27368

MICs were determined using custom made Sensititre plates (Thermo Fisher Scientific, UK). Antibiotics tested were tylosin (concentration range 0.5–32 µg/mL), lincomycin (0.25–32 µg/mL), spectinomycin (2–128 µg/mL), enrofloxacin (0.03–2 µg/mL), and danofloxacin (0.03–2 µg/mL). Testing was done according to [15,16]. Briefly, a suspension containing 5% growth indicator alamarBlue (Thermo Fisher Scientific, United Kingdom) in Friis broth without antibiotics and *M. bovis* 5×10^5 CFU/mL was made, and 200 µL of the suspension was pipetted into each well of the Sensititre plate. Plates were sealed and incubated at 37 °C for 48 ± 1 h and read visually; blue indicating no growth and red indicating growth of the isolate. MIC was the lowest concentration of antibiotic completely suppressing growth (blue color).

Author Contributions: Conceptualization, T.P., N.V., T.A., and S.P.; methodology, T.P., N.V., and T.A.; formal analysis, T.P., N.V., and T.A.; investigation, N.V. and H.S.; resources, H.S.; writing—original draft preparation, T.P.; writing—review and editing, T.P., T.A., H.S., and S.P.; supervision, T.A.; project administration and funding acquisition, S.P. All authors have read and agreed to the published version of the manuscript.

Acknowledgments: We are grateful to Riikka Luukkanen and Petra Väisänen for excellent technical assistance. We thank DVM Kasia Kupisiewicz for critical reding of the manuscript.

References

1. Maunsell, F.P.; Woolums, A.R.; Francoz, D.; Rosenbusch, R.F.; Step, D.L.; Wilson, D.J.; Janzen, E.D. Mycoplasma bovis infections in cattle. *J. Vet. Intern. Med.* **2011**, *25*, 772–783. [CrossRef] [PubMed]
2. Perez-Casal, J.; Prysliak, T.; Maina, T.; Suleman, M.; Jimbo, S. Status of the development of a vaccine against Mycoplasma bovis. *Vaccine* **2017**, *35*, 2902–2907. [CrossRef] [PubMed]
3. Nicholas, R.A. Bovine mycoplasmosis: Silent and deadly. *Vet. Rec.* **2011**, *168*, 459–462. [CrossRef]
4. Pfützner, H.; Sachse, K. Mycoplasma bovis as an agent of mastitis, pneumonia, arthritis and genital disorders in cattle. *Rev. Sci. Tech.* **1996**, *15*, 1477–1494. [CrossRef]
5. Haapala, V.; Pohjanvirta, T.; Vähänikkilä, N.; Halkilahti, J.; Simonen, H.; Pelkonen, S.; Soveri, T.; Simojoki, H.; Autio, T. Semen as a source of Mycoplasma bovis mastitis in dairy herds. *Vet. Microbiol.* **2018**, *216*, 60–66. [CrossRef] [PubMed]
6. Hirth, R.S.; Nielsen, S.W.; Plastridge, W.N. Bovine salpingo-oophoritis produced with semen containing a Mycoplasma. *Pathol. Vet.* **1966**, *3*, 616–632. [CrossRef]
7. Kissi, B.; Juhász, S.; Stipkovits, L. Effect of mycoplasma contamination of bull semen on fertilization. *Acta Vet. Hung.* **1985**, *33*, 107–117.
8. Wentink, G.H.; Frankena, K.; Bosch, J.C.; Vandehoek, J.E.D.; van den Berg, T. Prevention of disease transmission by semen in cattle. *Livest. Prod. Sci.* **2000**, *62*, 207–220. [CrossRef]
9. OIE Terrestrial Animal Health Code, Chapter 4.7. Available online: https://www.oie.int/index.php?id=169&L=0&htmfile=chapitre_coll_semen.htm (accessed on 5 August 2020).
10. Shin, S.J.; Lein, D.H.; Patten, V.H.; Ruhnke, H.L. A new antibiotic combination for frozen bovine semen 1. Control of mycoplasmas, ureaplasmas, Campylobacter fetus subsp. venerealis and Haemophilus somnus. *Theriogenology* **1988**, *29*, 577–591. [CrossRef]
11. CSS—National Association of Animal Breeders. Available online: https://www.naab-css.org/uploads/userfiles/files/CSSMinReq-Jan2014201607-ENG.pdf (accessed on 5 August 2020).
12. Visser, I.J.R.; ter Laak, E.A.; Jansen, H.B.; Gerard, O. The effect of antibiotic mixtures on Haemophilus somnus, Campylobacter fetus spp. venerealis, Mycoplasma bovis, and Ureaplasma diversum in frozen bovine semen. *Reprod. Domest. Anim.* **1995**, *30*, 55–59. [CrossRef]
13. Visser, I.J.; ter Laak, E.A.; Jansen, H.B. Failure of antibiotics gentamycin, tylosin, lincomycin and spectinomycin to eliminate Mycoplasma bovis in artificially infected frozen bovine semen. *Theriogenology* **1999**, *51*, 689–697. [CrossRef]
14. Rehman, F.; Zhao, C.; Shah, M.A.; Qureshi, M.S.; Wang, X. Semen extenders and artificial insemination in ruminants. *Veterinaria* **2013**, *1*, 1–8.
15. Ayling, R.D.; Rosales, R.S.; Barden, G.; Gosney, F.L. Changes in antimicrobial susceptibility of Mycoplasma bovis isolates from Great Britain. *Vet. Rec.* **2014**, *175*, 486. [CrossRef] [PubMed]
16. Heuvelink, A.; Reugebrink, C.; Mars, J. Antimicrobial susceptibility of Mycoplasma bovis isolates from veal calves and dairy cattle in the Netherlands. *Vet. Microbiol.* **2016**, *189*, 1–7. [CrossRef]
17. Klein, U.; de Jong, A.; Youala, M.; El Garch, F.; Stevenin, C.; Moyaert, H.; Rose, M.; Catania, S.; Gyuranecz, M.; Pridmore, A.; et al. New antimicrobial susceptibility data from monitoring of Mycoplasma bovis isolated in Europe. *Vet. Microbiol.* **2019**, *238*, 108432. [CrossRef]
18. Gloria, A.; Contri, A.; Wegher, L.; Vignola, G.; Dellamaria, D.; Carluccio, A. The effects of antibiotic additions to extenders on fresh and frozen-thawed bull semen. *Anim. Reprod. Sci.* **2014**, *150*, 15–23. [CrossRef] [PubMed]

19. Vähänikkilä, N.; Pohjanvirta, T.; Haapala, V.; Simojoki, H.; Soveri, T.; Browning, G.F.; Pelkonen, S.; Wawegama, N.K.; Autio, T. Characterisation of the course of Mycoplasma bovis infection in naturally infected dairy herds. *Vet. Microbiol.* **2019**, *231*, 107–115. [CrossRef]
20. Vähänikkilä, N.; Pohjanvirta, T.; Vaahtoranta, L.; Silvennoinen, M.; Skovgaard Jensen, S.K.; Pelkonen, S.; Autio, T. Detection of Mycoplasma bovis in bovine semen—An interlaboratory trial. In Proceedings of the 22nd Congress of the International Organization for Mycoplasmology, Portsmouth, NH, USA, 9–12 July 2018; Brown, D., Wells, N., Eds.; p. 143.
21. Sulyok, K.M.; Kreizinger, Z.; Fekete, L.; Hrivnák, V.; Magyar, T.; Jánosi, S.; Schweitzer, N.; Turcsányi, I.; Makrai, L.; Erdélyi, K.; et al. Antibiotic susceptibility profiles of Mycoplasma bovis strains isolated from cattle in Hungary, Central Europe. *BMC Vet. Res.* **2014**, *10*, 256. [CrossRef]
22. Gautier-Bouchardon, A.V.; Ferré, S.; Le Grand, D.; Paoli, A.; Gay, E.; Poumarat, F. Overall decrease in the susceptibility of Mycoplasma bovis to antimicrobials over the past 30 years in France. *PLoS ONE* **2014**, *9*, e87672. [CrossRef]
23. Parker, A.M.; House, J.K.; Hazelton, M.S.; Bosward, K.L.; Sheehy, P.A. Comparison of culture and a multiplex probe PCR for identifying Mycoplasma species in bovine milk, semen and swab samples. *PLoS ONE* **2017**, *12*, e0173422. [CrossRef]
24. McDonald, K.M. The Development of a Dual Target Mycoplasma Bovis TaqMan Real-Time PCR System for Rapid Analysis of Bovine Semen. Master's Thesis, The Ohio State University, Columbus, OH, USA, 2012.
25. Ball, H.J.; Logan, E.F.; Orr, W. Isolation of mycoplasmas from bovine semen in Northern Ireland. *Vet. Rec.* **1987**, *121*, 322–324. [CrossRef] [PubMed]
26. Bölske, G. Survey of mycoplasma infections in cell cultures and a comparison of detection methods. *Zentralbl. Bakteriol. Mikrobiol. Hyg. Ser. A* **1988**, *269*, 331–340. [CrossRef]
27. Sachse, K.; Salam, H.S.H.; Diller, R.; Schubert, E.; Hoffmann, B.; Hotzel, H. Use of a novel real-time PCR technique to monitor and quantitate Mycoplasma bovis infection in cattle herds with mastitis and respiratory disease. *Vet. J.* **2010**, *186*, 299–303. [CrossRef] [PubMed]
28. Fricker, M.; Messelhäußer, U.; Busch, U.; Schere, S.; Ehling-Schultz, M. Diagnostic real-time PCR assays fot the detection of emetic Bacillus cereus strains in food and recent food-borne outbreaks. *Appl. Environ. Microbiol.* **2007**, *73*, 1892–1898. [CrossRef] [PubMed]

Permissions

All chapters in this book were first published by MDPI; hereby published with permission under the Creative Commons Attribution License or equivalent. Every chapter published in this book has been scrutinized by our experts. Their significance has been extensively debated. The topics covered herein carry significant findings which will fuel the growth of the discipline. They may even be implemented as practical applications or may be referred to as a beginning point for another development.

The contributors of this book come from diverse backgrounds, making this book a truly international effort. This book will bring forth new frontiers with its revolutionizing research information and detailed analysis of the nascent developments around the world.

We would like to thank all the contributing authors for lending their expertise to make the book truly unique. They have played a crucial role in the development of this book. Without their invaluable contributions this book wouldn't have been possible. They have made vital efforts to compile up to date information on the varied aspects of this subject to make this book a valuable addition to the collection of many professionals and students.

This book was conceptualized with the vision of imparting up-to-date information and advanced data in this field. To ensure the same, a matchless editorial board was set up. Every individual on the board went through rigorous rounds of assessment to prove their worth. After which they invested a large part of their time researching and compiling the most relevant data for our readers.

The editorial board has been involved in producing this book since its inception. They have spent rigorous hours researching and exploring the diverse topics which have resulted in the successful publishing of this book. They have passed on their knowledge of decades through this book. To expedite this challenging task, the publisher supported the team at every step. A small team of assistant editors was also appointed to further simplify the editing procedure and attain best results for the readers.

Apart from the editorial board, the designing team has also invested a significant amount of their time in understanding the subject and creating the most relevant covers. They scrutinized every image to scout for the most suitable representation of the subject and create an appropriate cover for the book.

The publishing team has been an ardent support to the editorial, designing and production team. Their endless efforts to recruit the best for this project, has resulted in the accomplishment of this book. They are a veteran in the field of academics and their pool of knowledge is as vast as their experience in printing. Their expertise and guidance has proved useful at every step. Their uncompromising quality standards have made this book an exceptional effort. Their encouragement from time to time has been an inspiration for everyone.

The publisher and the editorial board hope that this book will prove to be a valuable piece of knowledge for researchers, students, practitioners and scholars across the globe.

List of Contributors

Paul C. Bartlett, Vickie J. Ruggiero and Bo Norby
College of Veterinary Medicine, Michigan State University, East Lansing, MI 48824, USA

Holden C. Hutchinson
USDA, Fort Collins, CO 80526, USA

Kelly R. B. Sporer and Casey J. Droscha
CentralStar Cooperative, East Lansing, MI 48910, USA

Tasia M. Taxis
Department of Animal Science, Michigan State University, East Lansing, MI 48824, USA

Shahid Khalfan
School of Animal and Veterinary Sciences, Charles Sturt University, Wagga Wagga, NSW 2650, Australia

Claire McMorrow, Allan J. Gunn, Marta Hernandez-Jover and Victoria J. Brookes
School of Animal and Veterinary Sciences, Charles Sturt University, Wagga Wagga, NSW 2650, Australia
Graham Centre for Agricultural Innovation (NSW Department of Primary Industries and Charles Sturt University), Wagga Wagga, NSW 2650, Australia

Zafer Yazici, Cuneyt Tamer, Hanne Nur Kurucay, Ahmed Eisa Elhag, Semra Gumusova and Harun Albayrak
Department of Veterinary Virology, Faculty of Veterinary Medicine, Ondokuz Mayis University, 55139 Samsun, Turkey

Emre Ozan and Bahadir Muftuoglu
Department of Veterinary Experimental Animals, Faculty of Veterinary Medicine, Ondokuz Mayis University, 55139 Samsun, Turkey

Gerald Barry
Veterinary Science Centre, School of Veterinary Medicine, University College of Dublin, Dublin 4, Ireland

Abdurrahman Anil Cagirgan
Bornova Veterinary Control Institute, Veterinary Control Institute Directorates, Ministry of Agriculture and Forestry, 35010 Izmir, Turkey

Andrew J. Read, Sarah Gestier, Kate Parrish, Deborah S. Finlaison, Xingnian Gu, Tiffany W. O'Connor and Peter D. Kirkland
Virology Laboratory, Elizabeth Macarthur Agriculture Institute, Woodbridge Road, Menangle, New South, Wales 2568, Australia

Alexandra Kiesler, Kerstin Seitz, Katharina Buczolich, Helga Petznek, Christiane Riedel, Hann-Wei Chen, Marlene Mötz, Till Rümenapf and Benjamin Lamp
Institute of Virology, Department for Pathobiology, University of Veterinary Medicine, Veterinaerplatz 1, 1210 Vienna, Austria

Lukas Schwarz, Elena Sassu, Sophie Dürlinger and Andrea Ladinig
Department for Farm Animals and Veterinary Public Health, University Clinic for Swine, University of Veterinary Medicine, Veterinaerplatz 1, 1210 Vienna, Austria

Sandra Högler, Andrea Klang and Herbert Weissenböck
Institute of Pathology and Forensic Veterinary Medicine, Department of Pathobiology, University of Veterinary Medicine, Veterinaerplatz 1, 1210 Vienna, Austria

Peter Kirkland
Virology Laboratory, Elizabeth Macarthur Agriculture Institute, Woodbridge Rd, Menangle, New South Wales 2568, Australia

Andrea Kinnear, Matthew Waldner, Sarah Parker, Janet E. Hill and Murray D. Jelinski
Western College of Veterinary Medicine, University of Saskatchewan, Saskatoon, SK S7N 5B4, Canada

Tim A. McAllister, Rahat Zaheer and Sara Andrés-Lasheras
Lethbridge Research and Development Centre, Agriculture and Agri-Food Canada, Lethbridge, AB T1J 4B1, Canada

Antonio C. Ruzzini
Western College of Veterinary Medicine, University of Saskatchewan, Saskatoon, SK S7N 5B4, Canada
College of Medicine, Department of Biochemistry, Microbiology and Immunology, University of Saskatchewan, Saskatoon, SK S7N 5E5, Canada

Kevin P. Szillat, Susanne Koethe, Kerstin Wernike, Dirk Höper and Martin Beer
Institute of Diagnostic Virology, Friedrich-Loeffler-Institut, Federal Research Institute for Animal Health, 17493 Greifswald-Insel Riems, Germany

Enrica Sozzi, Cristian Salogni, Davide Lelli, Ilaria Barbieri, Ana Moreno, Giovanni Loris Alborali and Antonio Lavazza
Istituto Zooprofilattico Sperimentale della Lombardia e dell'Emilia Romagna "Bruno Ubertini" (IZSLER), Via Antonio Bianchi 7/9, 25124 Brescia, Italy

Anja Dalmann and Ilona Reimann
Institute of Diagnostic Virology, Friedrich-Loeffler-Institut, 17493 Greifswald-Insel Riems, Germany

Eric J. Snijder and Nadia Oreshkova
Molecular Virology Laboratory, Department of Medical Microbiology, Leiden University Medical Center, 2333 ZA Leiden, The Netherlands

Mette Bisgaard Petersen
Department of Veterinary Clinical Sciences, University of Copenhagen, Agrovej 5A, 2630 Taastrup, Denmark

Lars Pedersen
SEGES, 8200 Aarhus, Denmark

Lone Møller Pedersen
Eurofins Milk Testing Denmark, 6600 Vejen, Denmark

Liza Rosenbaum Nielsen
Department of Animal and Veterinary Sciences, University of Copenhagen, Grønnegårdsvej 8, 1870 Frederiksberg, Denmark

Karim Abdelsalam
Department of Veterinary and Biomedical Sciences, South Dakota State University, Brookings, SD 57007, USA
Faculty of Veterinary Medicine, Zagazig University, Zagazig 44519, Egypt

Mrigendra Rajput, Jacob Sobraske, Neelu Thakur and Christopher C. L. Chase
Department of Veterinary and Biomedical Sciences, South Dakota State University, Brookings, SD 57007, USA

Hossam Abdallah, Ahmed A. H. Ali and Gamal Elmowalid
Faculty of Veterinary Medicine, Zagazig University, Zagazig 44519, Egypt

Carlos G. das Neves
Norwegian Veterinary Institute, N-0106 Oslo/N-9010 Tromsø, Norway
Faculty of Health Sciences, UiT The Arctic University of Norway, N-9037 Tromsø, Norway

Stefan Alenius and Jonas Johansson Wensman
Department of Clinical Sciences, Swedish University of Agricultural Sciences, SE-75007 Uppsala, Sweden

Ingebjørg Helena Nymo
Norwegian Veterinary Institute, N-0106 Oslo/N-9010 Tromsø, Norway
Department of Arctic and Marine Biology, UiT The Arctic University of Norway, N-9037 Tromsø, Norway

Morten Tryland
Department of Arctic and Marine Biology, UiT The Arctic University of Norway, N-9037 Tromsø, Norway

Eystein Skjerve
Centre for Epidemiology and Biostatistics, Faculty of Veterinary Sciences, Norwegian University of Life Sciences, N-0033 Oslo, Norway

Katarzyna Dudek, Ewelina Szacawa and Dariusz Bednarek
Department of Cattle and Sheep Diseases, National Veterinary Research Institute, 57 Partyzantów Avenue, 24100 Pulawy, Poland

Robin A. J. Nicholas
The Oaks, Nutshell Lane, Farnham, Surrey GU9 0HG, UK

Robin van den Braak, Bartjan Simmelink and Ad de Groof
Department Discovery & Technology, MSD Animal Health, Wim de Körverstraat 35, 5830AA Boxmeer, The Netherlands

Alba Folgueiras-González
Department Discovery & Technology, MSD Animal Health, Wim de Körverstraat 35, 5830AA Boxmeer, The Netherlands
Laboratory of Experimental Virology, Department of Medical Microbiology, Amsterdam UMC Location AMC, University of Amsterdam, Meibergdreef 9, 1105AZ Amsterdam, The Netherlands

Martin Deijs and Lia van der Hoek
Laboratory of Experimental Virology, Department of Medical Microbiology, Amsterdam UMC Location AMC, University of Amsterdam, Meibergdreef 9, 1105AZ Amsterdam, The Netherlands

Natália Sobreira Basqueira, Jean Silva Ramos, Fabricio Dias Torres and Viviani Gomes
Department of Internal Medicine, College of Veterinary Medicine and Animal Science, University of São Paulo, São Paulo 05508-270, Brazil

Liria Hiromi Okuda
Biological Institute, 1252 Conselheiro Rodrigues Alves Ave, Vila Mariana, São Paulo 04014-900, Brazil

David John Hurley
Food Animal Health and Management Program, College of Veterinary Medicine, University of Georgia, Athens, GA 30602, USA

Anny Raissa Carolini Gomes
Department of Veterinary Medicine, Federal University of Paraná, Curitiba 80040-380, Brazil

Tarja Pohjanvirta, Nella Vähänikkilä, Sinikka Pelkonen and Tiina Autio
Finnish Food Authority, Laboratory and Research Division, Veterinary Bacteriology and Pathology Unit, Neulaniementie 4, 70210 Kuopio, Finland

Henri Simonen
VikingGenetics, Korpikyläntie 77, 15870 Hollola, Finland

Index

www.ingramcontent.com/pod-product-compliance
Lightning Source LLC
LaVergne TN
LVHW080946210926
848485LV00004B/783

* 9 7 8 1 6 4 1 1 6 7 7 0 3 *